Yoshiaki Toyama • Atsushi Miyawaki
Masaya Nakamura • Masahiro Jinzaki
Editors

Make Life Visible

Editors
Yoshiaki Toyama
Department of Orthopaedic Surgery
Keio University, School of Medicine
Shinjuku, Tokyo, Japan

Atsushi Miyawaki
RIKEN, Center for Brain Science
Laboratory for Cell Function Dynamics
Wako, Saitama, Japan

Masaya Nakamura
Department of Orthopaedic Surgery
Keio University, School of Medicine
Shinjuku, Tokyo, Japan

Masahiro Jinzaki
Department of Diagnostic Radiology
Keio University, School of Medicine
Shinjuku, Tokyo, Japan

https://doi.org/10.1007/978-981-13-7908-6

Preface

In recent years, marked advances in imaging technology have enabled the visualization of phenomena formerly believed to be completely impossible. These technologies have made major contributions to the elucidation of the pathology of diseases as well as to their diagnosis and therapy. Adding further promise for future development are imaging tools in the broad sense, such as optics and optogenetics – the revolutionary use of light to control cells and organisms.

From molecular imaging to clinical images, the Japanese are world leaders in basic and clinical research of visualization. We strive to foster innovative, creative, advanced research that gives full play to imaging technology in the broad sense while exploring cross-disciplinary areas in which individual research fields interact and pursuing the development of new techniques where they fuse together.

The 9th Specific Research Project, "Make Life Visible," was established by the Uehara Memorial Foundation as a 3-year research project to support such research. In this Special Project, three areas (Sessions 1–3) were targeted from basic research to clinical application. Nineteen Japanese researchers were selected, and research was begun in 2015.

Session 1. Visualizing and Controlling Molecules for Life
Session 2. Imaging Disease Mechanisms
Session 3. Imaging-Based Diagnosis and Therapy

The 12th Uehara International Symposium 2017, entitled "Make Life Visible," was convened in Tokyo from June 12 to 14, 2017. In this international symposium, we have built on the outcomes of the 9th Special Project, with presentations focusing on the cutting-edge findings of visualization technologies by the Japanese Special Project members as well as ten leading researchers invited from overseas.

The aim of this symposium was to be a forum for the presentation of the latest research outcomes, future prospects, and new strategies in visualization technology, from basic research to the clinical front lines (diagnosis and treatment).

Thanks to the speakers, most of the chapters contain a video file of this symposium, and we are very pleased to be able to publish the proceedings of this exiting symposium.

Tokyo, Japan	Yoshiaki Toyama
Saitama, Japan	Atsushi Miyawaki
Tokyo, Japan	Masaya Nakamura
Tokyo, Japan	Masahiro Jinzaki

Contents

Part I
Visualizing and Controlling Molecules for Life

Chapter 1
Photoacoustic Tomography: Deep Tissue Imaging by Ultrasonically Beating Optical Diffusion

Lihong V. Wang

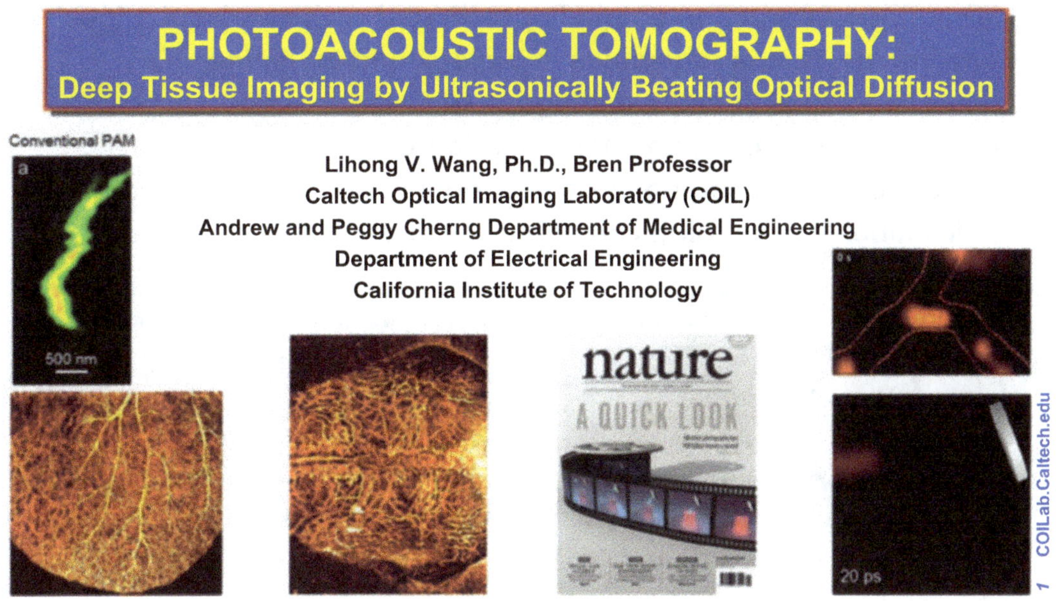

Photoacoustic tomography has been developed for in vivo functional, metabolic, molecular, and histologic imaging by physically combining optical and ultrasonic waves. Broad applications include early-cancer detection and brain imaging. High-resolution optical imaging—such as confocal microscopy, two-photon microscopy, and optical coherence tomography—is limited to superficial imaging within the optical diffusion limit (~1 mm in the skin) of the surface of scattering tissue. By synergistically combining light and sound, photoacoustic tomography provides deep penetration at high ultrasonic resolution and high optical contrast.

Electronic Supplementary Material The online version of this chapter (https://doi.org/10.1007/978-981-13-7908-6_1) contains supplementary material, which is available to authorized users.

L. V. Wang (✉)
California Institute of Technology, Pasadena, CA, USA
e-mail: LVW@Caltech.edu; http://COILab.Caltech.edu

Y. Toyama et al. (eds.), *Make Life Visible*,
https://doi.org/10.1007/978-981-13-7908-6_1

In photoacoustic computed tomography, a pulsed broad laser beam illuminates the biological tissue to generate a small but rapid temperature rise, which leads to emission of ultrasonic waves due to thermoelastic expansion. The unscattered pulsed ultrasonic waves are then detected by ultrasonic transducers. High-resolution tomographic images of optical contrast are then formed through image reconstruction. Endogenous optical contrast can be used to quantify the concentration of total hemoglobin, the oxygen saturation of hemoglobin, and the concentration of melanin. Exogenous optical contrast can be used to provide molecular imaging and reporter gene imaging as well as glucose-uptake imaging.

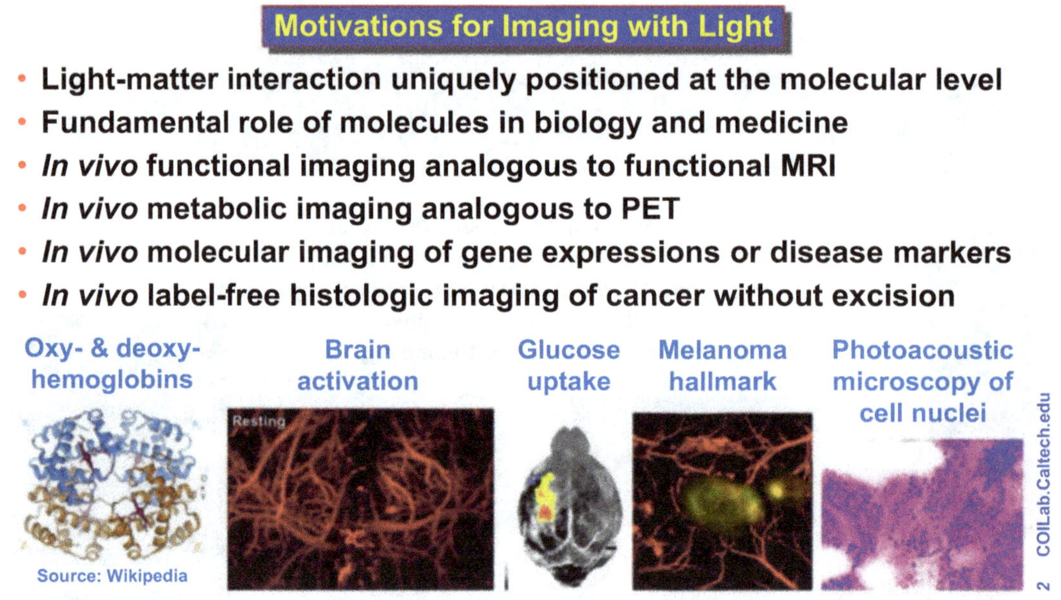

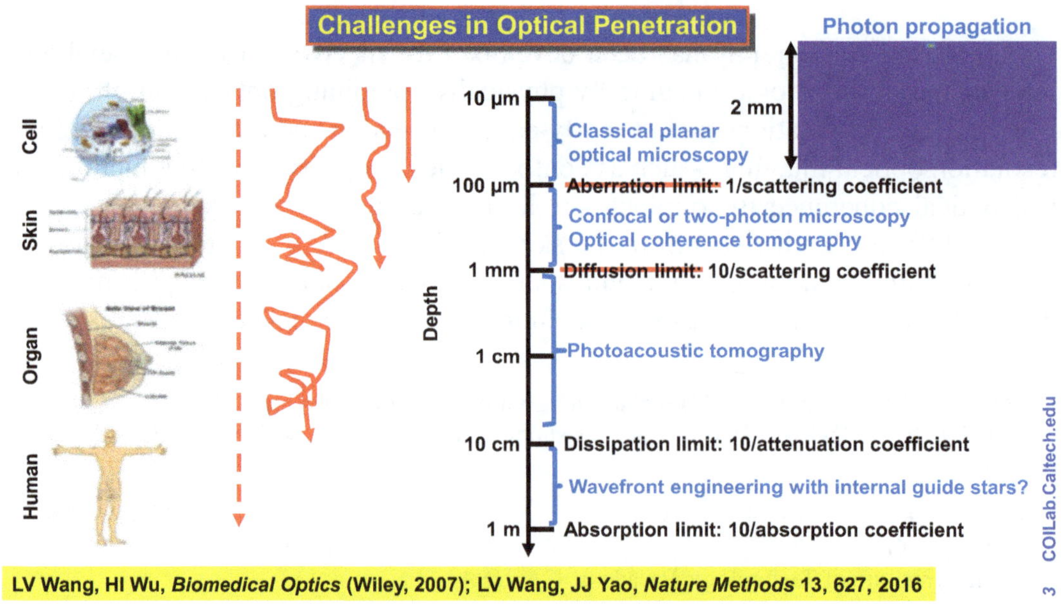

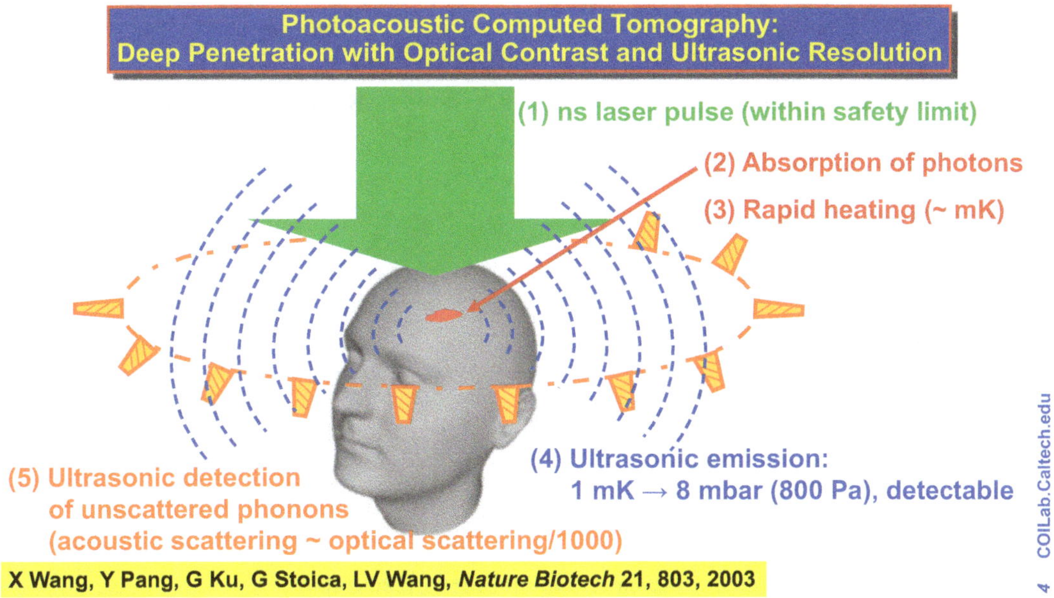

In photoacoustic microscopy, a pulsed laser beam is delivered into the biological tissue to generate ultrasonic waves, which are then detected with a focused ultrasonic transducer to form a depth resolved 1D image. Raster scanning yields 3D high-resolution tomographic images. Super-depths beyond the optical diffusion limit have been reached with high spatial resolution. The following image of a mouse brain was acquired in vivo with intact skull using optical-resolution photoacoustic microscopy.

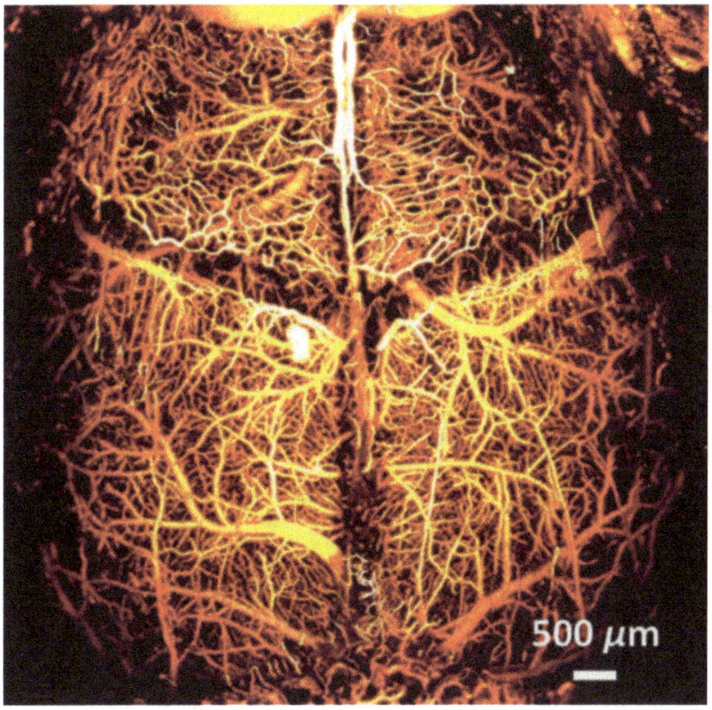

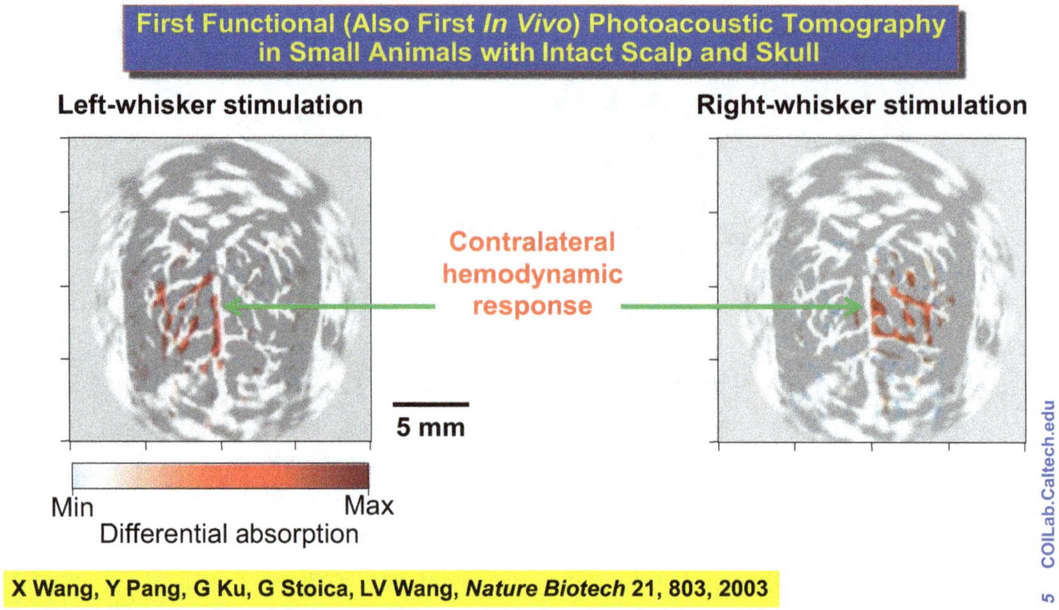

The annual conference on photoacoustic tomography has become the largest in SPIE's 20,000-attendee Photonics West since 2010.

Wavefront engineering and compressed ultrafast photography will be touched upon.

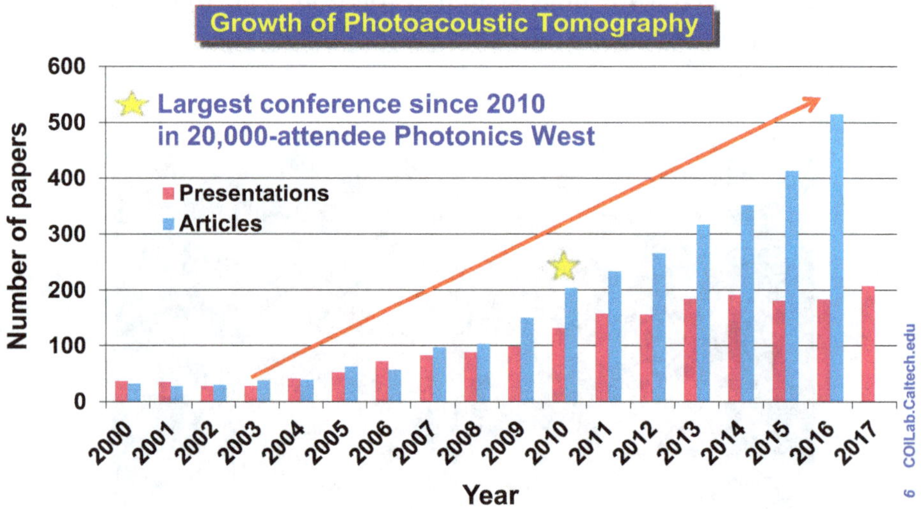

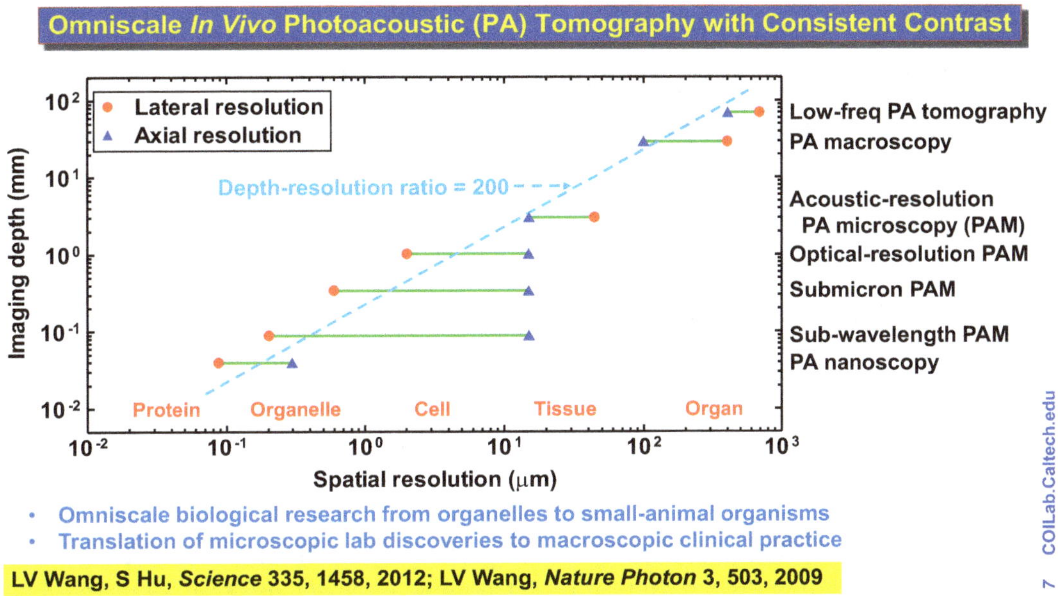

Selected Publications:

1. Nature Biotechnology 21, 803 (2003).
2. Nature Photonics 5, 154 (2011).
3. Science 335, 1458 (2012).
4. Nature Methods 13, 67 (2016).

Chapter 2
Regulatory Mechanism of Neural Progenitor Cells Revealed by Optical Manipulation of Gene Expressions

Itaru Imayoshi, Mayumi Yamada, and Yusuke Suzuki

The basic-helix-loop-helix (bHLH) transcription factors Hes1, Ascl1/Mash1 and Olig2 facilitate the fate determination of astrocytes, neurons and oligodendrocytes, respectively (Imayoshi and Kageyama 2014). However, these bHLH transcription factors are co-expressed in multipotent self-renewing neural progenitor cells even before cell fate choice (Imayoshi et al. 2013). This finding indicates that these fate determination factors are differentially expressed between self-renewing and differentiating neural progenitor cells with unique expression dynamics. Live imaging analysis with fluorescent and bioluminescent proteins is a powerful strategy for monitoring expression dynamics. Our imaging results indicate that bHLH transcription factors are expressed in an oscillatory manner by neural progenitor cells, and that one of them becomes dominant in fate choice. We propose that the multipotent state of neural progenitor cells correlates with the oscillatory expression of several

Electronic Supplementary Material The online version of this chapter (https://doi.org/10.1007/978-981-13-7908-6_2) contains supplementary material, which is available to authorized users.

I. Imayoshi (✉)
Graduate School of Biostudies, Kyoto University, Kyoto, Japan

Institute for Frontier Life and Medical Sciences, Kyoto University, Kyoto, Japan

World Premier International Research Initiative–Institute for Integrated Cell-Material Sciences, Kyoto University, Kyoto, Japan

The Hakubi Center, Kyoto University, Kyoto, Japan

Japan Science and Technology Agency, Precursory Research for Embryonic Science and Technology, Saitama, Japan

Medical Innovation Center/SK Project, Graduate School of Medicine, Kyoto University, Kyoto, Japan
e-mail: imayoshi.itaru.2n@kyoto-u.ac.jp; iimayosh@virus.kyoto-u.ac.jp

Y. Toyama et al. (eds.), *Make Life Visible*,
https://doi.org/10.1007/978-981-13-7908-6_2

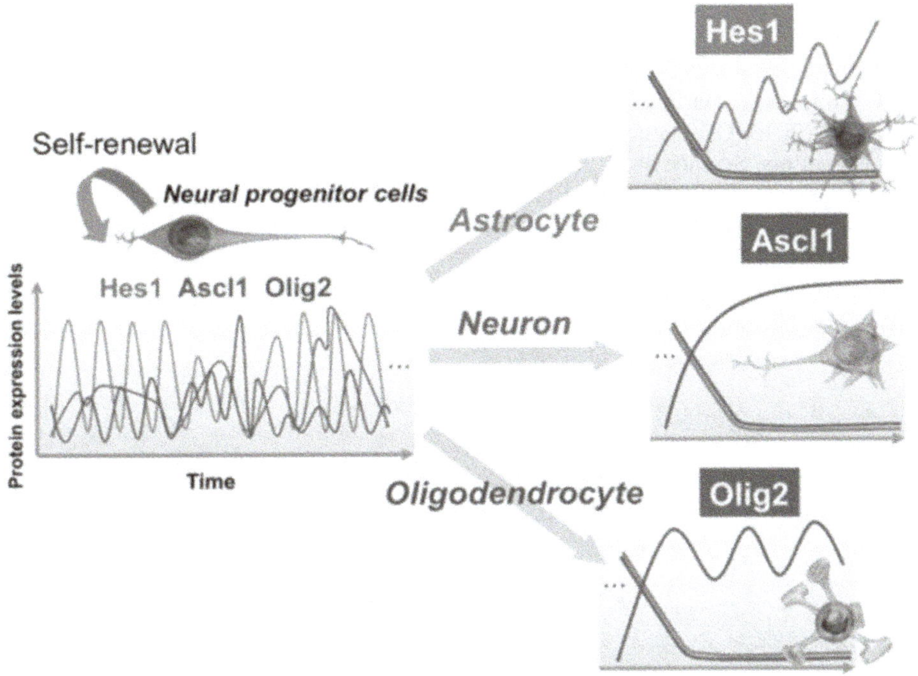

Fig. 2.1 Expression dynamics of bHLH factors in multipotency and cell fate determination. (This figure was modified from Figure 5 of Imayoshi and Kageyama 2014)

bHLH transcription factors, whereas the differentiated state correlates with the sustained expression of a single bHLH transcription factor.

To address the cousal relationships between the expression dynamics (oscillatory versus sustained) and functional outcomes (cell proliferation versus fate differentiation), the optogenetic approach has been employed to control the expression patterns of bHLH transcription factors (Imayoshi et al. 2013). We applied a novel optogenetic method (photo-activatable Gal4/UAS system) to manipulate the expression patterns of bHLH transcription factors using blue light illumination, showing that oscillatory expression activates the cell proliferation of neural progenitor cells, whereas sustained expression induces cell fate determination (Fig. 2.1).

M. Yamada
Graduate School of Biostudies, Kyoto University, Kyoto, Japan

Institute for Frontier Life and Medical Sciences, Kyoto University, Kyoto, Japan

World Premier International Research Initiative–Institute for Integrated Cell-Material Sciences, Kyoto University, Kyoto, Japan

Medical Innovation Center/SK Project, Graduate School of Medicine, Kyoto University, Kyoto, Japan

Y. Suzuki
Graduate School of Biostudies, Kyoto University, Kyoto, Japan

Institute for Frontier Life and Medical Sciences, Kyoto University, Kyoto, Japan

Medical Innovation Center/SK Project, Graduate School of Medicine, Kyoto University, Kyoto, Japan

References

Imayoshi I, Isomura A, Harima Y, Kawaguchi K, Kori H, Miyachi H, Fujiwara T, Ishidate F, Kageyama R (2013) Oscillatory control of factors determining multipotency and fate in mouse neural progenitors. Science 342:1203–1208

Imayoshi I, Kageyama R (2014) bHLH factors in self-renewal, multipotency, and fate choice of neural progenitor cells. Neuron 82:9–23

Chapter 3
Eavesdropping on Biological Processes with Multi-dimensional Molecular Imaging

Andrey Andreev, Scott E. Fraser, and Sara Madaan

3.1 Intravital Imaging

A more complete understanding of biological processes at cellular and molecular levels requires the ability to study them in time and space. Such observation became increasingly easy with the use of genetically encoded fluorescent markers, such as GFP, and the latest developments in optical microscopy. This combination of tools permits the structure and function of biological tissues to be imaged in zebrafish non-invasively. For example, it has become possible to image cardiac structure when GFP is fused to cytoskeletal elements, such as alpha-catenin; similarly, neural activity can be followed when genetically encoded calcium sensors are used to eavesdrop on sets of neurons. Such intravital imaging has furthered our understanding of the relationships between cardiac structure and function, as well as between neuronal activity patterns and complex behaviors such as sleep. Imaging these processes in 3 dimensions – at whole tissue scale and at subcellular resolution – is challenging to perform at sufficient speeds to capture the dynamics under study. Here we review some emerging approaches that combine the speed of Light Sheet microscopy with sets of computational image processing and image analysis tools, offering clear paths to overcome these challenges. We will take advantage of the zebrafish as an excellent system for imaging, and offer examples drawn from recent

A. Andreev · S. Madaan
Translational Imaging Center, Department of Molecular and Computational Biology, University of Southern California, Los Angeles, CA, USA

S. E. Fraser (✉)
Translational Imaging Center, Department of Molecular and Computational Biology, University of Southern California, Los Angeles, CA, USA

Department of Biomedical Engineering, University of Southern California, Los Angeles, CA, USA
e-mail: sfraser@provost.usc.edu

Y. Toyama et al. (eds.), *Make Life Visible*,
https://doi.org/10.1007/978-981-13-7908-6_3

efforts to perform 3D imaging at single-cell resolution of the beating heart, and of whole-brain neural activity.

3.2 Volumetric Cardiac Imaging in Embryonic Zebrafish

3.2.1 Zebrafish As a Model System for Cardiovascular Research

Congenital heart diseases (CHDs), not only represent the most prevalent birth defects in humans but also one of the leading causes of infant mortality and morbidity (Pierpont et al. 2007). Although several vertebrate model systems allow mechanistic investigations of cardiac development and of cardiac diseases, zebrafish (*Danio rerio*) offers a powerful model organism for cardiovascular development studies using imaging tools. Because of its small size, passive diffusion of oxygen can support the normal development of zebrafish embryos that are completely lacking a functional cardiovascular system or blood circulation; this permits analyses of embryos with severe cardiovascular defects that would be impossible in other systems (Stainier et al. 1996). Because zebrafish embryos develop externally and are optically transparent, they are ideal for live, in vivo imaging of cellular and physiologic processes involved in cardiac morphogenesis (Hove et al. 2003). The zebrafish heart is small enough in size (~250 μm × 200 μm × 150 μm) to be imaged in its entirety at sub-cellular resolution.

Zebrafish and mammalian hearts exhibit several well conserved structures including atria, ventricles, cardiac valves and a cardiac conduction system which coordinates the contractions of the atrial and ventricular chambers and maintains a normal heart rate (Beis et al. 2005; Chi et al. 2008; Sedmera et al. 2003; Stainier et al. 1993). These conserved features make zebrafish studies of cardiac development (e.g. valve development) and physiology (e.g. cardiac conduction studies) relevant to human cardiac development and pathologies.

The rapid development and large offspring numbers make zebrafish ideal for forward genetic screens, which have identified numerous cardiovascular mutant phenotypes. These mutants provide excellent model systems to understand human cardiac disease mechanisms, and the similarities of the mutant phenotypes to key features of some human cardiomyopathies, have resulted in the identification of novel candidate genes responsible for human cardiomyopathies. Zebrafish cardiac mutants have identified regulatory mechanisms that play crucial roles during cardiogenic specification and differentiation, migration of cardiac progenitor cells, heart tube morphogenesis, and cardiac function. For instance, the zebrafish weak atrium (*wea*) mutant has shed light on the importance of blood flow through the developing ventricle for the establishment of proper ventricle morphology (Auman et al. 2007).

Reverse genetic approaches allow functional tests of genes suspected to play important roles in cardiac function, development or pathology. For example, several potential genetic risk markers for atrio-ventricular (AV) valve and septum defects, identified from a study of 190 heart disease patients, result in malformation of the AV canal and other defects when expressed in the zebrafish (Vermot et al. 2009; Wienholds et al. 2003).

3.2.2 Cardiac Development: Symbiosis of Function and Form

Examining the relationship between function and form of the heart can offer important insights into cardiac morphogenesis as well as late-onset or acquired cardiac diseases (Hove et al. 2003; Bartman and Hove 2005; Beis et al. 2005). Since the anatomy of the heart is not fully formed until several days after its function has been initiated, it seems likely that the heart's early mechanical function plays a role in its own morphogenesis. The beating of the heart generates several types of forces at different spatial and temporal scales. While both endocardial and myocardial cells undergo cyclical compression and expansion at the tissue scale, individual endothelial cells directly experience the shear stresses and oscillatory flows generated by moving blood (Vermot et al. 2009). Several studies have suggested that changes in myocardial function result in cardiac remodeling (Hove et al. 2003; Bartman and Hove 2005; Beis et al. 2005).

3D imaging of fixed heart tissue has prompted the proposal of models for how cardiac function affects cardiac development. For example, Auman et al. used confocal imaging of fixed zebrafish to propose (Auman et al. 2007) that cardiomyocyte contractility, in addition to previously suggested hemodynamics (Hove et al. 2003), plays a role in determining the structures of cardiomyocytes in different parts of the zebrafish heart. Because stopping the heart can lead to changes in cardiac cell morphology, imaging of fixed or immobile hearts is not an ideal means to accurately assess changes in cell shape and size. Similarly, 3D Ca^{2+} –mapping in heart tissue using light sheet microscopy has improved our understanding of cardiac conduction patterns, but in cells of an immobilized heart (Weber et al. 2017). The development of techniques that allow visualization of the cardiac chambers as well as the blood flow through the heart in 3 dimensions over the time-period of the heart development would best advance our understanding of how the proper functioning of the developing heart affects cardiac morphology and vice versa.

3.2.3 Cardiac Imaging Is a 4-Dimensional Challenge

Visualizing the beating heart by using *in vivo* dynamic imaging has become possible due to the availability of several stable transgenic zebrafish lines expressing fluorescent proteins in defined cardiac and blood cells. To study cardiac developmental mechanisms, in vivo dynamic imaging methods must provide high spatial and temporal resolution, and must allow imaging of an individual zebrafish embryos throughout significant fractions of their development. Only then will it become possible to address the relationship between blood flow, shear stress, wall motion and normal cardiac development.

Despite the flexibility offered by the small size and transparent tissues of zebrafish embryos, it is still a fundamental challenge to create four-dimensional (4D) images (i.e. a volumetric (3D) movie of the beating embryonic zebrafish heart through the full depth of the beating organ) at volume rates sufficient to resolve fast cardiac motion. In order to create a high spatial resolution 3D volume rendering, data from every voxel (up to several million voxels) must be acquired in a sequential fashion. The fluorescent labeling used to visualize the tissues imposes its own limitations. For example, the excitation needed to stimulate the dye can also bleach the dyes and cause other potential photo-toxic events. Image contrast results from the detected fluorescence from the sample (often called signal) against the autofluorescence of the tissue and detector signal due to electrical noise in the absence of fluorescence (often called noise). The signal to noise ratio (SNR) must be high enough to allow the observer to differentiate labeled tissue from the background. A large number of photons must be recorded per pixel to accurately image the sample, as fluorescence emission is a Poisson process and the probability that the actual intensity at a pixel is equal to the expected intensity is proportional to $\sqrt{N}$, where N is the number of photons generated by fluorescence excitation. Typically, these concerns favor longer detection times so that signal can be collected per pixel; however, this makes the acquisition of a single volumetric image an inordinately slow process (Vermot et al. 2008).

Creating a volumetric movie of the beating heart, requires the acquisition of many high spatial resolution volumetric images at a high temporal resolution. High temporal resolution is required because cardiac walls move at velocities up to 2 mm/s and blood cells flow at velocities up to 17 mm/s. To maintain subcellular resolution, each volumetric image must be acquired in a time-period so short that the cardiac motion does not blur the image. This predicts a required volume acquisition rate of more than 1000 volumes/s. Even if such high imaging speeds were possible, the extremely short detector integration time would require an extremely high fluorescence signal rate, which would, in turn, require a very bright fluorescence excitation light. As this would lead to photobleaching and phototoxicity, such an approach would likely compromise the imaging quality and, more importantly, perturb the developing organism (Taylor et al. 2012).

Confocal Slit Microscopy made it possible to reach imaging speeds of 120 frames/s through parallel acquisition of data from a line of voxels at a time (Liebling et al. 2005). In this technique the high Numerical Aperture (NA) detection objective is used to create a blade shaped illumination beam focused to a line (instead of a single point in a conventional confocal laser scanning microscope) and all the pixels in this illuminated line are imaged in parallel. Axial sectioning is achieved by using a pinhole slit. As with other confocal microscopy techniques, the imaging speed is mostly limited by significant photobleaching due to excitation of fluorescence outside the detection plane.

The imaging speed provided by Confocal Slit microscopy (up to 3 volumes/s) is still nowhere near the speeds required (~1000 volumes/s) to capture the entire beating embryonic zebrafish heart without blurring due to wall motion or blood flow. One approach to imaging the heart is to slow down the heart wall motion and the blood flow by using chemical agents; however, this can't provide an accurate measure of the role of cardiac function on cardiac development at realistic heart rates. A better approach is to use computational techniques that utilize the quasi-periodic nature of the heart to reconstruct a volumetric representation of the beating heart from images acquired at speeds greater than 60 frames/s.

We have elected to combine computational reconstruction approaches with the fast imaging provided by Selective Plane Illumination Microscopy (SPIM), as it offers the speed of Confocal Slit Microscopy, but is dramatically less bleaching. SPIM provides diffraction limited (sub-micron resolution) imaging at high frame rates (up to 200 frames/s) and sufficient Signal to Noise ratio, by parallelizing the detection of all the voxels in a single optical section. Optical sectioning is achieved by illuminating the sample with a thin sheet of light created by a separate objective lens along a path orthogonal to the optical axis of the detection objective, thus eliminating fluorescence excitation outside of the imaged optical section. The limitation of SPIM lies in the requirement that the sample must be optically accessible from two orthogonal directions.

3.2.4 Principles of Cardiac Gated Imaging in Zebrafish

To build a 3D representation of the beating heart using SPIM or other fast 2D imaging techniques, multiple images of 2D optical slices in a volume are acquired sequentially over a period spanning multiple heartbeat periods. The different strategies for collecting a 4D rendering (3D over time) can be understood if we consider the needs for capturing a sequence of 3-dimensional images representing the different phases of the cardiac cycle. Each 3D image is composed of 2D image slices; thus, a 4D movie of the heart is a 2D matrix containing one 2D image in each cell (Fig. 3.1). The two axes of this matrix are the phase (φ) of the beating heart and the axial position (z) of the image slice. The cells in this matrix could be filled with images that are acquired in almost any order, as long as computational algorithms can utilize the quasi-periodic nature of the heart's motion to assign the 2D slices into the correct cell in the matrix. Once the matrix has been filled, the 2D cardiac images acquired during different heart beat periods are stitched into a single cardiac volume image at a single phase of the beating heart. The 4D rendering is derived from the 3D cardiac images for each phase point during the cardiac cycle, stitched. 4D cardiac imaging strategies can be classified into three groups: prospective cardiac gating, retrospective cardiac gating, and phase stamping.

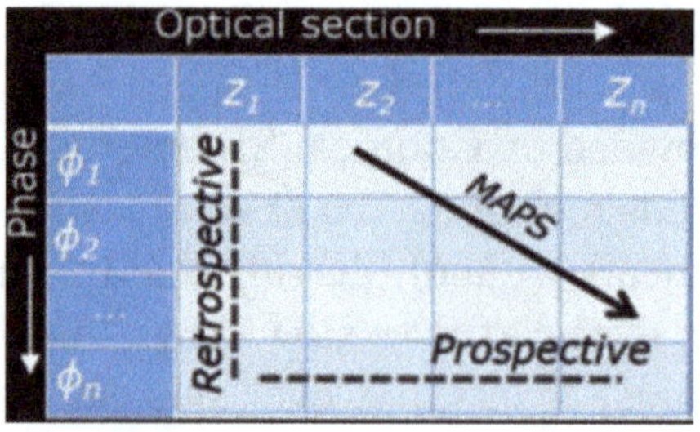

Fig. 3.1 Spatiotemporal Phase (φ) – slice position (z) representation of a 4D (3D + time) heart. If each cell in the 2-dimensional φ – z matrix consists one 2D image slice corresponding to that phase and slice position, then the matrix can be used to generate a volumetric movie of the beating heart. There are three ways to fill up this matrix with 2D image slices: prospective, retrospective and Macroscopic Phase Stamping (MaPS). In prospective gating images corresponding to entries along one column are acquired sequentially, creating a 3D image of heart at one phase point. In retrospective gating images corresponding to one row are acquired sequentially, creating a movie (2D + time) of the heart at one z plane. In MaPS, sequentially acquired images correspond to entries along diagonal lines of the matrix, thus filling the matrix with the least amount of photobleaching and hardware complexity

3.2.4.1 Prospective Gating

In prospective gating a reference signal is used to identify exactly when the heart will be in a desired phase in its cycle (Taylor et al. 2012). The reference signal could be frame data streamed from a bright-field imaging camera (Taylor et al. 2012), laser Doppler velocimetry data from a non-invasive needle probe (Jenkins et al. 2007), or scattered light modulated in intensity by the heartbeat collected from a region of tissue (such as esophagus or thorax) using a fiber optic cable (Brau et al. 2002; Sablong et al. 2014). Real-time analysis of this signal allows image acquisition of each 2D "z-slice", required to build up a 3D image for a given phase (φ) point (time point in the heartbeat), to be triggered when the heart is in that desired position. Thus, if we represent the 4D beating heart as a φ-z matrix (with phases along the columns and z along the rows) where each entry is a 2D z-slice, then prospective gating collects images corresponding to entries along one column at a time, creating a 3D image of heart, one phase point at a time (Fig. 3.1).

Taylor et al. (2012) used prospective gating of SPIM images to generate volumetric movies of an embryonic zebrafish heart and observed peak cardiac wall velocities of 160 μm/s. The authors used brightfield images of the heart acquired using the SPIM detection objective as the reference signal for gating. By using one heartbeat period worth of frames as the representative frames, they determined the phase of the heartbeat for each brightfield frame, as it was acquired, by comparing it with these representative frames, to trigger the acquisition of a fluorescent frame at the desired phase point. The number of fluorescent frames acquired is exactly equal to the number of fluorescent frames used in the final 3D reconstruction which minimizes the photodamage. The phase prediction module can also be used to trigger an ablation laser for high precision targeting of moving cells within a normally-beating heart while observing the effects of ablation.

3.2.4.2 Retrospective Gating

In retrospective gating, movies are acquired for each 2D slice, over the course of multiple heart beat cycles and relative temporal shifts between adjacent 2D slices are calculated in order to temporally align movies from neighboring slices (Liebling et al. 2005). The 2D slice movies are first truncated to an integer number of heartbeats. Then pairwise correlation between the wavelet coefficients of frames of neighboring movies are used to determine the phase offset between neighboring 2D movies (Liebling et al. 2005). While, prospective gating collects images along the columns of the φ-z matrix, retrospective gating collects images along the rows (Fig. 3.1). Liebling et al. later improved upon their technique by using "temporal warping" of slice sequences by taking the variability of the cardiac rate between different slice sequences into account. The improved approach could reduce the quantization error introduced while assigning a discrete phase to any frame in one slice sequence based on the phase of the most similar frames in the neighboring slice sequence.

The simplicity of the imaging hardware in retrospective gating makes it a desirable technique for cardiac imaging. Retrospective gating has been combined with 2-photon SPIM to achieve high penetration depth while maintaining the high imaging speed required for cardiac imaging (Trivedi et al. 2015). This could allow imaging of older zebrafish embryos that have a more complex cardiac structure. Retrospective gating requires higher number of acquired frames (~2–5 min of continuous recording at 100 frames/s) compared to prospective gating; however, the total elapsed imaging time is generally shorter for retrospective approaches. With prospective gating, only one point in the phase-z matrix is acquired per heartbeat, which can extend elapsed imaging times up to 20 min, depending upon the number of desired z-slices.

3.2.4.3 Macroscopic Phase Stamping

Both gating techniques have been used in cardiac imaging using modalities other than fluorescence microscopy (Thompson and McVeigh 2004; Larson et al. 2004; Grass et al. 2003; Treece et al. 2002). Despite being widely used, both these techniques suffer from limitations arising from the need to create 3D volumes from 2D slices in the absence of an imaging modality that can capture a 3D volume at a rate sufficient to minimize the motion of the heart to sub-pixel amounts. For the retrospective approach, the assumption of sample continuity in the z direction can break down in case of a peristaltic wave propagating through the cardiac tube along the imaging axis. Retrospective gating also lacks simultaneous and independent acquisition of the phase of the acquired images. The primary limitation for the prospective approach is the hardware complexity and the inability to trigger accurately off less distinct phase points due to the slower motion of cardiac tissue in the brightfield frames during the start of atrial and ventricular contraction, which leads to jitter in the final φ-z reconstruction.

We have developed Macroscopic Phase Stamping (MaPS) to provide a more robust reconstruction, by jointly refining low resolution brightfield images acquired synchronously with optically sectioned fluorescent images acquired with SPIM (Truong et al. 2014; Truong 2017). The brightfield images allow us to determine the macroscopic spatio-temporal phase of the beating heart in the fluorescent images in post-processing. In MaPS, the sample is repeatedly scanned along the axial direction, while the imaging plane is kept stationary during the synchronized fluorescent + brightfield image acquisition. Since both the z position and the phase of the beating heart advance from one image to the next, the phase-z matrix is filled diagonally (Fig. 3.1). The z position for the fluorescent frames is assigned based on the stage position.

MaPS combines the simplicity of the hardware needed for retrospective gating with the advantage of an independent phase channel in prospective gating, providing an improvement over both approaches. The hardware complexity is minimized because both cameras are synchronized only to each other and not to a cardiac event. The availability of the synchronized bright field images provides an independent channel to determine the periodicity of the heartbeat on which any type of cardiac gating relies. The brightfield images allow us to synchronize fluorescent images that are adjacent to each other in the z direction without using the fluorescent images themselves, resulting in more accurate reconstructions of the 3D structure of the heart.

The high resolution of the individual 2D slices afforded by SPIM added with the more accurate reconstruction process provides high spatial resolution 3D reconstruction volumes, in which individual cardiac cell boundaries are easily resolvable (Fig. 3.2a). The high spatio-temporal resolution has allowed us to segment individual

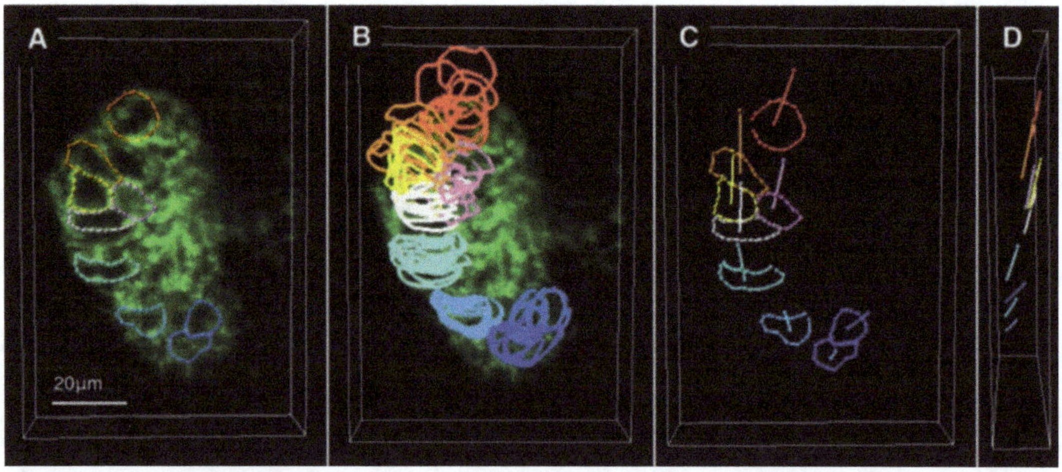

Fig. 3.2 (**a**) Macroscopic Projection of a 3D rendering of a 4D reconstructed cardiac movie at 84 hpf where the cardiac boundaries are visible through endogenous expression of citrine labeled alpha-catenin. The 4D cardiac movie was reconstructed through Macroscopic Phase Stamping of SPIM images. (**b**) Selectively segmented cell boundaries at different phases in the heart beat. (**c**) Selectively segmented cell boundaries along with their displacement during the heart beat (straight lines) from ventral (**c**) and lateral (**d**) views

cardiac cells and determine their displacement over the course of a heartbeat period (Fig. 3.2b–d). This will enable cardiac researchers to understand of how individual cell biomechanics relates to the overall biomechanics of the beating heart. Recent improvements in MaPS have reduced the error introduced due to phase assignments by using a finer quantization of the phase, reducing artefacts that might otherwise appear in the volumetric renderings when the heart wall moves at its fastest speeds.

Aperiodically beating mutant zebrafish hearts, which represent some of the best tools for understanding the causes and effects of human cardiac diseases such as arrhythmias, are also the most challenging to image with cardiac gating-based techniques described above. Imaging individual blood cells that flow aperiodically through a periodically beating heart is another goal that future developments in cardiac imaging tools would attempt to accomplish.

3.3 Large Scale *In Vivo* Brain Imaging with Two-Photon Light-Sheet Microscopy

One of the important characteristics of the brain is its ability to constantly change and adapt, driven in large part by its combined evoked and spontaneous activity, typically without any periodic pattern. Brain activity observation allows insight into these dynamic changes of the nervous system. Complex animal behaviors often involve activity that spans many brain regions. If we want to advance our understanding of complex behaviors such as learning or sleep, we necessarily have to look at multiple regions of the brain with single-cell resolution. This remains a challenge to overcome, as most current tools for functional brain imaging lack either resolution or field of view. For example, one of the best tools to study the activity of the roughly 100 billion neurons human brain, functional MRI using BOLD (blood-oxygen-level dependent) contrast, produces striking three-dimensional images; however, the signal presented in each voxel of thousands of neurons. At the other end of the spectrum are microscopy techniques, where the best light imaging instruments collect data from only a small fraction of the cortical neurons in mice. The best experiments collect data from a thousand out of the four million cortical neurons: merely 0.025% of the cells.

Zebrafish, with its compact brain, offers the potential of optical imaging that can observe neural activity at whole-brain scale with single-cell resolution. Functional imaging can be achieved using genetically-encoded fluorescent calcium indicators as an indicator of neuronal activity, as calcium is elevated in most neurons when they fire action potentials. Genetically encoded calcium indicators change their fluorescence intensity depending on calcium ion concentration in the neuron. Some dyes change fluorescence efficiency (intensity-based), while other sensors change spectral parameters (shifting emission spectra from green to red, for example). Fast imaging techniques, such as light-sheet microscopy or laser scanning microscopy, are need to capture these signals. The advantages and limitations of these imaging tools will be discussed below.

3.3.1 Brain Activity Monitoring in Behaving Zebrafish

The zebrafish larva offers an important compromise, as it is a vertebrate model relevant to higher animals and mammals, in which almost all of its 100,000 neurons of the central nervous system can be imaged. While such imaging is still challenging and requires the application of advanced optical light sheet microscopy (to be discussed later), it is the feasibility of in toto imaging that drives our choice to focus on the zebrafish nervous system here.

The benefits of zebrafish larva as model organism stem from the combination of its compact size and optical transparency, thus permitting high-resolution optical microscopy. In order to visualize neural activity, transgenic animals, positionally expressing a gene encoding a calcium-sensitive fluorophore (cf. GCaMP or its variants) have been used. These genetically encoded fluorescent calcium indicators change their color or their brightness when a cell's calcium level increases, as it does following even single action potentials. GCaMP indicators, based on a fusion of a modified GFP fluorescent protein and the calmodulin calcium-binding domain, offer a large change in signal with changes in calcium levels. In addition, they offer the ability to use multiple colors, since GFP and other colored fluorescent proteins permit the creation of whole palette of calcium sensors, from blue to deep-red (Akerboom et al. 2013). GCaMP sensors are intensity-based, that is, they change their intensity as the calcium level changes. This is in contrast to other ratiometric calcium sensors, which change their fluorescent spectrum as the calcium level changes. Ratiometric indicators offer more accurate measurements of calcium concentration, but the need to measure the spectrum of the dye, or the ratio of its intensity at two emission (or excitation) wavelengths limits the number of simultaneous labels that can be deployed simultaneously. Several limitations should be considered, including temporal resolution of these sensors. While action potentials have duration of 10's of milliseconds or less, calcium sensors give a signal in response to neuronal activity that lasts 100 ms/s. The speed of the signal can decline when sensor is concentrated in the cell soma, away from synapses where neural-related calcium transients are generated. In vertebrates that is not a general issue, the soma is electrically involved in the neural processing; however, in some invertebrate species, the soma can be physically and electrically distant from the synaptic activity. Currently, sensors of the GCaMP6 family are best option for imaging neural activity, when a single color is enough and two-photon excitation is required.

Modern bioengineering techniques allow labeling of neurons in specific brain region by expressing the reporter using a vector, an artificial DNA sequence, containing a tissue-specific promoter sequence, followed by protein coding sequence for one of the calcium sensors. A common zebrafish promoter used to drive gene in the nervous system is the promoter of the *HuC* gene, also known as *elavl3*. Often, the sensor fused with nuclear-localization sequence (as nls-GCaMP) (Kim et al. 2014), in order to increase the concentration of protein in nuclei, and hence increase signal-to-noise ratio. Concentration of the fluorescence signal in a discrete location such as the nuclei can be helpful for downstream image processing, as images of nuclear-localized fluorescent molecules are bright focal spots, easily segmented computationally. Concentrating the sensor molecules in nuclei decreases temporal resolution, as changes in calcium across the cell must propagate from its release site to the nucleus in order to affect sensor's fluorescence, which can take up to a second. Faster dynamics are possible by localization of the sensor to other cellular compartments, such as synapses, by fusing it with synaptophysin (Li et al. 2011). This concentrates the sensor in compartment of interest (synapse) because synaptophysin is naturally localized there by the cell's own machinery. However, such fusions also raise the possibility of perturbing the local environment of the synapse, since the synapse is a very crowded and tightly regulated compartment; furthermore, the protein molecule fused to the sensor might be perturbed and lose its original functionality.

Brain imaging using calcium indicators has been successfully applied to study zebrafish brain activity. For example, fluorescent calcium indicator dyes have been useful to investigate distribution of spontaneous activity-independent calcium transients in zebrafish spinal cord (Ashworth and Bolsover 2002). Intensity-based sensors, primarily members of GCaMP family, were used to observe neural activity while the animal is performing complex behaviors, such as prey capture (Muto et al. 2013), visual or auditory responses (Thompson and Scott 2016), optokinetic responses (Vladimirov et al. 2014), or spontaneous activity reorganization during development (Avitan et al. 2017).

An excellent demonstration of the power of in vivo brain imaging in zebrafish, was the description of the activity in the visual system (optic tectum) during prey capture (Muto et al. 2013) using wide field microscopy with visible light illumination. By observing the freely swimming fish surrounded by several paramecia, the authors were able to record calcium activity in tectal neurons and create maps of activity corresponding to the particular position of prey in the fish's visual field. By simultaneous imaging of prey movement and calcium activity authors were able to map how prey's trajectory maps onto optic tectum: the prey's ventral-dorsal movement resulted in distinct tectal activity than prey movement in anterior-posterior direction. This work not only demonstrated the promise of brain imaging in zebrafish, but also revealed limitations of the particular imaging technique. First of all, the resolution of the imaging was low, averaging signals from tens of neurons. More importantly, this imaging approach used visible light to excite fluorescence, and hence potentially perturbed the animal's visually-guided behaviors, as animal continuously illuminated with very bright blue light.

The optic tectum or its equivalent, the superior colliculus in the mammalian midbrain, is present in all vertebrates and responsible for the animal's orientation toward a subject and attention. In larval zebrafish, the optic tectum is only about 100 um thick and is positioned at the dorsal surface of the brain, making it an accessible system for studying neural function. This allowed Avitan et al (2017) to follow changes in functional mapping during development in larval zebrafish. Observing spontaneous activity in animals of age 4–7 days post fertilization (dpf), the authors discovered changes in single-cell as well as group activity patterns during development. Immobilization of the animal and use of two-photon laser scanning microscopy (LSM) allowed imaging with single-cell resolution, thus making it possible to robustly identify cellular communities containing as small as a few cells.

Advancements in imaging techniques, behavioral protocols, and genetic tools, as well as image analysis algorithms, allow whole-brain imaging of behaving zebrafish with single-cell resolution. These achievements prove how useful zebrafish and brain imaging can be together. More importantly it supports the use of zebrafish model and imaging for detailed studies of more complex behaviors, such as learning and sleep. Sleep behavior in particular requires careful approach, since it occurs over long period of time; hence we need a tool that would allow longitudinal (up to 24 h) imaging of brain activity in behaving zebrafish. Combined with already established sleep behavioral models, such as narcolepsy or insomnia models, such toolbox would be immensely useful for more detailed examination of underlying neural substrate of these disorders, as well as natural sleep.

3.3.2 Principles and Successes of Light-Sheet Microscopy for Zebrafish Brain Imaging

Light-sheet microscopy, or selective-plane illumination microscopy (SPIM), solves previous limitations by providing tool to collect large-scale imaging data with cellular resolution (Huisken 2004). Photo-toxicity is lower because only imaged volume is illuminated, thus allowing imaging either with higher signal-to-noise, or greater speed. SPIM imaging has reached a 1 volume per second imaging rate, sufficient for whole-brain GCaMP activity mapping. Light-sheet mode also provides opportunity to use two-photon illumination, using light invisible to the fish. This removes artifacts of high-power visible light illumination, such as visual system stimulation, and allows better use of optogenetic tools.

Even though a number of commercial SPIM systems are available, many labs choose to build their own light-sheet microscopes, often following designs available in numerous research publications. A project dedicated to creation of an open-source light-sheet microscope, OpenSPIM, provides detailed designs and step-by-step instructions for the assembly of a relatively cheap home-built microscope with a small footprint. For more flexible solutions it is important that the software for running microscopes is open source and free. The popular microscopy program, Micro-Manager provides a package that supports a myriad of hardware components, allowing robust control of almost any part of a microscope.

First experiments with whole-brain SPIM imaging in zebrafish larvae were performed on paralyzed animals (Ahrens et al. 2012) during adaptation of motor behavior. This work was further developed (Vladimirov et al. 2014) to show how ablation of particular neurons changes fictive whole-animal behavior. One limitation of these experiments is that study of such "fictive" behavior in a paralyzed animal, when motor response is not observed but rather recorded by measuring motor neurons' activity, is achieved by inducing irreversible paralysis. This preparation limits experiment time, as animals can survive such treatment for only a few hours.

Sample preparation is important for experiments in living animals. Imaging of zebrafish brain using SPIM can be achieved with immobilization, but without total paralysis (Keller et al. 2008). Often soft agarose gel is used to restrict animal head under detection objective to perform long-term observation of neural activity with single-cell resolution. Such restraining can be deleterious from several points of view. For longer imaging in young animals, agarose embedding impedes proper development (Kaufmann et al. 2012). Such immobilization can also possibly change behavior by stimulating efferent neurons, neurons of the lateral line, and other sensory circuits. New methods are being developed in order to overcome this limitation and image freely swimming larval zebrafish (Kim et al. 2017), but only using high power visible light as fluorescence excitation source. When sufficiently advanced, these would provide much needed tool to observe neural activity while animal performs unrestricted behavior. Such experiments would allow observation of movement and prey capture behavior in real time, as well as long-term imaging, necessary for studying development or learning. Applied to imaging compact and accessible zebrafish brain, this would allow observation of brain activity in behaving vertebrate at unprecedented scale, unavailable to rodent model systems.

High temporal resolution is important for fast-pacing action potentials, as discussed above. In light-sheet microscopy pixels in different axial planes are acquired at different times, limiting temporal resolution. Light-field microscopy (LFM) offers a potential solution to this problem. LFM (Levoy et al. 2009) uses a microlens array interposed between the image plane and the camera to re-image light of sources from different axial positions to different sets of pixels on the camera. Computational deconvolution is used to reconstruct 3-dimensional image of the sample. This comes at a price of lower spatial resolution, but it allows the capturing of events at millisecond time scales across large volumes, extending to as large as nearly the entire zebrafish brain. LFM is a promising tool as it would allow imaging of very fast events across the brain, such as propagation of action potentials along axons.

In our work, we were able to observe neural activity during sleep and wake in zebrafish (Fig. 3.3) for more than 24 h for the first time (Lee et al. 2017). Application of two-photon light-sheet microscopy and opto- and chemo-genetic activation of sleep-promoting NPVF circuit, allowed us to demonstrate how sleep behavior manifest itself on brain activity level in natural and induced sleep (Fig. 3.3c). Light-sheet imaging though allows extension of this simple analysis in order to quantify functional inter-neuronal connections, correlation of activity between neurons, and other metrics that are usually used to understand functionality of the brain. Extension of this work (presented at the Society for Neuroscience Annual Meeting, 2017),

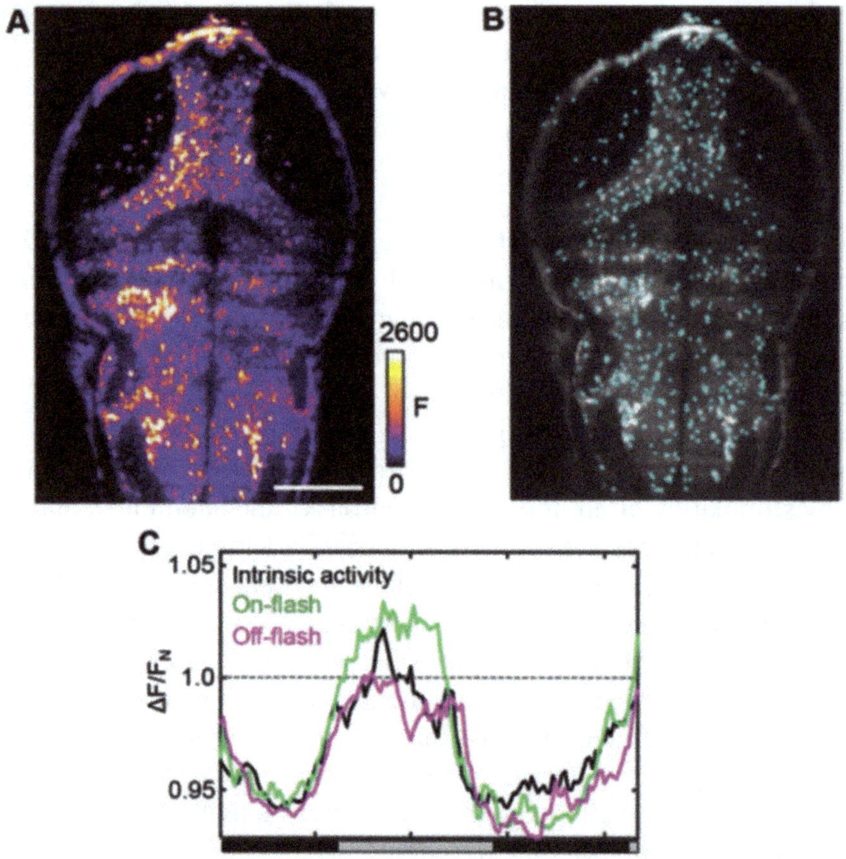

Fig. 3.3 (**a**) Single-plane imaging of brain in 6dpf zebrafish *Tg*(HuC:H2B-GCaMP6s). Neurons are labeled with nuclei-concentrated calcium indicator GCaMP6s. (**b**) Neurons are localized using PCA/ICA toolbox (Mukamel et al. 2009). (**c**) Day/night oscillation in fluorescent signals across whole brain of the animal. Imaging does not perturb circadian clock and allows observation of spontaneous and light-induced activity

shows that functional correlation between regions differs in sleep and wake. In particular we observed that activity of cerebellum lobes becomes more correlated during sleep, suggesting a pathway to study role of sleep in memory consolidation in zebrafish. Another exciting application allowed by development of this toolbox is the investigation of effects of melatonin and other hypnotic chemicals on brain activity during sleep and wake. This should permit comparative analyses of chemically-induced sleep with natural healthy sleep.

3.4 Conclusion

The development of imaging tools, discussed here, allows unprecedented access to biological processes in living zebrafish. Light-sheet and light-field imaging provide information about anatomy and function of rapidly beating heart with subcellular resolution and permit whole-brain mapping of activity with single-neuron resolution. Future work will benefit from combination of large-scale, high-resolution imaging with genomics and other genome-scale methods. Many of these tools are already available, but a collaborative environment where biologists who can maintain optimal conditions for sample survival, physicists and engineers who can create the imaging instruments, and mathematicians who can design analytical tools can work together in order to foresee the possible challenges and find alternative solutions, will be required to carry out interesting and meaningful experiments.

References

Ahrens MB, Li JM, Orger MB et al (2012) Brain-wide neuronal dynamics during motor adaptation in zebrafish. Nature 485:471–477. https://doi.org/10.1038/nature11057

Akerboom J, Carreras Calderón N, Tian L et al (2013) Genetically encoded calcium indicators for multi-color neural activity imaging and combination with optogenetics. Front Mol Neurosci 6(2). https://doi.org/10.3389/fnmol.2013.00002

Ashworth R, Bolsover SR (2002) Spontaneous activity-independent intracellular calcium signals in the developing spinal cord of the zebrafish embryo. Brain Res Dev Brain Res 139:131–137

Auman HJ, Coleman H, Riley HE et al (2007) Functional modulation of cardiac form through regionally confined cell shape changes. PLoS Biol 5:e53. https://doi.org/10.1371/journal.pbio.0050053

Avitan L, Pujic Z, Mölter J et al (2017) Spontaneous activity in the zebrafish tectum reorganizes over development and is influenced by visual experience. Curr Biol CB 27:2407–2419.e4. https://doi.org/10.1016/j.cub.2017.06.056

Bartman T, Hove J (2005) Mechanics and function in heart morphogenesis. Dev Dyn 233:373–381. https://doi.org/10.1002/dvdy.20367

Beis D, Bartman T, Jin S-W et al (2005) Genetic and cellular analyses of zebrafish atrioventricular cushion and valve development. Dev Camb Engl 132:4193–4204. https://doi.org/10.1242/dev.01970

Brau ACS, Wheeler CT, Hedlund LW, Johnson GA (2002) Fiber-optic stethoscope: a cardiac monitoring and gating system for magnetic resonance microscopy. Magn Reson Med 47:314–321

Chi NC, Shaw RM, Jungblut B, Huisken J, Ferrer T, Arnaout R, Scott I, Beis D, Xiao T, Baier H, Jan LY, Tristani-Firouzi M, Stainier DYR, Hogan BLM (2008) Genetic and physiologic dissection of the vertebrate cardiac conduction system. PLoS Biol 6(5):e109

Grass M, Manzke R, Nielsen T et al (2003) Helical cardiac cone beam reconstruction using retrospective ECG gating. Phys Med Biol 48:3069–3084

Hove JR, Köster RW, Forouhar AS et al (2003) Intracardiac fluid forces are an essential epigenetic factor for embryonic cardiogenesis. Nature 421:172–177. https://doi.org/10.1038/nature01282

Huisken J (2004) Optical sectioning deep inside live embryos by selective plane illumination microscopy. Science 305:1007–1009. https://doi.org/10.1126/science.1100035

Jenkins MW, Chughtai OQ, Basavanhally AN et al (2007) In vivo gated 4D imaging of the embryonic heart using optical coherence tomography. J Biomed Opt 12:030505. https://doi.org/10.1117/1.2747208

Kaufmann A, Mickoleit M, Weber M, Huisken J (2012) Multilayer mounting enables long-term imaging of zebrafish development in a light sheet microscope. Dev Camb Engl 139:3242–3247. https://doi.org/10.1242/dev.082586

Keller PJ, Schmidt AD, Wittbrodt J, Stelzer EHK (2008) Reconstruction of zebrafish early embryonic development by scanned light sheet microscopy. Science 322:1065–1069. https://doi.org/10.1126/science.1162493

Kim CK, Miri A, Leung LC et al (2014) Prolonged, brain-wide expression of nuclear-localized GCaMP3 for functional circuit mapping. Front Neural Circuits 8:138. https://doi.org/10.3389/fncir.2014.00138

Kim DH, Kim J, Marques JC et al (2017) Pan-neuronal calcium imaging with cellular resolution in freely swimming zebrafish. Nat Methods 14:1107–1114. https://doi.org/10.1038/nmeth.4429

Larson AC, White RD, Laub G et al (2004) Self-gated cardiac cine MRI. Magn Reson Med 51:93–102. https://doi.org/10.1002/mrm.10664

Lee DA, Andreev A, Truong TV et al (2017) Genetic and neuronal regulation of sleep by neuropeptide VF. eLife 6. https://doi.org/10.7554/eLife.25727

Levoy M, Zhang Z, McDowall I (2009) Recording and controlling the 4D light field in a microscope using microlens arrays. J Microsc 235:144–162. https://doi.org/10.1111/j.1365-2818.2009.03195.x

Li H, Foss SM, Dobryy YL et al (2011) Concurrent imaging of synaptic vesicle recycling and calcium dynamics. Front Mol Neurosci 4:34. https://doi.org/10.3389/fnmol.2011.00034

Liebling M, Forouhar AS, Gharib M et al (2005) Four-dimensional cardiac imaging in living embryos via postacquisition synchronization of nongated slice sequences. J Biomed Opt 10:054001. https://doi.org/10.1117/1.2061567

Mukamel EA, Nimmerjahn A, Schnitzer MJ (2009) Automated analysis of cellular signals from large-scale calcium imaging data. Neuron 63:747–760. https://doi.org/10.1016/j.neuron.2009.08.009

Muto A, Ohkura M, Abe G et al (2013) Real-time visualization of neuronal activity during perception. Curr Biol CB 23:307–311. https://doi.org/10.1016/j.cub.2012.12.040

Pierpont ME, Basson CT, Benson DW et al (2007) Genetic basis for congenital heart defects: current knowledge: a scientific statement from the American Heart Association Congenital Cardiac Defects Committee, Council on Cardiovascular Disease in the Young: endorsed by the American Academy of Pediatrics. Circulation 115:3015–3038. https://doi.org/10.1161/CIRCULATIONAHA.106.183056

Sablong R, Rengle A, Ramgolam A et al (2014) An optical fiber-based gating device for prospective mouse cardiac MRI. IEEE Trans Biomed Eng 61:162–170. https://doi.org/10.1109/TBME.2013.2278712

Sedmera D, Reckova M, deAlmeida A, Sedmerova M, Biermann M, Volejnik J, Sarre A, Raddatz E, McCarthy RA, Gourdie RG, Thompson RP (2003) Functional and morphological evidence for a ventricular conduction system in zebrafish and hearts. Am J Phys Heart Circ Phys 284(4):H1152–H1160

Stainier DY, Lee RK, Fishman MC (1993) Cardiovascular development in the zebrafish. I. Myocardial fate map and heart tube formation. Dev Camb Engl 119:31–40

Stainier DY, Fouquet B, Chen JN et al (1996) Mutations affecting the formation and function of the cardiovascular system in the zebrafish embryo. Dev Camb Engl 123:285–292

Taylor JM, Girkin JM, Love GD (2012) High-resolution 3D optical microscopy inside the beating zebrafish heart using prospective optical gating. Biomed Opt Express 3:3043–3053. https://doi.org/10.1364/BOE.3.003043

Thompson RB, McVeigh ER (2004) Flow-gated phase-contrast MRI using radial acquisitions. Magn Reson Med 52:598–604. https://doi.org/10.1002/mrm.20187

Thompson AW, Scott EK (2016) Characterisation of sensitivity and orientation tuning for visually responsive ensembles in the zebrafish tectum. Sci Rep 6:34887. https://doi.org/10.1038/srep34887

Treece GM, Prager RW, Gee AH, Berman L (2002) Correction of probe pressure artifacts in freehand 3D ultrasound. Med Image Anal 6:199–214

Trivedi V, Truong TV, Trinh LA, Holland DB, Liebling M, Fraser SE (2015) Dynamic structure and protein expression of the live embryonic heart captured by 2-photon light sheet microscopy and retrospective registration. Biomed Opt Express 6(6):2056

Truong TV (2017) Optimized live volumetric imaging with light sheet microscopy and related strategies. Microsc Microanal 23:2320–2321. https://doi.org/10.1017/S1431927617012260

Truong TV, Trivedi V, Trinh L et al (2014) Live 4D imaging of the embryonic vertebrate heart with two-photon light sheet microscopy and simultaneous optical phase stamping. Biophys J 106:435a–436a. https://doi.org/10.1016/j.bpj.2013.11.2453

Vermot J, Fraser SE, Liebling M (2008) Fast fluorescence microscopy for imaging the dynamics of embryonic development. HFSP J 2:143–155. https://doi.org/10.2976/1.2907579

Vermot J, Forouhar AS, Liebling M et al (2009) Reversing blood flows act through klf2a to ensure normal valvulogenesis in the developing heart. PLoS Biol 7:e1000246. https://doi.org/10.1371/journal.pbio.1000246

Vladimirov N, Mu Y, Kawashima T et al (2014) Light-sheet functional imaging in fictively behaving zebrafish. Nat Methods 11:883–884. https://doi.org/10.1038/nmeth.3040

Weber M, Scherf N, Meyer AM et al (2017) Cell-accurate optical mapping across the entire developing heart. eLife 6. https://doi.org/10.7554/eLife.28307

Wienholds E, van Eeden F, Kosters M et al (2003) Efficient target-selected mutagenesis in zebrafish. Genome Res 13:2700–2707. https://doi.org/10.1101/gr.1725103

Chapter 4
Apical Cytoskeletons Help Define the Barrier Functions of Epithelial Cell Sheets in Biological Systems

Sachiko Tsukita, Tomoki Yano, and Elisa Herawati

4.1 Introduction

Epithelial cells adhere to each other by tight junctions (TJs) to form cell sheets, which is a critical step in epithelial barrier creation and the morphogenesis of vertebrate tissues (Fleming et al. 2000; Tsukita et al. 2001; Anderson et al. 2004; Furuse and Moriwaki 2009; Van Itallie and Anderson 2014; Tanaka et al. 2017). The apical surface of an epithelial cell sheet faces the outer environment, such as the lumen in the intestinal tract or the environment outside the skin surface. In the sheet, the cells' apical membranes are regarded as a continuous, connected surface, in which the cell-cell adhesion sites are cemented by TJs. Notably, each epithelial cell exhibits basolateral polarity, and therefore the apical surface of an epithelial cell sheet differs from the basolateral one, and possesses specific features that relate to its roles in a particular biological functional system (Nelson 2009; Apodaca 2017). Apical differentiation is a popular topic of study, and includes microvilli, cilia, circumferential rings (Nelson 2009; Apodaca 2017), and ratchet structures, which have been described in *Drosophila* but not yet in vertebrates (Martin et al. 2009).

Electronic Supplementary Material The online version of this chapter (https://doi.org/10.1007/978-981-13-7908-6_4) contains supplementary material, which is available to authorized users.

S. Tsukita (✉) · T. Yano
Laboratory of Biological Science, Graduate School of Frontier Biosciences and Graduate School of Medicine, Osaka University, Osaka, Japan
e-mail: atsukita@biosci.med.osaka-u.ac.jp

E. Herawati
Laboratory of Biological Science, Graduate School of Frontier Biosciences and Graduate School of Medicine, Osaka University, Osaka, Japan

Faculty of Mathematics and Natural Sciences, Biology Study Program, Universitas Sebelas Maret, Surakarta, Indonesia

Y. Toyama et al. (eds.), *Make Life Visible*,
https://doi.org/10.1007/978-981-13-7908-6_4

Consistent with the critical and varied roles of the apical surface, we recently identified a 3-layered cytoskeletal network of actin filaments, intermediate filaments, and microtubules that exists just below the apical membrane of epithelial cell sheets. The apical cytoskeletons are presumably organized under the control of the TJs and regulate epithelial morphogenesis and barrier functions in conjunction with TJ formation and TJ-based cell signaling. Thus, we propose to define this set of structures as a system called the "TJ-apical complex" (Yano et al. 2017).

A natural question is why this apical cytoskeletal system was not discovered until recently. It is a very thin-layered structure mainly composed of actin filaments, intermediate filaments, and microtubules, which appear as a continuous structure extending horizontally just beneath the apical plasma membrane. We discovered this network using an advanced imaging system, including ultrahigh voltage electron microscopic tomography and confocal super-resolution microscopy, that we developed (Kunimoto et al. 2012; Yano et al. 2013; Tateishi et al. 2017). Although the molecular mechanisms and physiological roles of the "TJ-apical complex" remain to be elucidated, we recently identified four TJMAPs (TJ Microtubule-associated Proteins; previously called J-MAPs), including cingulin which are TJ-associated proteins that bind to the apical cytoskeletons (Yano et al. 2013). During the morphogenesis of epithelial cell sheets, apical constriction and the size of the apical area defined by TJs must be kept in balance. Our recent data suggest that TJMAPs may constitute a platform on which the apical cytoskeletons and TJs associate to organize biological systems, although more study is needed to examine this possibility (Fig. 4.1).

Regarding the functions of the "TJ-apical complex," multiciliated cells represent a highly specific case in which the apical microtubules are particularly highly developed. In tracheal multiciliated cells (MCCs), the apical microtubules have a specific role in establishing the regular arrangement of basal bodies (BBs), which generate cilia in the apical membranes (Kunimoto et al. 2012; Herawati et al. 2016; Tateishi

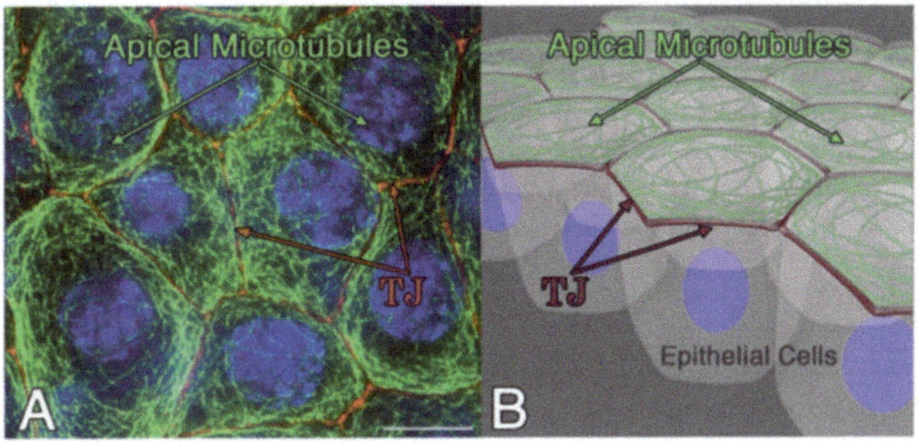

Fig. 4.1 Immunofluorescence image (**a**) and schematic drawing (**b**) of the apical microtubule network existing beneath the apical membrane of epithelial cells. Microtubules (α-tubulin-staining), green; Tight junctions (ZO1-staining) red; Nuclei (DAPI-staining), blue. Scale, 10 μm. TJ, tight junction. Bar, 10 μm

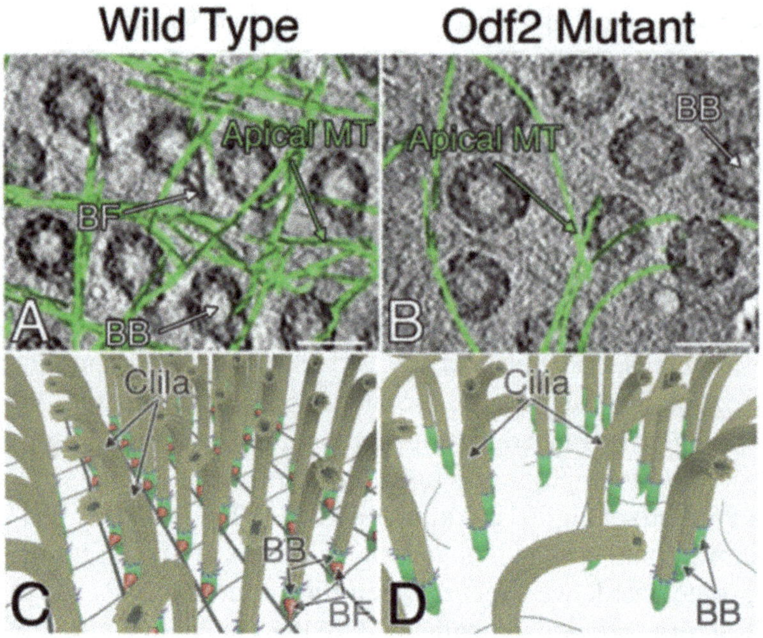

Fig. 4.2 Ultra high-voltage electron-microscopy images (**a**, **b**) of basal bodies and schematic drawing (**c**, **d**) of multi-ciliated epithelial cells. The apical microtubules (green) between basal bodies (BBs) in the wild-type mice and Odf2-mutant (Kunimoto et al. 2012). In the Odf2 mutant mice, the BB (basal body) alignment was perturbed by the loss of BFs (basal feet: the accessory structure of BBs) and of the regular apical microtubule network. Bar, 100 nm

et al. 2017). To explore the differentiation mechanism leading to the regular BB alignment, we examined tracheal MCCs expressing GFP-centrin, a BB-associated protein, using our new long-term, high-resolution, live-imaging system. The microtubule-dependent regular arrangement of BBs is critical for the synchronous beating and metachronal waves of hundreds of motile cilia on the apical membrane of MCCs (Guirao and Joanny 2007; Elgeti and Gompper 2013). Thus, the physiological role of the apical cytoskeleton that we revealed in this case is likely to be essential for tissue function (Fig. 4.2).

By comparing the findings for various epithelial cells, both the common and unique characteristics of the apical cytoskeletal structures are being revealed. In the following sections, we discuss the roles of the apical cytoskeletons, especially microtubules, in epithelial cell sheets that have specific functional relevance (Fig. 4.3).

4.2 The Apical Cytoskeletons in General Epithelial Cells

In confluent epithelial cell sheets, each cell is highly polarized in the apico-basal direction, and the cells' apical membranes are regarded as a continuous surface connected by TJs. Although the mechanism by which TJs are positioned at the most apical part of the lateral membrane is not understood, the TJs determine the edges

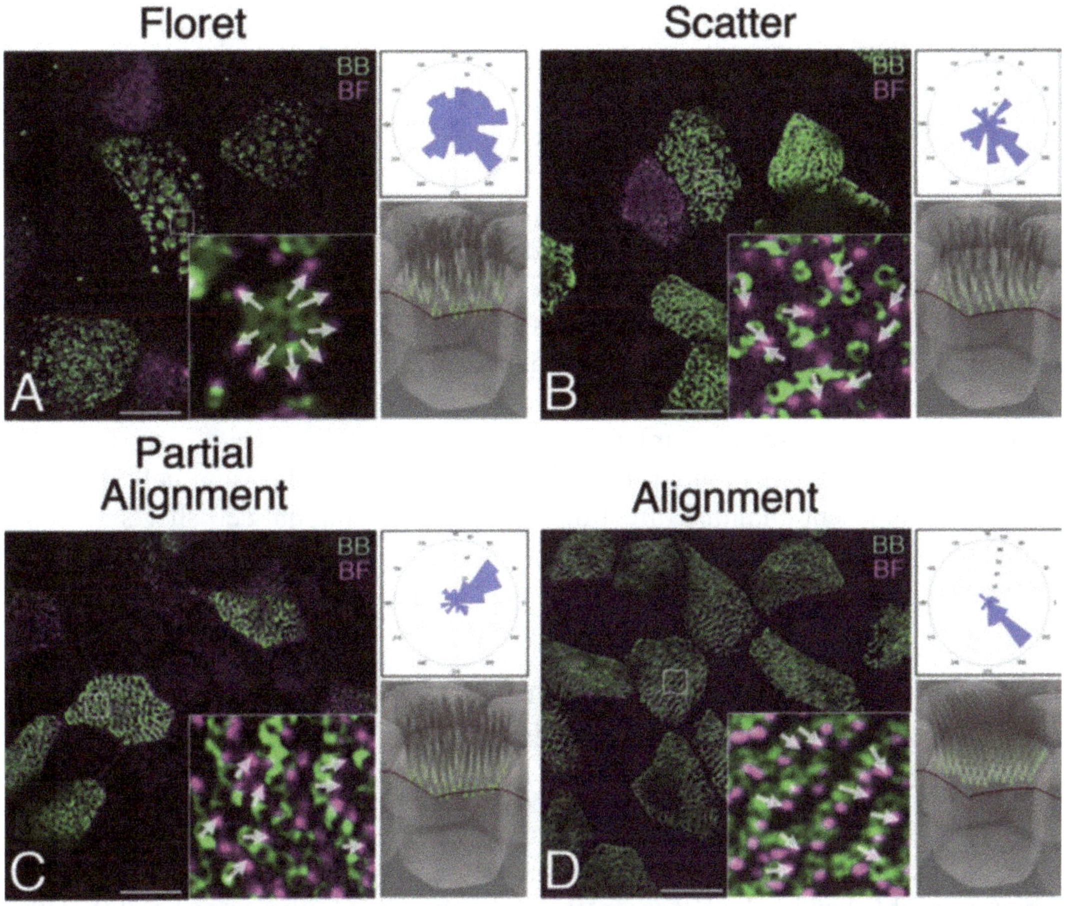

Fig. 4.3 Immunofluorescence images, circular diagrams, and schematic drawing of basal bodies (BBs) and basal feet (BF) during BB pattern development of Floret (**a**), Scatter (**b**), Partial Alignment (**c**) and Alignment (**d**). Orientation of each BB is shown by an arrow connecting the center of a BB marker (green) to the center of a BF marker (red) (insets) and by the circular diagrams of ciliary orientation (direction of white arrows in the immunofluorescence image). (Bottom) Illustration of cilia. Bar, 10 μm

of each cell's apical membrane when the cell sheet is viewed from the top (the apical view). Distinct, specific differentiation mechanisms occur in the apical area. Well-known classical examples of apical differentiation are the circumferential ring at cell-cell boundaries and the terminal web (Leblond et al. 1960; Hull and Staehelin 1979; Owaribe et al. 1981; Burgess 1982; Keller et al. 1985). In *Drosophila* epithelial cells, a "ratchet structure" consisting of actin filaments exists in the medial area of apical membranes (Martin et al. 2009), although no similar structure has been clearly identified in mammalian epithelial cells. By applying our super-resolution microscopy system to cultured epithelial cell sheets, we discovered the detailed structure of the apical cytoskeleton, which was previously unknown and uniquely distributed beneath the apical membrane like a shell (Yano et al. 2013). This location led us to propose that the apical cytoskeletal network is associated with TJs, which are located at the most apical part of the lateral membrane, and that these structures form a system called the "TJ-apical complex." However, to establish this new point of view, we needed to acquire evidence at the molecular level for the association of the apical cytoskeleton with the TJs.

We further examined the apical cytoskeleton in detail, by performing ultra-high voltage electron microscopy experiments in which the microtubules and intermediate filaments were tracked. In general epithelial cells in culture, the apical microtubules and intermediate filaments were distributed in the apical plane in rather uniformly scattered patterns and partly overlapped each other, without any specific patterns in their distribution (Tateishi et al. 2017). In this respect, it is notable that we identified four microtubule-associated proteins, which also associate with TJs, in our recent findings, TJ-associated microtubule-binding proteins. We believe that analyses of the TJ-associated microtubule-binding proteins, which may form the platform for associations among the apical cytoskeletons, TJs, and cell signaling molecules, represent a unique direction for studying epithelial cell sheets and epithelial barriers.

4.3 The Apical Cytoskeletons in Multiciliated Cells, a Possible Extreme Example of a "TJ-Apical Complex" with a Clear Function

MCCs drive fluid transport through coordinated ciliary beating, the direction of which is established by the BB orientation of hundreds of cilia on one cell (Salathe 2007). In airway MCCs, the BBs are uniformly oriented and linearly aligned by an unknown mechanism. To explore the mechanism for BB alignment, we observed GFP-centrin2-labeled BBs in mouse tracheal MCCs in primary culture using our long-term, high-resolution, live-imaging method (Herawati et al. 2016). We found that the differentiating BB arrays sequentially adopted four stereotyped patterns: a clustering "Floret," "Scatter," "Partial alignment," and linear "Alignment" pattern. During this acquisition of regularity, we particularly noted that the patterns and densities of microtubules in the apical plane of the MCCs were well correlated with the BB patterning. In addition, the BB alignment was perturbed by disrupting the apical microtubules with nocodazole or by a basal foot (BF)-depleting Odf2 mutation. Based on these experimental results, we explored the development of BB alignment from random to the final well-ordered pattern biotheoretically. We found that the self-organization could be explained by applying hydrodynamic theories in which the apical cytoskeletons were treated as a two-dimensional viscous fluid that underwent a contractile force mediated by cytoskeletal motors and filament polymerization (Marchetti et al. 2013; Prost et al. 2015; Herawati et al. 2016). These results revealed the functional importance of the cytoskeletal components that exist in the apical plane of the epithelial cell sheet in tracheal MCCs. Although the relationship between the apical cytoskeletons and TJs remains to be elucidated, their locations and binding molecules suggest that they are closely related both physically and functionally in MCCs. How the apical cytoskeleton is built by the TJ and its related signaling is another critical issue that remains to be explored.

4.4 Perspective

Epithelial cell sheets with a differentiated apical side are formed and organized by mechanisms involving apicobasal polarity, the details of which have been well addressed in other reviews (Shin et al. 2006; Nelson 2009; Rodriguez-Boulan and Macara 2014; Apodaca 2017). In general, to establish the apicobasal polarization in epithelial cell sheets, polarity proteins generate asymmetric membrane domains that form the basis for establishing the cell–cell adhesive TJs and adherens junctions (AJs), which combine to form apical junctional complexes (AJCs). In addition, planar cell polarity (PCP), which forms in the apical plane of epithelial cell sheets, is arranged perpendicular to the basolateral polarity. The actin filaments of the circumferential ring also lie horizontally along the apical membrane at cell boundaries. The "TJ-apical complex" expands horizontally below the apical membrane in an almost evenly scattered pattern. Since it includes TJs, it is likely to play a role in the paracellular barrier. On the other hand, since it is directly or indirectly associated with the apical membranes of epithelial cells, it probably also has a role in the transcellular barrier. Thus, the epithelial barrier is created and regulated by the combination of paracellular and transcellular barriers, which are determined, at least in part, by the "TJ-apical complex." Our continued investigation of the "TJ-apical complex" in ciliated and non-ciliated epithelial cells is expected to unveil its physiological significance in a variety of biological epithelial barrier systems.

References

Anderson JM, Van Itallie CM, Fanning AS (2004) Setting up a selective barrier at the apical junction complex. Curr Opin Cell Biol 16:140–145. https://doi.org/10.1016/j.ceb.2004.01.005

Apodaca G (2017) Role of polarity proteins in the generation and organization of apical surface protrusions. Cold Spring Harb Perspect Biol:a027813. https://doi.org/10.1101/cshperspect.a027813

Burgess DR (1982) Reactivation of intestinal epithelial cell brush border motility: ATP-dependent contraction via a terminal web contractile ring. J Cell Biol 95:853–863

Elgeti J, Gompper G (2013) Emergence of metachronal waves in cilia arrays. Proc Natl Acad Sci 110:4470–4475. https://doi.org/10.1073/pnas.1218869110/-/DCSupplemental.www.pnas.org/cgi/doi/10.1073/pnas.1218869110

Fleming TP, Papenbrock T, Fesenko I, Hausen P, Sheth B (2000) Assembly of tight junctions during early vertebrate development. Semin Cell Dev Biol 11:291–299. https://doi.org/10.1006/scdb.2000.0179

Furuse M, Moriwaki K (2009) The role of claudin-based tight junctions in morphogenesis. Ann N Y Acad Sci 1165:58–61. https://doi.org/10.1111/j.1749-6632.2009.04441.x

Guirao B, Joanny JF (2007) Spontaneous creation of macroscopic flow and metachronal waves in an array of cilia. Biophys J 92:1900–1917. https://doi.org/10.1529/biophysj.106.084897

Herawati E, Taniguchi D, Kanoh H, Tateishi K, Ishihara S, Tsukita S (2016) Multiciliated cell basal bodies align in stereotypical patterns coordinated by the apical cytoskeleton. J Cell Biol 214:571–586. https://doi.org/10.1083/jcb.201601023

Hull BE, Staehelin LA (1979) The terminal web. A reevaluation of its structure and function. J Cell Biol 81:67–82. https://doi.org/10.1083/jcb.81.1.67

Keller TCS, Conzelman KA, Chasan R, Mooseker MS (1985) Role of myosin in terminal web contraction in isolated intestinal epithelial brush borders. J Cell Biol 100:1647–1655

Kunimoto K, Yamazaki Y, Nishida T, Shinohara K, Ishikawa H, Hasegawa T, Okanoue T, Hamada H, Noda T, Tamura A, Tsukita S, Tsukita S (2012) Coordinated ciliary beating requires Odf2-mediated polarization of basal bodies via basal feet. Cell 148:189–200. https://doi.org/10.1016/j.cell.2011.10.052

Leblond CP, Puchtler H, Clermont Y (1960) Structures corresponding to terminal bars and terminal web in many types of cells. Nature 186:784–788

Marchetti MC, Joanny JF, Ramaswamy S, Liverpool TB, Prost J, Rao M, Simha RA (2013) Hydrodynamics of soft active matter. Rev Mod Phys 85:1143–1189. https://doi.org/10.1103/RevModPhys.85.1143

Martin AC, Kaschube M, Wieschaus EF (2009) Pulsed contractions of an actin-myosin network drive apical constriction. Nature 457:495–499. https://doi.org/10.1038/nature07522

Nelson WJ (2009) Remodeling epithelial cell organization: transitions between front-rear and apical-basal polarity. Cold Spring Harb Perspect Biol 1:1–19. https://doi.org/10.1101/cshperspect.a000513

Owaribe K, Kodama R, Eguchi G (1981) Demonstration of contractility of circumferential actin bundles and its morphogenetic significance in pigmented epithelium in vitro and in vivo. J Cell Biol 90:507–514. https://doi.org/10.1083/jcb.90.2.507

Prost J, Jülicher F, Joanny J (2015) Active gel physics. Nat Phys 11:111–117. https://doi.org/10.1038/nphys3224

Rodriguez-Boulan E, Macara IG (2014) Organization and execution of the epithelial polarity programme. Nat Rev Mol Cell Biol 15:225–242. https://doi.org/10.1038/nrm3775

Salathe M (2007) Regulation of mammalian ciliary beating. Annu Rev Physiol 69:401–422. https://doi.org/10.1146/annurev.physiol.69.040705.141253

Shin K, Fogg VC, Margolis B (2006) Tight junctions and cell polarity. Annu Rev Cell Dev Biol 22:207–235. https://doi.org/10.1146/annurev.cellbio.22.010305.104219

Tanaka H, Tamura A, Suzuki K, Tsukita S (2017) Site-specific distribution of claudin-based paracellular channels with roles in biological fluid flow and metabolism. Ann N Y Acad Sci 1405:44–52. https://doi.org/10.1111/nyas.13438

Tateishi K, Nishida T, Inoue K, Tsukita S (2017) Developmental cell three-dimensional organization of layered apical cytoskeletal networks associated with mouse airway tissue development. Sci Rep 7:1–10. https://doi.org/10.1038/srep43783

Tsukita S, Furuse M, Itoh M (2001) Multifunctional strands in tight junctions. Nat Rev Mol Cell Biol 2:285–293. https://doi.org/10.1038/35067088

Van Itallie CM, Anderson JM (2014) Architecture of tight junctions and principles of molecular composition. Semin Cell Dev Biol 36:157–165. https://doi.org/10.1016/j.semcdb.2014.08.011

Yano T, Matsui T, Tamura A, Uji M, Tsukita S (2013) The association of microtubules with tight junctions is promoted by cingulin phosphorylation by AMPK. J Cell Biol 203:605–614. https://doi.org/10.1083/jcb.201304194

Yano T, Kanoh H, Tamura A, Tsukita S (2017) Apical cytoskeletons and junctional complexes as a combined system in epithelial cell sheets. Ann N Y Acad Sci 1405:32–43. https://doi.org/10.1111/nyas.13432

Chapter 5
Neural Circuit Dynamics of Brain States

Karl Deisseroth

1. In 1972, Karl Hartmann enumerated the reasons that light is a uniquely suited tool for probing living systems. Though coming from the perspective of spectroscopy, his perceptive list holds true even for systems as complex as the adult mammalian brain.
2. The brain, like other living systems, tolerates light, which can be delivered flexibly over a range of wavelengths and irradiance values. Crucially, working with the instantaneous speed and inertia-less nature of light, at least as far as biological spatial and temporal scales are concerned, brings immense value for using light as a control and readout tool in biology. And the fact that most cells do not respond to light provides an enormous signal-to-noise advantage—if any light sensitivity can be conferred.
3. Our efforts on using light to illuminate brain structure and function have taken us from the basic science investigation of microbial protein crystal structures, to optical probing of brainwide wiring and gene expression patterns, to optogenetics (development and application of methods for using light delivered via fiberoptics to control single cells or kinds of cells in the brains of behaving mammals).

Electronic Supplementary Material The online version of this chapter (https://doi.org/10.1007/978-981-13-7908-6_5) contains supplementary material, which is available to authorized users.

K. Deisseroth (✉)
Stanford University, Stanford, CA, USA

Howard Hughes Medical Institute (HHMI), Stanford, CA, USA
e-mail: deissero@stanford.edu

Y. Toyama et al. (eds.), *Make Life Visible*,
https://doi.org/10.1007/978-981-13-7908-6_5

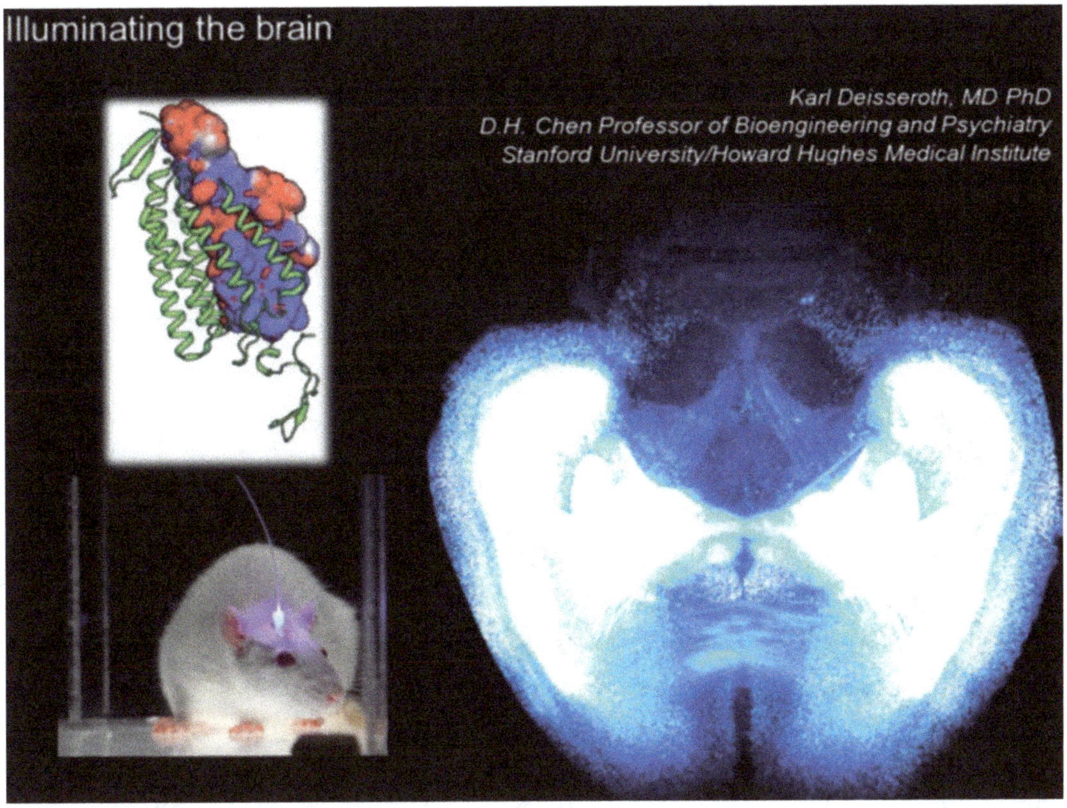

4. The biggest challenge facing us now is integrating the following datastreams at cellular resolution across the brain: (1) natural activity during behavior (with fluorescence Ca^{2+} imaging), (2) causal activity during behavior (with optogenetics), and (3) local/global wiring with gene expression (via hydrogel-tissue chemistry methods such as CLARITY).

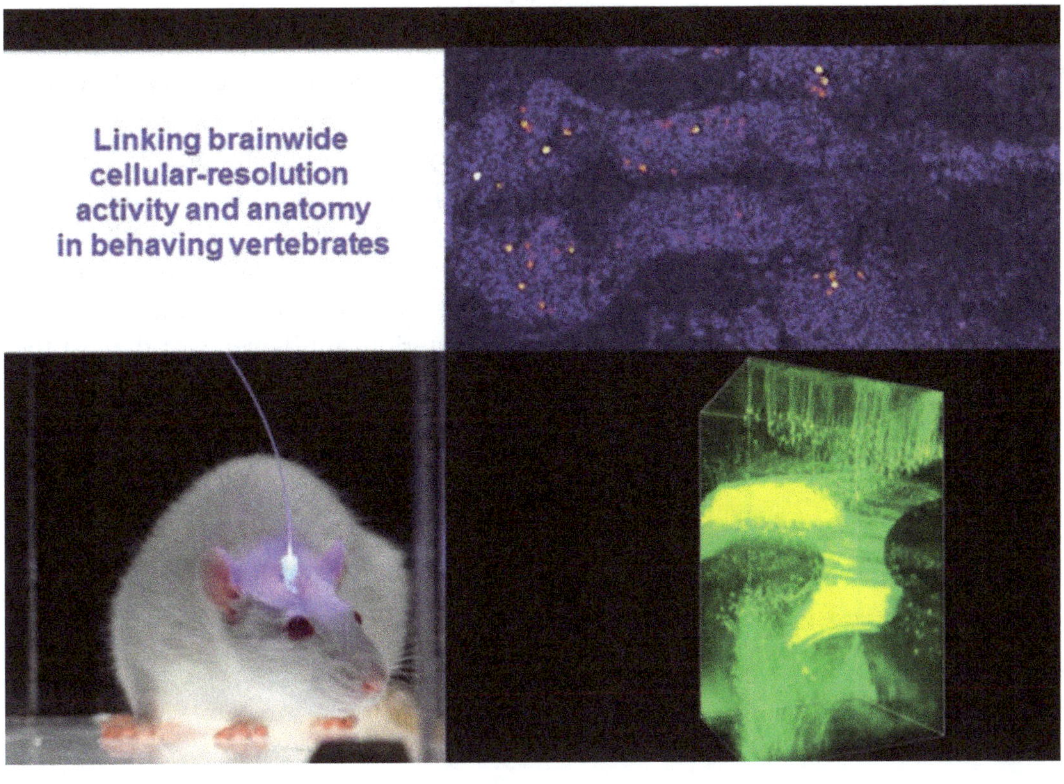

5. Electrical and magnetic interventions, while fast, cannot readily provide cell-type specificity—since all neurons respond to these signals. Optogenetics is a way of providing cellular resolution with cell-type specificity by expressing a light transducer in targeted cells—which allows use of a vastly more tractable signal since virtually no neurons respond to light under normal conditions.

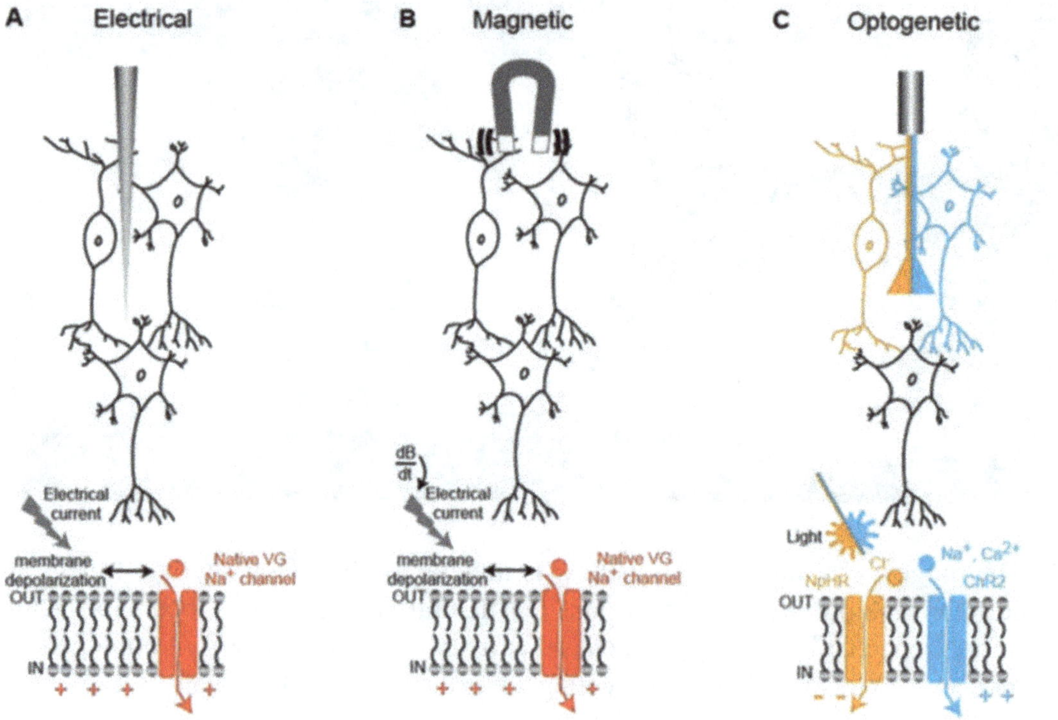

Cell 2016 (with P. Rajasethupathy and E. Ferenczi)

6. This method works well if the light transducer is also a cell-activity effector—thus all-in-one microbial opsin proteins provided the optimal solution, since their single polypeptide chain (bound to a naturally-present chromophore) can both absorb a photon and generate current. The channelrhodopsin is an interesting member of this family since it can move many ions across the membrane, in response to light by opening its channel pore. But while structural information on non-channel (pump) members of this protein family has been available for decades, the channelrhodopsins remained mysterious until events of the last few years.

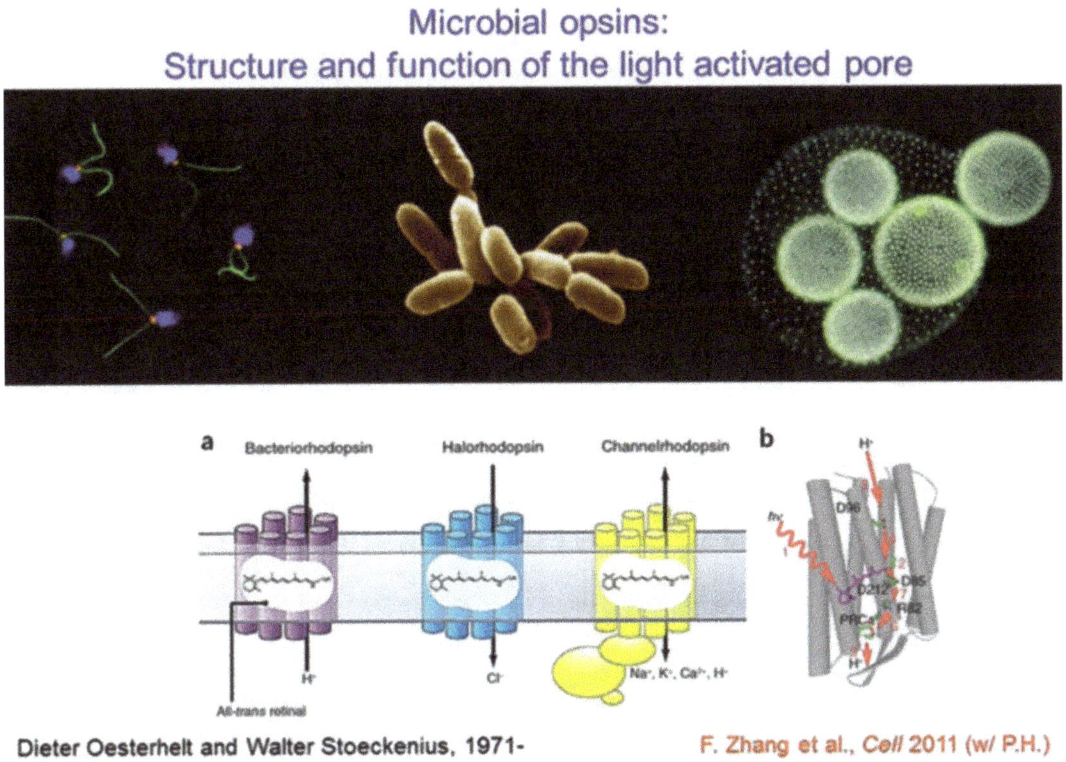

7. Detailed protein biophysics and chemistry, involving crystal-structure determination, molecular dynamics modeling, and structure/model-guided redesign, have given rise to fundamentally distinct forms of photon-spike coupling. In 2010, ultrafast coupling was created that allowed control of spiking at 200 Hz or more. In 2011, control of spiking with red light was implemented. In 2008, bistable cellular control of excitation was implemented, in which single pulses of light cause stable excitation (which can last many minutes until reversed with a pulse of redshifted light). And in 2014 bistable cellular inhibition was implemented, via creation of anion-conducting channelrhodopsins (through pore redesign for chloride flux followed by porting the bistability mutations onto the anion-conducting backbone). Each of these variants was designed and implemented using atomic-structure-level modeling and understanding.

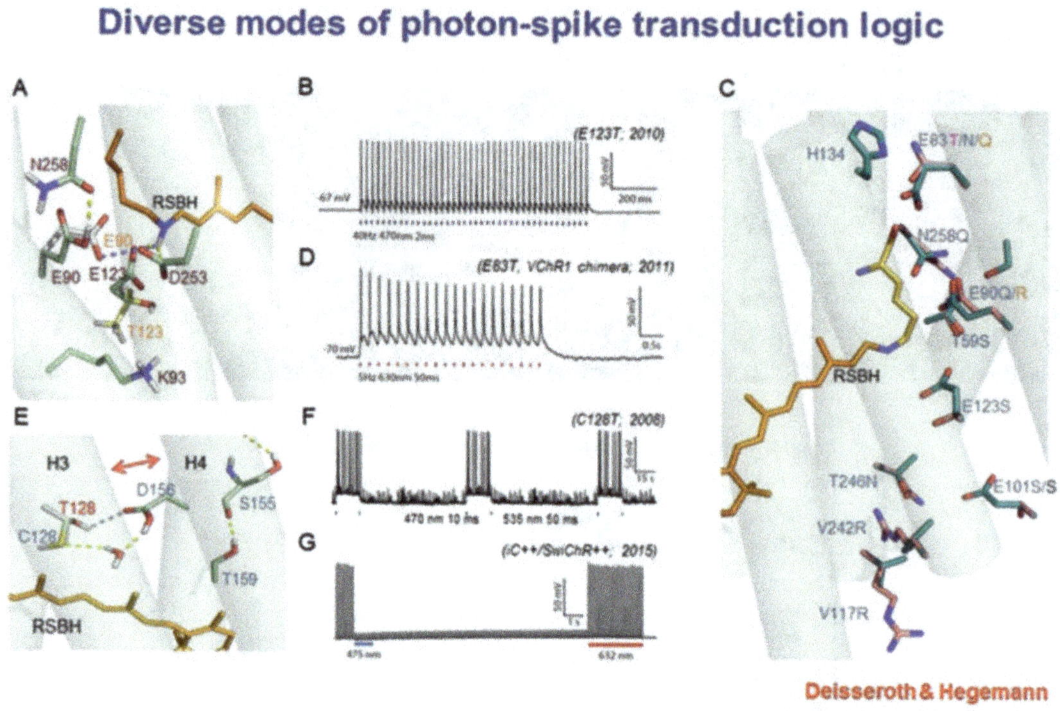

8. The ChETA mutations of channelrhodopsins allowed the first ultrafast spiking over hundreds of Hz in fast-spiking neurons, *in vitro* and *in vivo*, and also corrected some fidelity breakdown issues that occur even at low spike rates.

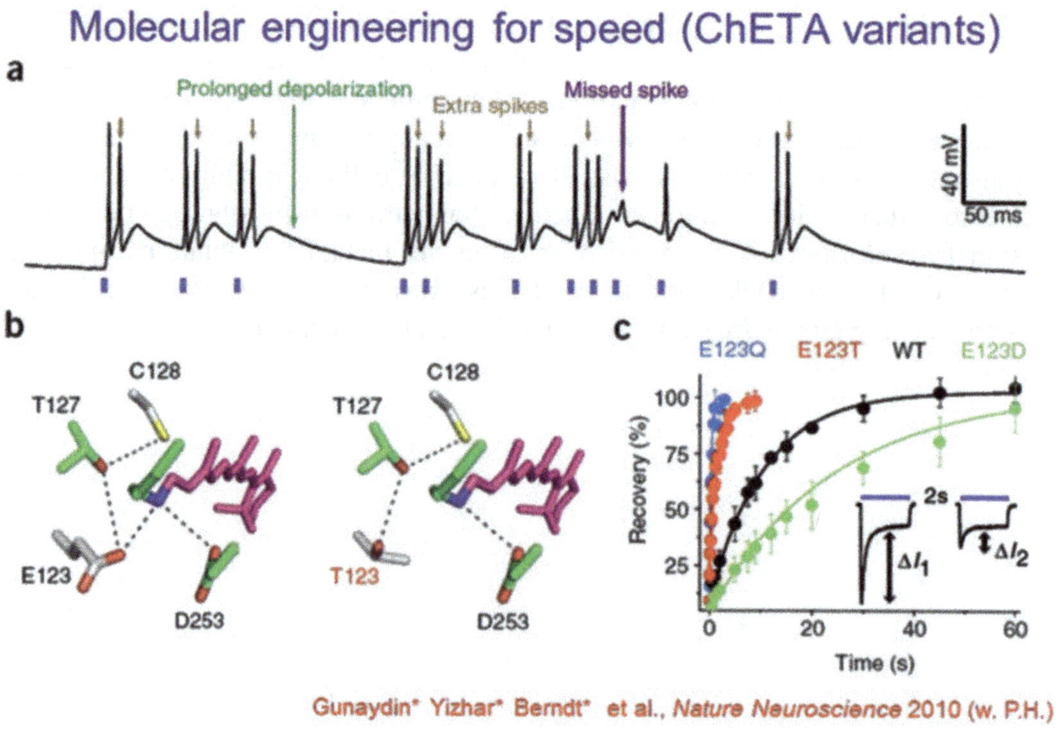

9. The SFO mutants represent the bistable type described above. The normally-fast (10 ms) deactivation after light-off of wild-type channelrhodospins can be extended to 30 min or more with mutations at the "DC bridge" (C128 and D156). Orders-of-magnitude greater operational light sensitivity in expressing cells is also achieved.
10. Resolution of the crystal structure finally demonstrated the nature of the pore, residing within each 7-TM monomer and not at the dimer interface as had been suggested by a low-resolution cryo-EM paper.
11. Obtaining the pore structure allow for redesign for new function. It was noted that a preponderance of electronegativity characterized the inner lining of the pore for these naturally cation-selective channels, suggesting a strategy to test a hypothesis for selectivity and create a new tool, by replacing these residues to create electropositivity and perhaps anion flux, which would be of great value for inhibitory optogenetics.

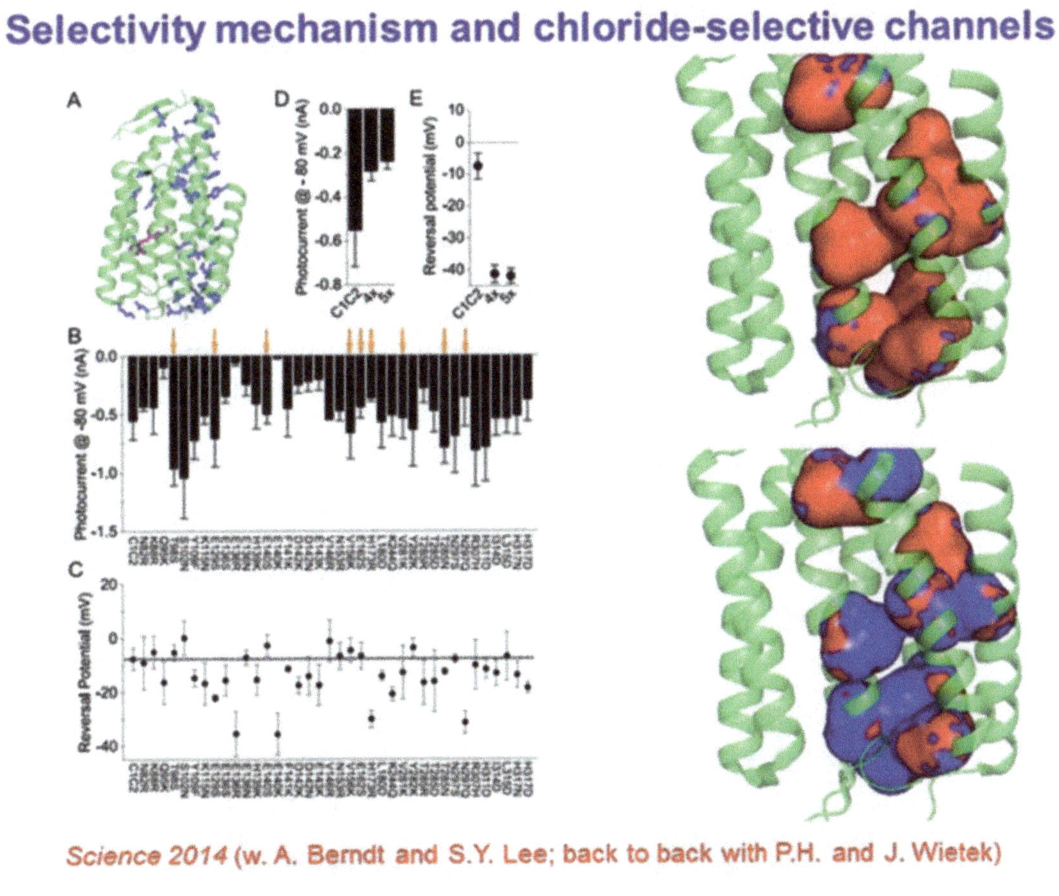

12. Surprisingly, this experiment was successful, and inhibitory channels became available which could shut down spiking in response to blue light, rather than drive spiking.
13. Bistable inhibition (a long-sought property for biologists doing optogenetics) then was enabled by porting the bistability mutations onto this new backbone.

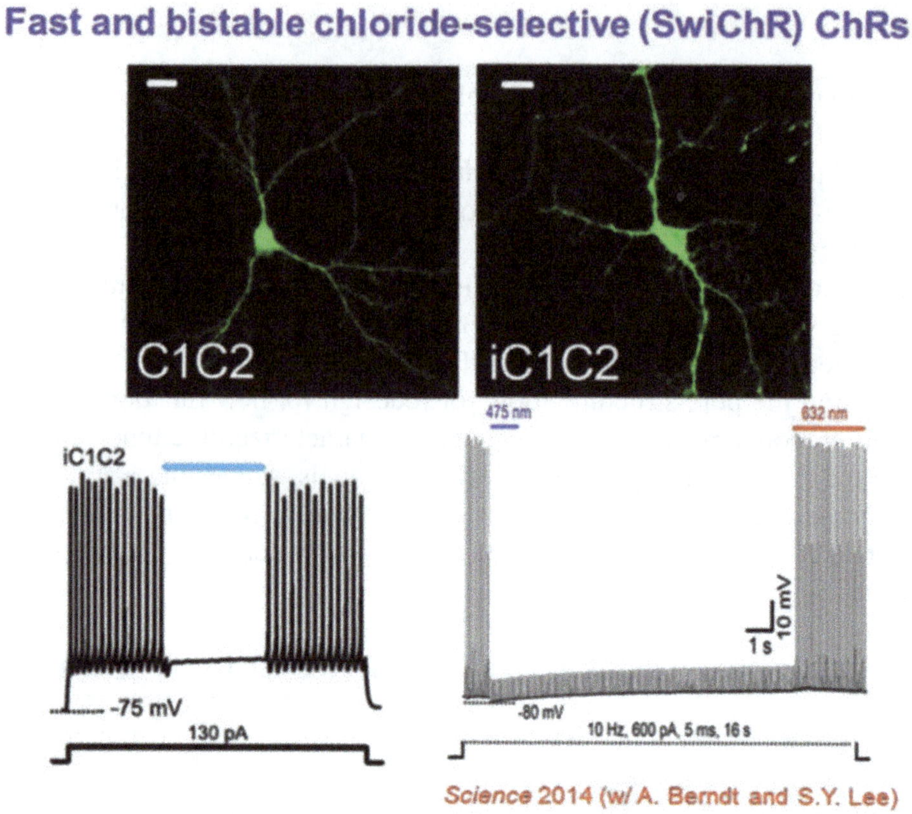

14. A year later, naturally-occurring light-activated chloride channels were discovered in the *Guillardia theta* algae. Validating yet further the structure-guided mutagenesis that had created the initial anion-conducting channelrhodopsins, the internal pore electrostatics of the naturally-occurring channels were predicted to be largely positive, similar to the redsigned channelrhodopsins.

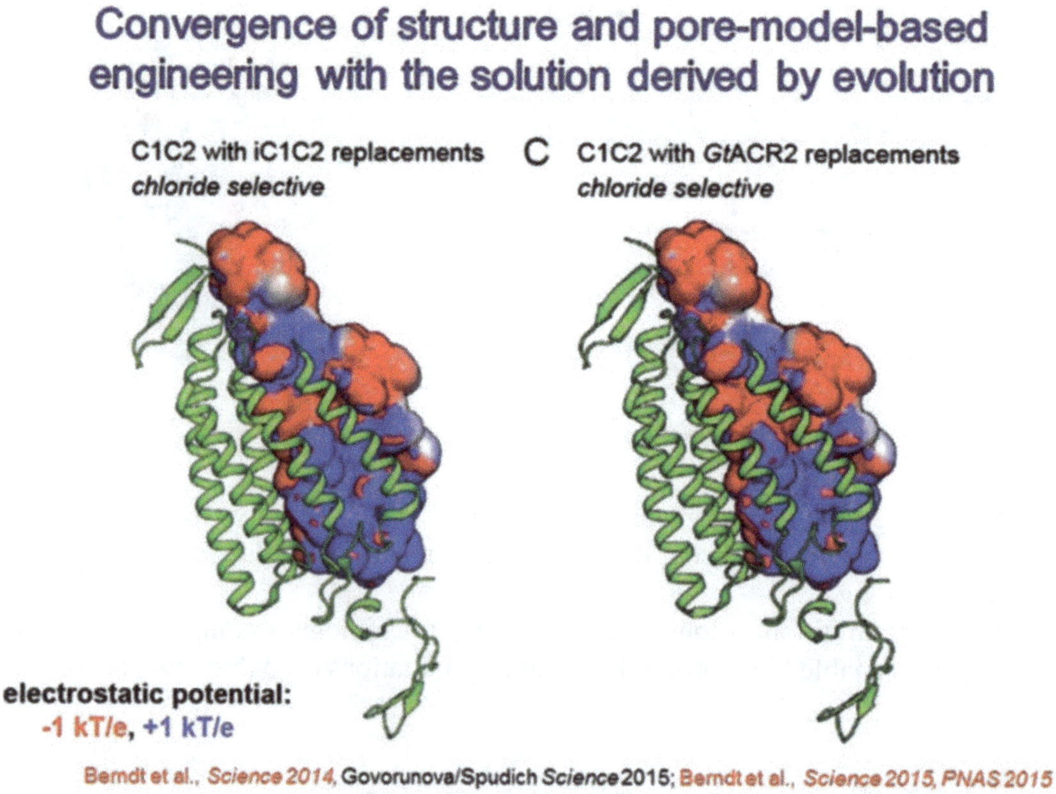

15. Color shifting is more challenging, but was ultimately achieved beginning in 2008 when a naturally-occurring redshifted variant called VChR1 was identified from the multicellular green alga *Volvox carteri*.
16. With additional mutagenesis of VChR1 (including creating a chimera with ChR1, and improving cellular trafficking) by 2011 red light-driven spiking was enabled with C1V1.
17. The greatest value of C1V1 and subsequent other red-driven opsins has been in integration with blue light-driven Ca^{2+} imaging at cellular resolution—resulting in all-optical experimentation. This can be done at the cellular level with single-cell-directed light guidance, or at the population level with fiber photometry. Either way, naturally-occurring activity as seen during behavior within defined cells or cell types can now be mimicked (or adjusted) in terms of timing and magnitude—allowing rigorous assessment of causal significance of naturally-occurring signals.
18. Regarding applications to such questions, optogenetics has been applied to a very broad range of natural and disease-relevant behaviors. A well-studied example is anxiety; the cells and projections across the brain that recruit the various features of anxiety, such as risk-avoidance, altered respiratory rate, and negative subjective valence, can all be now assigned to contributory specific projections defined by origin and target, with specificity arising from optogenetics. Brain states could be shown (with optogenetics) to be assembled from these features defined by brainwide projections.

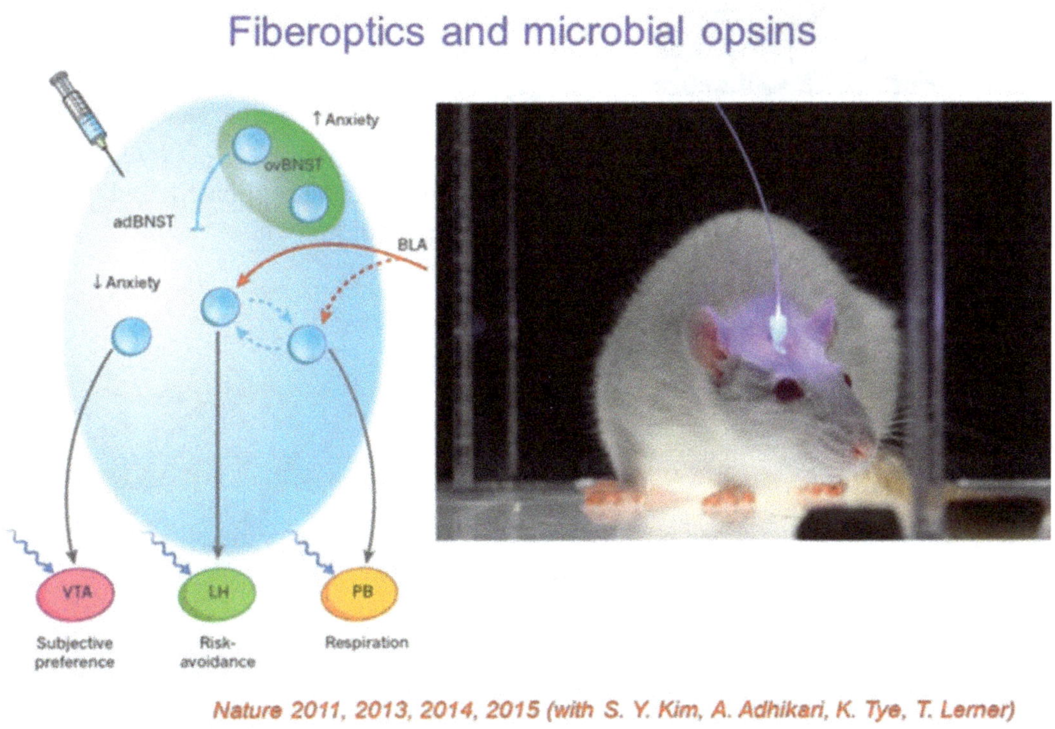

19. Another example of both basic and disease-relevant interest is the behavioral state transition from active-coping to passive-coping in response to a challenge. This is a naturally adaptive transition, but also in extreme forms can be problematic in human clinical states such as depression. This process has been studied in rats in the forced swim test (FST), and optogenetics has been used to test causal significance of cells and projections across the brain in this very important (and often adaptive) state transition.

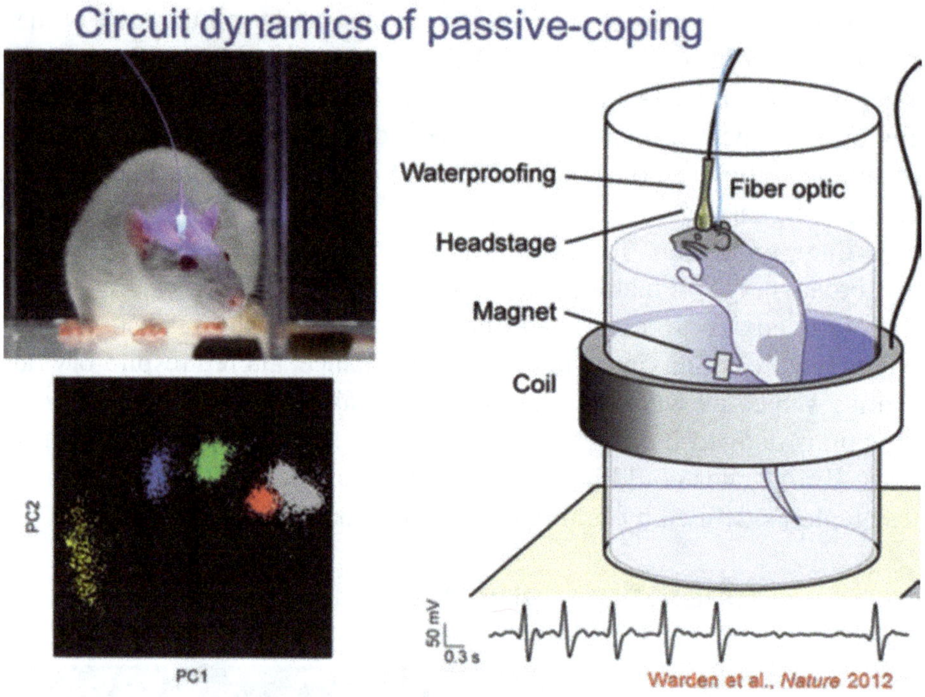

20. Many individual regions across the brain had been implicated, but specific causal projections and pathways involved were not known.

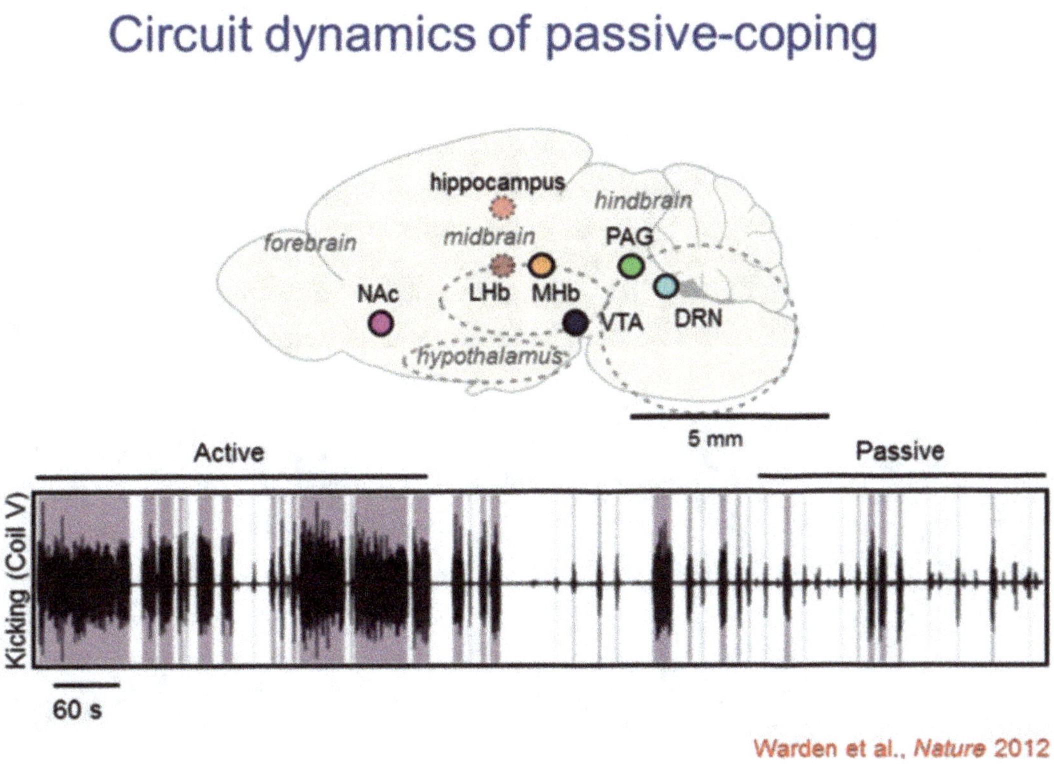

21. Driving the projection from the medial prefrontal cortex (mPFC) to the lateral habenula favored the passive-coping state, quantified as reduced kicking and swimming in the FST. These effects were not seen in non-challenging situations (no psychomotor changes in the open-field locomotion test for example) and were not seen with nonspecific optogenetic drive of all mPFC neurons, nor of mPFC projections to basolateral amygdala.
22. In contrast, driving the projection from the mPFC to the dorsal raphe nucleus favored the active-coping state (again with no effect in the open field). However, these point-by point investigations may miss unanticipated loci of control, and do not represent brainwide joint statistics. We therefore are seeking to develop brainwide cellular-resolution assays.
23. Zebrafish provide a valuable approach for initially exploring this avenue, particularly since we have developed truly brainwide cellular-resolution Ca^{2+} imaging assays.
24. This two-photon imaging approach provides the bona fide cellular resolution needed for linking cellular activity to cellular identity. In headfixed zebrafish (with tail free to assess direction and vigor of exertion) the brainwide cellular activity patterns relevant to behavior can be assessed without regional bias or preconception.

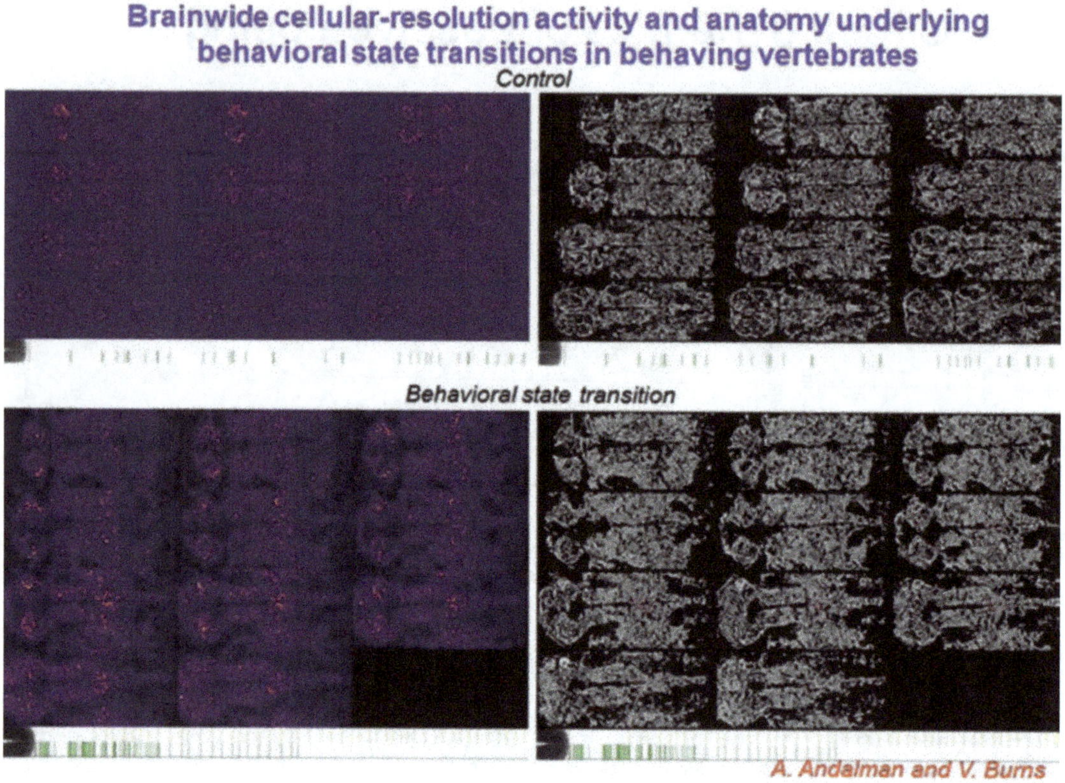

25. Moreover, with technology recently developed in our group, those same cells can be then further interrogated for detailed molecular phenotyping, including gene expression and neurotransmitter identity. This requires computational approaches to morph the during-life activity-dataset to the post-life molecular-phenotype-datasets, which do not readily align without the computational warping approach (termed MultiMAP and recently published in *Cell* 2017 from Matt Lovett-Barron and co-workers in my lab).
26. This method in the end has finally enabled our linkage of brainwide anatomical identity/molecular phenotype, to cellular-resolution activity during behavior, an approach that will open the door to a very wide array of investigations in neuroscience (both basic and preclinical). The final piece of the puzzle is local and global wiring of these same cells, now addressable with hydrogel-tissue chemistry methods such as CLARITY.

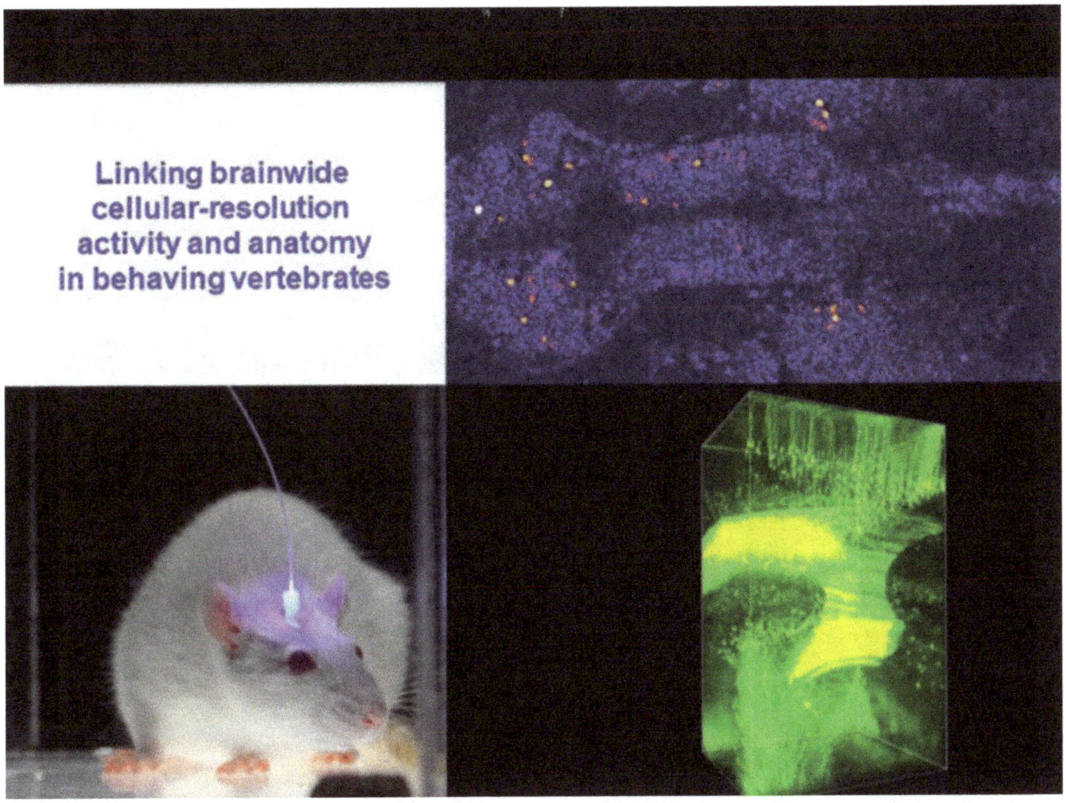

27. With hydrogel-tissue chemistry, specific classes of native biomolecules in tissue are immobilized or covalently anchored (for example through individualized interface molecules to gel monomer molecules) and precisely-timed polymerization causing tissue-gel hybrid formation is triggered within all the cells across the tissue in an ordered and controlled process to create an optically and chemically accessible biomolecular matrix. Indeed, when the biomolecules of interest are thereby transferred to the polymer lattice, a robust new composite hydrogel-tissue material results, which becomes the substrate for future chemical and optical interrogation that can be probed and manipulated in new ways. Moderate tissue expansion occurs as was shown in 2013 and 2014, but this can be reversed if needed with a refractive index matching solution.
28. Hydrogel-tissue chemistry is particularly well suited for nucleic acid interrogation, especially with the EDC CLARITY method—important for rich typology labeling.
29. This approach also opens the door to immediate-early gene tracking at cellular resolution for genes such as Arc, as well as noncoding RNAs such as microRNAs.

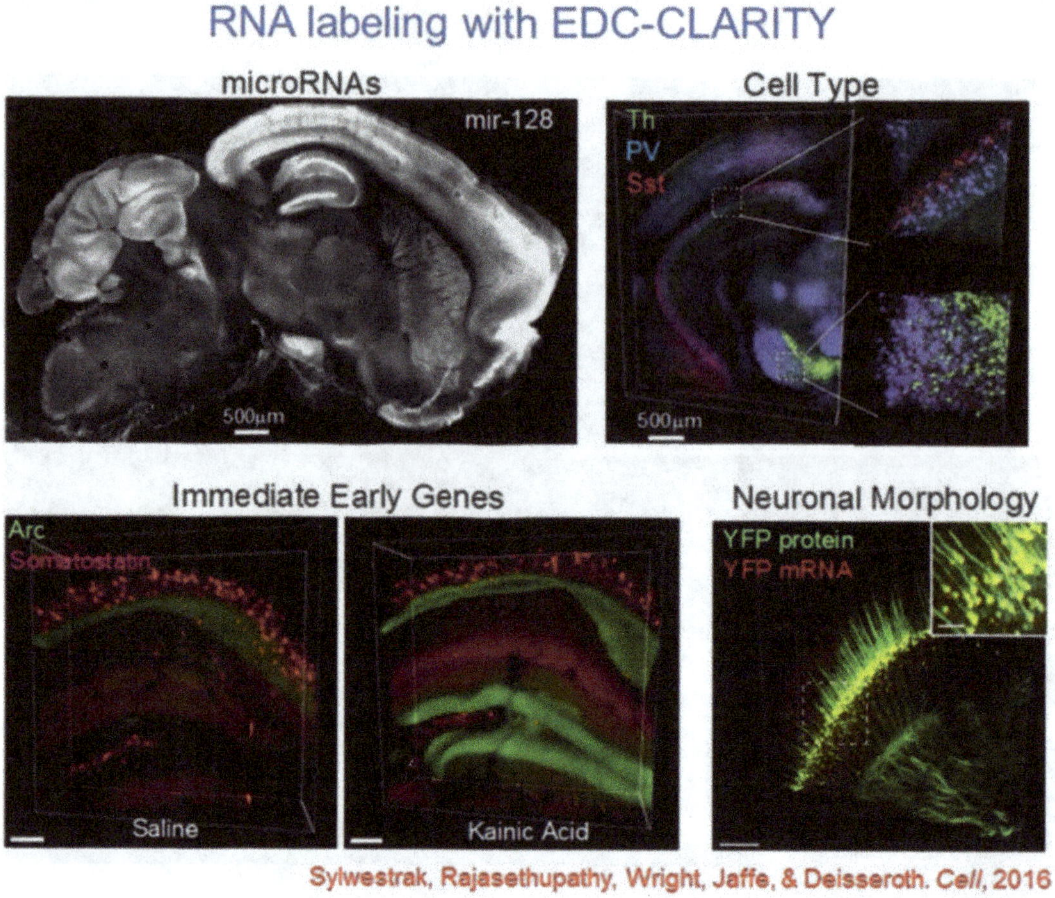

30. A bottleneck initially was imaging speed; high-resolution imaging of large intact volumes of tissue was a new opportunity but created a new challenge. To wit, simple point scanning approaches were translatable to transparent volumes (with the large reduction in light scattering) but were prohibitively slow, and also caused fluorophore bleaching issues since the entire tissue is illuminated as the imaging pinhole is slowly scanned. Fast lightsheet methods cracked this problem, allowing widefield cell-resolution imaging of large transparent volumes with speed suitable for quantitating adult whole-brain cohorts.
31. A further innovation was linking these datasets with activity traces, so that all individual cells (and their brainwide projections) that had been strongly active during a specific experience (for example, a negative-valence mild shock, or a positive valence cocaine administration) could be automatically counted in large cohorts of adult mice. Projections across the brain, such as from mPFC to ventral striatum, could be identified from individual cells that furthermore could be molecularly phenotyped in the same volumes (as with the important immediate-early transcription factor NPAS4).
32. In general, these hydrogel-tissue chemistry methods, by virtue of their all-aqueous-solution implementation and robust tissue-gel composition, afford unique opportunities for rich phenotyping of both proteins and nucleic acids as well as other advantages, including preservation of native fluorophores—the latter particularly important for the goal of registering fluorescent activity signals observed during life with the molecular and wiring information (from the very same cells) that can only be acquired after life.

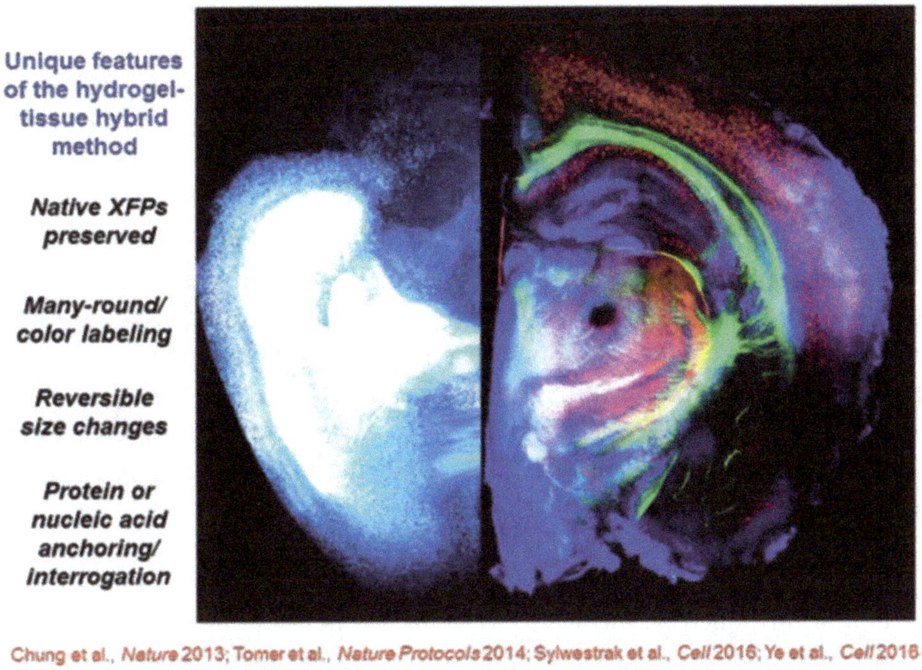

33. While this approach will always be fundamentally designed for basic science, examples of translation of ideas from optical control to the clinic are already occurring. For example, it has become clear in multiple clinical domains that elevated mPFC activity has been associated with reduced reward-seeking or experiencing, both in the context of anhedonia in depression and cocaine seeking in addiction treatment. An optogenetics-guided clinical trial has already found efficacy for treatment in cocaine addiction in studies led by Bonci and colleagues.

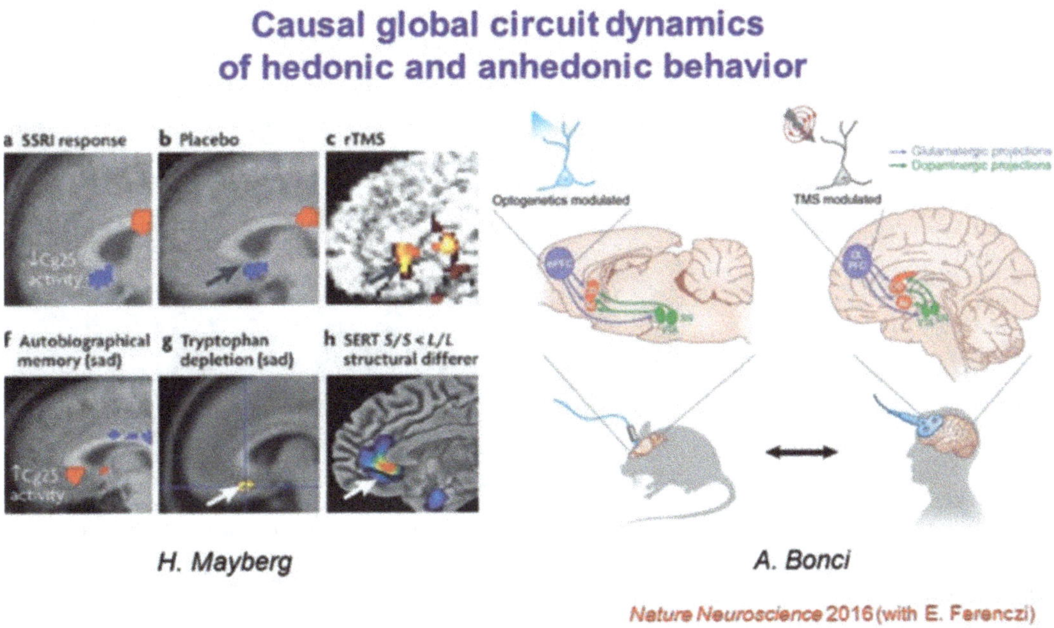

34. Furthermore, the combination of step-function and red-shifted opsins in fact allowed a causal, basic-science test of mechanisms by which elevated mPFC activity might suppress reward experience or motivation. First, the blue-light-driven step-function opsin SSFO was used to stably elevate mPFC activity in freely-moving rats; this intervention was observed to cause anhedonic behavior in these animals.
35. Second, the ventral tegmental area dopamine (VTA-DA) neuron population (source of a primary reward signal in these animals and likely in human beings as well) was optogenetically stimulated (with the red light-driven opsin C1V1 to avoid crosstalk with SSFO circuit elements); it was observed that in those epochs wherein the prefrontal SSFO had been recruited, the stimulated VTA-DA cells were much impaired in their ability to recruit downstream reward circuitry in the ventral striatum. These findings, requiring multiple redesigned microbial opsins to achieve, provided a brainwide circuit-dynamical mechanism for suppression of reward behavior as seen clinically.
36. It is remarkable to consider that some of the most ancient and challenging clinical conditions, such as those in psychiatry which admitted to medical-model description only 200 years ago, are now yielding to mechanistic studies that rely on atomic-scale structure-function studies of microscopic-plant proteins—a testament to basic science.
37. This work required an immensely talented team of students, postdoctoral fellows, esteemed collaborators, staff, and funding agencies, whose names are indicated here.

Antoine Adamantidis → McGill
Raag Airan → Stanford
Avishek Adhikari → UCLA
Will Allen
Polina Anikeeva → MIT
Alex Aravanis
Andre Berndt → U. Wash.
Ed Boyden → MIT
Kwanghun Chung → MIT
Tom Davidson
Lief Fenno
Emily Ferenczi
Inbal Goshen → Hebrew U.
Viviana Gradinaru → Caltech
Logan Grosenick
Lisa Gunaydin → UCSF
Christina Kim
Sung-Yon Kim → Seoul NU
Jin Hyung Lee → Stanford
Soo Yeun Lee
Talia Lerner → Northwestern
Priya Rajasethupathy → Rockefeller
Vikaas Sohal → UCSF
Emily Sylwestrak
Raju Tomer → Columbia
Kay Tye → MIT
Ilana Witten → Princeton
Melissa Warden → Cornell
Li Ye
Ofer Yizhar → Weizmann
Kelly Zalocusky
Feng Zhang → MIT

Resources
optogenetics.org
clarityresourcecenter.org

P. Hegemann; O. Nureki; S. Delp; A. Gottschalk; G. Nagel; K. Tanaka; E. Bamberg; A. Kreitzer; B. Roska; J. Sahel; E. Nestler; T. Hokfelt; O. Kiehn; S. Tonegawa; L. de Lecea; R. Malenka; M. Carlen; D. Meletis; M. Kokaia; A. Bonci; P. Janak; J. Henderson; M. Schnitzer; G. Augustine; G. Feng; L.H. Tsai; A. Graybiel

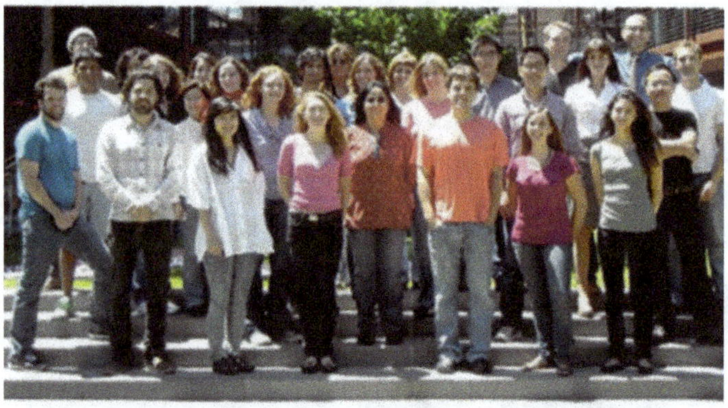

Charu Ramakrishnan, Cynthia Delacruz, Maisie Lo, Sally Pak, Minsuk Hyun, Chelsey Perry, Joel Finkelstein and Julie Mirzabekov

Funding: NIMH, NIDA, NINDS, NSF, Simons, DARPA, HHMI, Gatsby, Coulter, Wiegers, Snyder, Grosfeld, Woo, Yu, NARSAD/BBRF.

References

Primer with methods and references linking optogenetics to hydrogel-tissue chemistry and fluorescence activity imaging. https://web.stanford.edu/group/dlab/media/papers/kimNatureReviews2017.pdf

Resource links for hydrogel-tissue chemistry. http://clarityresourcecenter.org/pdfs/Table_S2_Transparency_Methods.pdf

Review on optogenetics. https://web.stanford.edu/group/dlab/media/papers/deisserothNatNeurosciCommentary2015.pdf

Review on channelrhodopsins. https://web.stanford.edu/group/dlab/media/papers/deisserothScience2017.pdf

Online Resources

www.clarityresourcecenter.org
www.optogenetics.org

Chapter 6
Optogenetic Reconstitution: Light-Induced Assembly of Protein Complexes and Simultaneous Visualization of Their Intracellular Functions

Tomomi Kiyomitsu

6.1 Introduction

To understand the basis of life, it is critical to visualize the dynamic behaviors of molecules within a cell. Since the discovery of green fluorescent protein (GFP) (Shimomura 1979), multiple fluorescent proteins or dyes have been developed (Rodriguez et al. 2017), and it has become possible to simultaneously visualize intracellular dynamics of multiple proteins in living cells. In addition, by combining recently developed genome editing technologies such as clustered regularly interspaced short palindromic repeats (CRISPR) (Ran et al. 2013), it is possible to monitor the dynamic behaviors of endogenous proteins even in animal cells, including human cultured cells.

In the last few decades, many genetic approaches, such as mutant screens and gene disruption, have been used in combination with live cell imaging to identify genes that code key proteins required for cellular functions (Hartwell 1978; Yanagida 2014; Goshima et al. 2007; Neumann et al. 2010). In addition, biochemical and proteomic approaches have defined functional protein complexes that underlie complicated cellular functions (Hutchins et al. 2010; Cheeseman et al. 2004; Obuse et al. 2004). Once key molecules or complexes are identified, biophysical and structural studies are performed to reveal the detailed molecular properties sufficient for their functions (Cheeseman et al. 2006; Dimitrova et al. 2016; Zhang et al. 2017; McKenney et al. 2014; Schlager et al. 2014). Furthermore, by combining mathematical simulations (Kimura and Onami 2005), nanodevices (Thery et al. 2005), and synthetic approaches (Good et al. 2013; Laan et al. 2012; Nguyen et al. 2014), novel molecular features that underlie complicated dynamic cellular events have been uncovered. However, it is still difficult to fully reconstitute macro-molecular

T. Kiyomitsu (✉)
Division of Biological Science, Graduate School of Science, Nagoya University, Nagoya, Japan
e-mail: kiyomitsu@bio.nagoya-u.ac.jp

Y. Toyama et al. (eds.), *Make Life Visible*,
https://doi.org/10.1007/978-981-13-7908-6_6

complexes, such as the mitotic spindle, which consists of hundreds of proteins (Goshima et al. 2007; Sauer et al. 2005), and to manipulate their functions under physiological condition.

Recently, several light-induced tools have been developed to manipulate intracellular localization of target proteins with a spatiotemporal precision in living cells (Levskaya et al. 2009; Kennedy et al. 2010; Strickland et al. 2012; Guntas et al. 2015). In combination with other techniques, this optogenetic technology has great potential to reconstitute functional protein complexes, which are otherwise difficult to reconstitute *in vitro*, and to directly assess their functions within a cell. Here, I have presented an optogenetic reconstitution system to achieve light-induced *in cell* reconstitution of protein complexes coupled with visualization and manipulation of their cellular functions.

6.2 Light-Induced Heterodimerization Tools

Since around 2009, several groups have developed light-induced protein–protein interaction tools using photoactivatable proteins/domains such as phytochrome B (Phy B) (Levskaya et al. 2009), cryptochrome 2 (CRY2) (Kennedy et al. 2010), and light, oxygen, and voltage (LOV) domains (Strickland et al. 2012; Guntas et al. 2015). In response to light, PhyB and CRY2 interact with their binding partners PIF and CIB1, respectively (Fig. 6.1). Thus, by tethering one module to appropriate sites, such as the plasma membrane, and by fusing the other module to the target protein as a tag, these tools work as a light-induced heterodimerization system (Fig. 6.1). In contrast, the LOV domain acts as a photoswitch that causes a conformational change in response to blue light and dissociates its C-terminal Jα helix from the core domain (Fig. 6.1). When a synthetic peptide is embedded in the Jα helix, this peptide is masked in the dark state but is exposed following light illumination. Thus, by designing the peptide and its binding partner, several light-induced dimerization tools have been developed, such as tunable light-controlled interacting protein tags (TULIP) (Strickland et al. 2012) and improved light-induced dimer (iLID) (Guntas et al. 2015). In iLID, SsrA peptide (seven residues) is embedded in the Jα helix and an SsrA-binding 13-kD protein, SspB, is used as the heterodimerization tag (Fig. 6.2). Although these photoactivatable proteins require cofactors, such as flavin mononucleotide, these cofactors exist in most mammalian cells or can be supplied externally in the culture medium (Zhang and Cui 2015). In addition to these photoactivatable proteins, photo-activated chemicals, such as photocaged dimerizer, have been recently developed to manipulate cell signaling with light (Fig. 6.1) (Ballister et al. 2014). Similar to GFP, these optogenetic tools are derived from plant and bacterial proteins and thus do not affect endogenous cellular functions in mammalian cells.

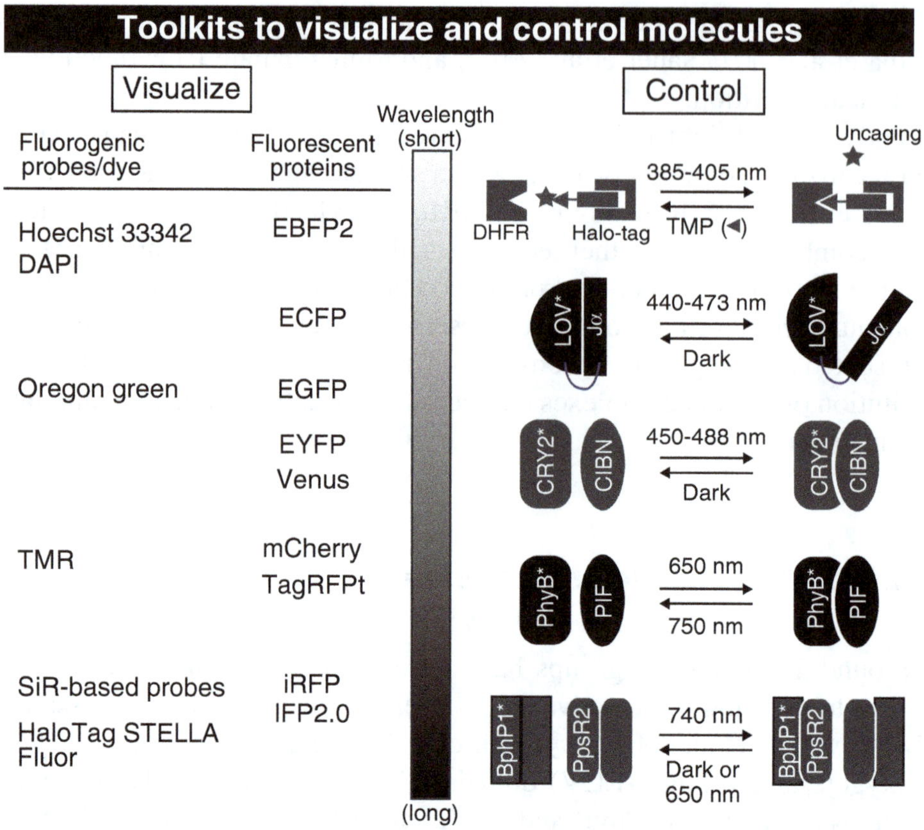

Fig. 6.1 Toolkits to visualize and control molecules with light. (Left) Fluorogenic probes/dyes and fluorescent proteins are summarized. There are several commercially available SiR-based probes and HaloTag STELLA Fluor™. (Right) Light-induced heterodimerization systems. Photocaged dimerizer cTMP-Htag, LOV domain-based conformational change, CRY2–CIBN, PhyB–PIF, and BphP1–PpsR2 interactions are summarized. ∗ indicates light-sensing proteins containing cofactors

These photoactivatable proteins and chemicals exhibit different characters and requirement for activation (Fig. 6.1; reviewed in (Zhang and Cui 2015)). Therefore, these characters must be considered for the experimental design. For example, to locally assemble protein complexes at the plasma membrane, optogenetic dimerizers with slow dissociation rate of target proteins may diffuse on the membrane following membrane targeting and fail to assemble the protein complexes at the specific site on the membrane. In contrast, to stably recruit signaling molecules on a specific organelle, such as kinetochore or centrosomes, optogenetic tools with slow dissociation rate would be more appropriate to generate robust cell signaling. Finally, simultaneous manipulation of two different target proteins is now possible by using different light-responsible tools such as blue- and near-infrared light-driven dimerizers (Kaberniuk et al. 2016).

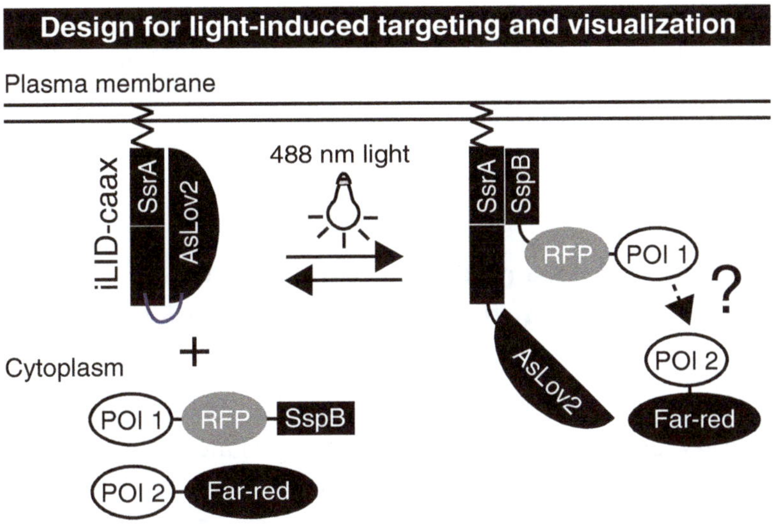

Fig. 6.2 A design for light-induced membrane targeting and visualization of its downstream events. Blue-light-responding iLID is tethered at the plasma membrane using CAAX motif. In response to blue-light (450–488 nm) illumination, iLID causes conformational change and exposes its Jα helix, containing the SsrA peptide, which interacts with SspB protein, resulting in membrane recruitment of cytoplasmic SspB-fusion proteins. By co-expressing SspB–RFP fused protein of interest 1 (POI 1) and far-red fluorescent protein/probe tagged POI 2, it can be simultaneously visualized how membrane recruited POI 1 protein affects POI 2 protein following light illumination

6.3 Visualization Tools Compatible with Optogenetic Manipulation

For simultaneous visualization of target protein and its downstream targets or events in response to light illumination, exciting fluorescent proteins or dyes without activating light-responsible proteins is required. For instance, when blue light is used to activate photoactivatable proteins, red or far-red light must be selected for visualization because shorter UV light also activates blue light-responsible elements (Fig. 6.2). To monitor the responses of the target protein and its downstream effectors following light illumination, at least two fluorescent proteins or dyes are required. Importantly, several far-red or near-infrared fluorescent proteins or cell permeable fluoregenic probes/dyes have been recently developed (Fig. 6.1), such as near-infrared fluorescent protein (iRFP) (Filonov et al. 2011), infrared fluorescent protein mutant (IFP2.0) (Yu et al. 2014), silicon–rhodamine-based fluorophore (SiR)-647 (Lukinavicius et al. 2014), SiR-700 (Lukinavicius et al. 2016), and HaloTag STELLA Fluor™ (http://www.promega.co.jp/halotag_imaging/). These fluoregenic probes/dyes are used in combination with SNAP-tag or HaloTag, or these dyes are directly conjugated with chemicals that bind to DNA, tubulin, or actin to visualize chromosomes (SiR–DNA) (Lukinavicius et al. 2015), tubulin (SiR–tubulin) (Lukinavicius et al. 2014), and actin cytoskeleton (SiR–actin) (https://spirochrome.com/). Thus, by combining these novel tools, simultaneous visualization of its downstream targets is now possible in parallel with light-induced manipulation of photoactivatable proteins. In contrast, when photocaged chemical dimerizer or near-infrared-activated proteins are used, GFP and other red fluorescent proteins or dyes can be used for multicolor imaging to visualize its downstream events and phenotypes.

6.4 Light-Induced Assembly/Reconstitution of Force-Generating Complexes During Mitosis

Recently, light-induced heterodimerization tools have been used to manipulate cell signaling and force-generating processes, such as organelle transport (van Bergeijk et al. 2015; Ballister et al. 2015) and cytokinesis (Wagner and Glotzer 2016). In these studies, protein complexes, including motor proteins such as dynein and myosin, are locally assembled following light illumination and their cellular functions are assessed within a cell. Another good target for optogenetic reconstitution is a cortical force-generating machinery (Kiyomitsu and Cheeseman 2012), which links the dynamic plus-end of astral microtubules emanating from the mitotic spindle with the plasma membrane and generates cortical pulling forces on astral microtubules to control spindle position and orientation during both symmetric and asymmetric cell division (Fig. 6.3a) (Kiyomitsu 2015; di Pietro et al. 2016). In most animal cells, this cortical machinery consists of evolutionally conserved protein complexes, including cytoplasmic dynein complex (Roberts et al. 2013), its binding partner dynactin complex, and cortically anchored nuclear mitotic apparatus protein (NuMA)–LGN–Gαi complex (Fig. 6.3b) (Kiyomitsu and Cheeseman 2012). Intrinsic or extrinsic polarity signals specify the cortical assembly site of the cortical machinery and drive the directional movement of the spindle (Fig. 6.3a, b) (Thery et al. 2005; Kiyomitsu and Cheeseman 2012). Although cortical microtubule interaction between dynein and dynamic microtubule end has been recently reconstituted in an *in vitro* system using purified dynein motor domain and micro-fabricated barriers (Laan et al. 2012), how functional force-generating machinery assembles in response to intrinsic and extrinsic signals (Fig. 6.3b, c) and generates large cortical spindle-pulling forces within a cell remains poorly understood.

Whereas dynein, dynactin and NuMA play other key roles in spindle assembly (Hueschen et al. 2017), LGN and Gαi specifically localize at the cell cortex and have no roles in functional spindle assembly (Kiyomitsu and Cheeseman 2012). Thus, depletion of LGN or Gαi by RNAi does not affect the integrity of the mitotic spindle and provides an appropriate condition to assemble cortical force-generating sub-complexes and directly assess their abilities in spindle positioning (Fig. 6.4a). Although the dynein heavy chain (~500 kD) and NuMA (~240 kD) are very large proteins, CRISPR-based genome editing enables to insert appropriate tags in their endogenous gene loci at either N- or C-terminal region (Natsume et al. 2016). In addition, by exogenously expressing truncation fragments, mutants, or siRNA-resistant proteins, it is also possible to assemble multiple different sub-complexes

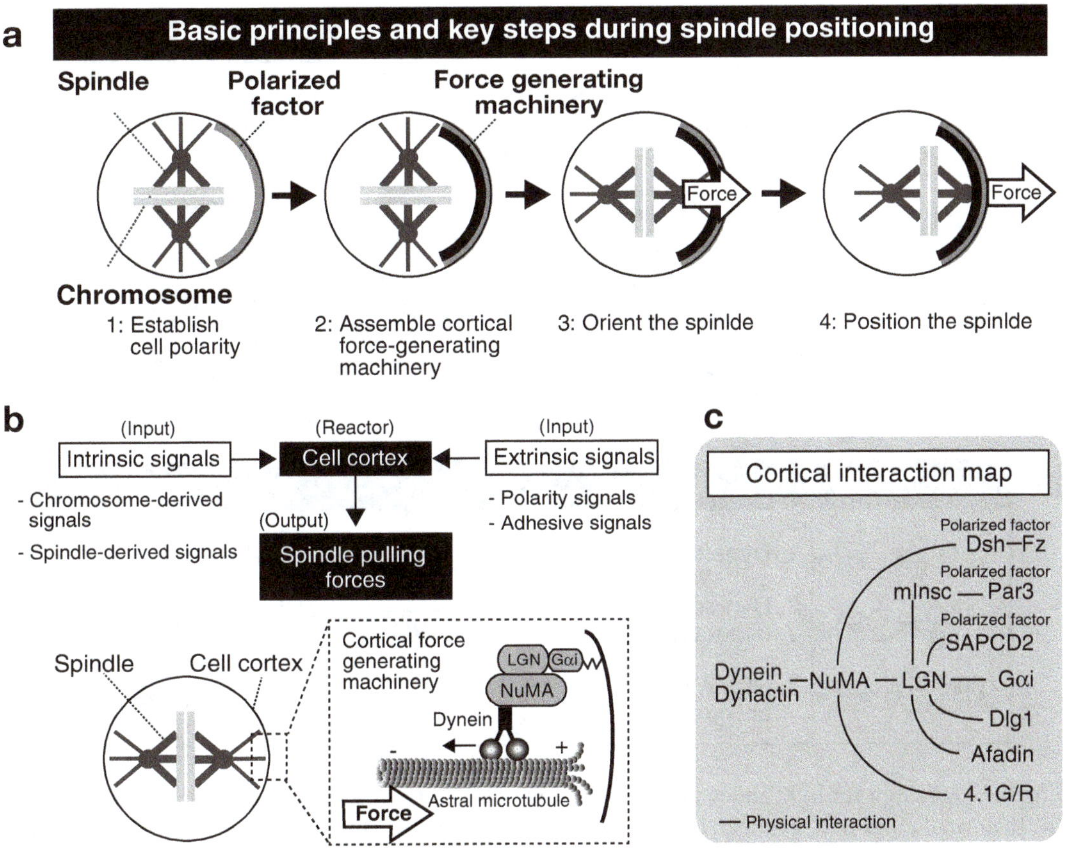

Fig. 6.3 Basic principles and essential steps to control spindle position and orientation. (**a**) A diagram summarizing the four key steps during spindle positioning. (**b**) A diagram showing how intrinsic and extrinsic signals are integrated at the cell cortex and generate cortical pulling forces to control spindle positioning. (**c**) Cortical interaction map of known cortical proteins. Line indicates physical interactions

and analyze their functions in spindle positioning (Fig. 6.4b). Furthermore, HeLa cells or other cultured human cell lines divide symmetrically and likely do not express polarized factors such as Dishevelled (Fig. 6.3c) (Segalen et al. 2010), which is required for controlling spindle orientation during oriented/asymmetric cell division. Thus, by artificially expressing these polarized factors in symmetrically dividing cells and manipulating their localization using light, it is possible to dissect their roles in the assembly of cortical force-generating complex and spindle orientation.

6.5 Perspectives

Previous studies have identified key macro-molecular complexes that play critical roles in diverse cellular functions (Cheeseman et al. 2004; Obuse et al. 2004; Kiyomitsu and Cheeseman 2012; Goshima et al. 2008). Hence, it is definitely

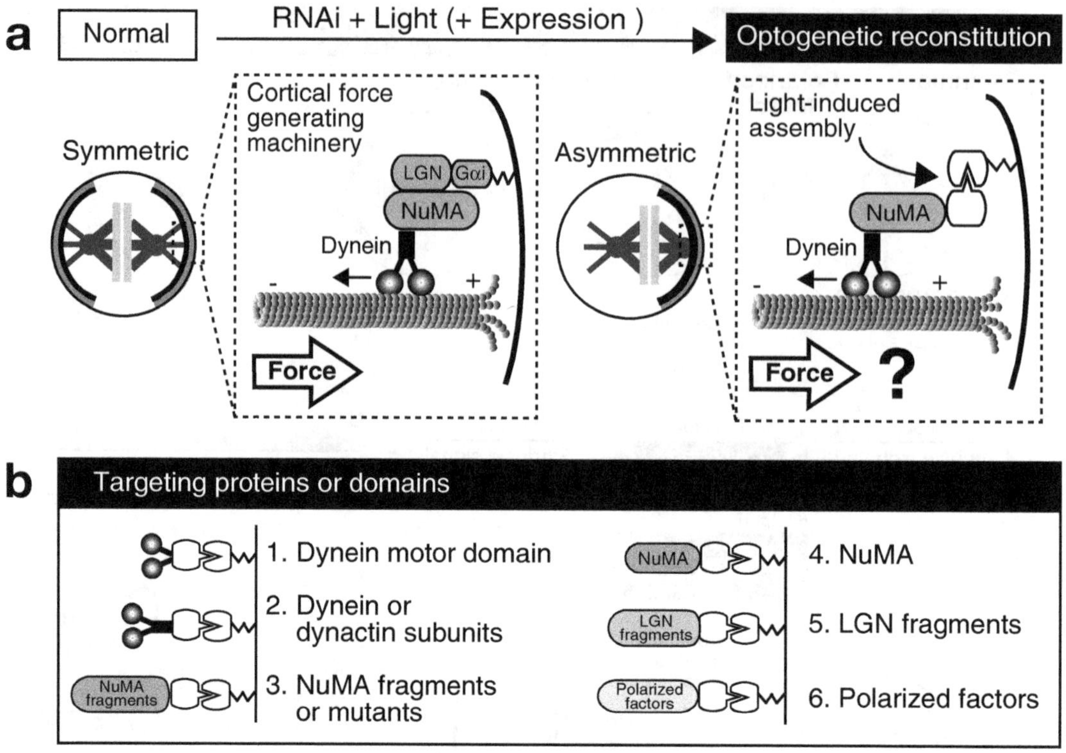

Fig. 6.4 A design for light-induced reconstitution of the cortical force-generating sub-complexes. (**a**) In normal condition, symmetrically dividing cultured cells display symmetric cortical localization of cortical force-generating machinery that includes dynein, dynactin, and NuMA–LGN–Gαi complexes. The metaphase spindle is placed at the center of the cell. Following depletion of cortically localized LGN or Gαi, upstream factors of NuMA, light-induced cortical targeting of NuMA recruits dynein and assembles the cortical force-generating sub-complex. The abilities of cortical puling-force generation by light-induced sub-complexes can be assessed by analyzing the dynamics of the spindle. (**b**) By expressing and targeting different modules, it is possible to reconstitute different sub-complexes and understand the sufficiency and requirement of cortical pulling-force generation

important to investigate their precise functions and structures in *in vitro* reconstitution systems. However, in many cases, it is difficult to fully reconstitute these macro-molecular complexes and their targets *in vitro*. Recent innovation of optogenetic tools has led to the development of *in vivo* reconstitution systems to understand the functional properties and structure of reconstituted sub-complexes within a cell. Light-induced targeting of proteins and their mutants is a powerful method to define both sufficiency and requirement of their molecular functions under more physiological conditions. Importantly, *in cell* reconstitution can be also used to manipulate cellular dynamics in a spatially and temporally controlled manner. For example, temporal reconstitution of force-generating sub-complex at specific cortical region during mitosis can induce spindle orientation or displacement and convert cell division mode from symmetric to asymmetric or vice versa in symmetrically or asymmetrically dividing cells. Such manipulation may lead to unexpected phenotypes and open new directions in the field of cell and developmental biology. Because light-based strategies have high penetrance, low toxicity, and high spatial and temporal precision, these characters and convenience are great advantages to manipulate target molecules in complicated *in vivo* situations, such as tissues in multicellular organisms.

References

Ballister ER, Aonbangkhen C, Mayo AM, Lampson MA, Chenoweth DM (2014) Localized light-induced protein dimerization in living cells using a photocaged dimerizer. Nat Commun 5:5475

Ballister ER, Ayloo S, Chenoweth DM, Lampson MA, Holzbaur ELF (2015) Optogenetic control of organelle transport using a photocaged chemical inducer of dimerization. Curr Biol 25:R407–R408

Cheeseman IM, Niessen S, Anderson S, Hyndman F, Yates JR 3rd, Oegema K, Desai A (2004) A conserved protein network controls assembly of the outer kinetochore and its ability to sustain tension. Genes Dev 18:2255–2268

Cheeseman IM, Chappie JS, Wilson-Kubalek EM, Desai A (2006) The conserved KMN network constitutes the core microtubule-binding site of the kinetochore. Cell 127:983–997

di Pietro F, Echard A, Morin X (2016) Regulation of mitotic spindle orientation: an integrated view. EMBO Rep 17:1106–1130

Dimitrova YN, Jenni S, Valverde R, Khin Y, Harrison SC (2016) Structure of the MIND complex defines a regulatory focus for yeast kinetochore assembly. Cell 167:1014–1027 e1012

Filonov GS, Piatkevich KD, Ting LM, Zhang J, Kim K, Verkhusha VV (2011) Bright and stable near-infrared fluorescent protein for in vivo imaging. Nat Biotechnol 29:757–761

Good MC, Vahey MD, Skandarajah A, Fletcher DA, Heald R (2013) Cytoplasmic volume modulates spindle size during embryogenesis. Science 342:856–860

Goshima G, Wollman R, Goodwin SS, Zhang N, Scholey JM, Vale RD, Stuurman N (2007) Genes required for mitotic spindle assembly in Drosophila S2 cells. Science 316:417–421

Goshima G, Mayer M, Zhang N, Stuurman N, Vale RD (2008) Augmin: a protein complex required for centrosome-independent microtubule generation within the spindle. J Cell Biol 181:421–429

Guntas G, Hallett RA, Zimmerman SP, Williams T, Yumerefendi H, Bear JE, Kuhlman B (2015) Engineering an improved light-induced dimer (iLID) for controlling the localization and activity of signaling proteins. Proc Natl Acad Sci U S A 112:112–117

Hartwell LH (1978) Cell division from a genetic perspective. J Cell Biol 77:627–637

Hueschen CL, Kenny SJ, Xu K, Dumont S (2017) NuMA recruits dynein activity to microtubule minus-ends at mitosis. elife 6. https://doi.org/10.7554/eLife.29328

Hutchins JR, Toyoda Y, Hegemann B, Poser I, Heriche JK, Sykora MM, Augsburg M, Hudecz O, Buschhorn BA, Bulkescher J et al (2010) Systematic analysis of human protein complexes identifies chromosome segregation proteins. Science 328:593–599

Kaberniuk AA, Shemetov AA, Verkhusha VV (2016) A bacterial phytochrome-based optogenetic system controllable with near-infrared light. Nat Methods 13:591–597

Kennedy MJ, Hughes RM, Peteya LA, Schwartz JW, Ehlers MD, Tucker CL (2010) Rapid blue-light-mediated induction of protein interactions in living cells. Nat Methods 7:973–975

Kimura A, Onami S (2005) Computer simulations and image processing reveal length-dependent pulling force as the primary mechanism for C. elegans male pronuclear migration. Dev Cell 8:765–775

Kiyomitsu T (2015) Mechanisms of daughter cell-size control during cell division. Trends Cell Biol 25:286–295

Kiyomitsu T, Cheeseman IM (2012) Chromosome- and spindle-pole-derived signals generate an intrinsic code for spindle position and orientation. Nat Cell Biol 14:311–317

Laan L, Pavin N, Husson J, Romet-Lemonne G, van Duijn M, Lopez MP, Vale RD, Julicher F, Reck-Peterson SL, Dogterom M (2012) Cortical dynein controls microtubule dynamics to generate pulling forces that position microtubule asters. Cell 148:502–514

Levskaya A, Weiner OD, Lim WA, Voigt CA (2009) Spatiotemporal control of cell signalling using a light-switchable protein interaction. Nature 461:997–1001

Lukinavicius G, Reymond L, D'Este E, Masharina A, Gottfert F, Ta H, Guther A, Fournier M, Rizzo S, Waldmann H et al (2014) Fluorogenic probes for live-cell imaging of the cytoskeleton. Nat Methods 11:731–733

Lukinavicius G, Blaukopf C, Pershagen E, Schena A, Reymond L, Derivery E, Gonzalez-Gaitan M, D'Este E, Hell SW, Gerlich DW et al (2015) SiR-hoechst is a far-red DNA stain for live-cell nanoscopy. Nat Commun 6:8497

Lukinavicius G, Reymond L, Umezawa K, Sallin O, D'Este E, Gottfert F, Ta H, Hell SW, Urano Y, Johnsson K (2016) Fluorogenic probes for multicolor imaging in living cells. J Am Chem Soc 138:9365–9368

McKenney RJ, Huynh W, Tanenbaum ME, Bhabha G, Vale RD (2014) Activation of cytoplasmic dynein motility by dynactin-cargo adapter complexes. Science 345:337–341

Natsume T, Kiyomitsu T, Saga Y, Kanemaki MT (2016) Rapid protein depletion in human cells by auxin-inducible degron tagging with short homology donors. Cell Rep 15:210–218

Neumann B, Walter T, Heriche JK, Bulkescher J, Erfle H, Conrad C, Rogers P, Poser I, Held M, Liebel U et al (2010) Phenotypic profiling of the human genome by time-lapse microscopy reveals cell division genes. Nature 464:721–727

Nguyen PA, Groen AC, Loose M, Ishihara K, Wuhr M, Field CM, Mitchison TJ (2014) Spatial organization of cytokinesis signaling reconstituted in a cell-free system. Science 346:244–247

Obuse C, Iwasaki O, Kiyomitsu T, Goshima G, Toyoda Y, Yanagida M (2004) A conserved Mis12 centromere complex is linked to heterochromatic HP1 and outer kinetochore protein Zwint-1. Nat Cell Biol 6:1135–1141

Ran FA, Hsu PD, Wright J, Agarwala V, Scott DA, Zhang F (2013) Genome engineering using the CRISPR-Cas9 system. Nat Protoc 8:2281–2308

Roberts AJ, Kon T, Knight PJ, Sutoh K, Burgess SA (2013) Functions and mechanics of dynein motor proteins. Nat Rev Mol Cell Biol 14:713–726

Rodriguez EA, Campbell RE, Lin JY, Lin MZ, Miyawaki A, Palmer AE, Shu X, Zhang J, Tsien RY (2017) The growing and glowing toolbox of fluorescent and photoactive proteins. Trends Biochem Sci 42:111–129

Sauer G, Korner R, Hanisch A, Ries A, Nigg EA, Sillje HH (2005) Proteome analysis of the human mitotic spindle. Mol Cell Proteomics 4:35–43

Schlager MA, Hoang HT, Urnavicius L, Bullock SL, Carter AP (2014) In vitro reconstitution of a highly processive recombinant human dynein complex. EMBO J 33:1855–1868

Segalen M, Johnston CA, Martin CA, Dumortier JG, Prehoda KE, David NB, Doe CQ, Bellaiche Y (2010) The Fz-Dsh planar cell polarity pathway induces oriented cell division via Mud/NuMA in Drosophila and zebrafish. Dev Cell 19:740–752

Shimomura O (1979) Structure of the chromophore of AEQUOREA green fluorescent protein. FEBS Lett 104:220–222

Strickland D, Lin Y, Wagner E, Hope CM, Zayner J, Antoniou C, Sosnick TR, Weiss EL, Glotzer M (2012) TULIPs: tunable, light-controlled interacting protein tags for cell biology. Nat Methods 9:379–384

Thery M, Racine V, Pepin A, Piel M, Chen Y, Sibarita JB, Bornens M (2005) The extracellular matrix guides the orientation of the cell division axis. Nat Cell Biol 7:947–953

van Bergeijk P, Adrian M, Hoogenraad CC, Kapitein LC (2015) Optogenetic control of organelle transport and positioning. Nature 518:111–114

Wagner E, Glotzer M (2016) Local RhoA activation induces cytokinetic furrows independent of spindle position and cell cycle stage. J Cell Biol 213:641–649

Yanagida M (2014) The role of model organisms in the history of mitosis research. Cold Spring Harb Perspect Biol 6:a015768

Yu D, Gustafson WC, Han C, Lafaye C, Noirclerc-Savoye M, Ge WP, Thayer DA, Huang H, Kornberg TB, Royant A et al (2014) An improved monomeric infrared fluorescent protein for neuronal and tumour brain imaging. Nat Commun 5:3626

Zhang K, Cui B (2015) Optogenetic control of intracellular signaling pathways. Trends Biotechnol 33:92–100

Zhang K, Foster HE, Rondelet A, Lacey SE, Bahi-Buisson N, Bird AW, Carter AP (2017) Cryo-EM reveals how human cytoplasmic dynein is auto-inhibited and activated. Cell 169:1303–1314 e1318

Chapter 7
^{19}F MRI Probes with Tunable Chemical Switches

Kazuya Kikuchi and Tatsuya Nakamura

7.1 Magnetic Resonance Imaging

MRI is the imaging technique based on nuclear magnetic resonance (NMR) phenomena. MRI offers high resolution, deep tissue imaging, and no radiation exposure (Louie et al. 2000). To acquire high contrast images, contrast agents such as Gd^{3+} complexes and superparamagnetic iron oxide nanoparticle (SPIO) are widely used in the field of clinical and research (Fig. 7.1) (Lee et al. 2008). Gd^{3+} complexes shorten the longitudinal relaxation time (T_1), results in enhancement of MRI signals. SPIO shorten the tranverse relaxation time (T_2), results in attenuation of MRI signal intensities. Figure 7.2 shows the switching OFF/ON type probes based on Gd^{3+} complexes and SPIO (Perez et al. 2002). However, ^1H MRI often suffers from high background signals derived from water and lipid etc. Therefore, there is a limitation of monitoring of biological signals.

Recently, heteronuclear MRI has been attracted considerable attentions as the alternative ^1H MRI. Several non proton MRI such as ^{13}C, ^{15}N, ^{19}F, ^{29}Si, ^{31}P, and ^{129}Xe has been utilized in biological analysis (Table 7.1) (Cassidy et al. 2013). Among these non proton MRI, ^{19}F MRI has considerable attentions, because fluorine has a 100% natural abundance and a high gyromagnetic ratio (Ahrens et al. 2005). In our bodies, there are a large amount of fluorine atoms in bones and teeth and almost no fluorine atoms in tissues. However, these fluorine atoms are immobilized in a solid state, exhibits very short T_2 which results in invisible MRI. Therefore, the ^{19}F MRI can acquire the image without the background signals.

Electronic Supplementary Material The online version of this chapter (https://doi.org/10.1007/978-981-13-7908-6_7) contains supplementary material, which is available to authorized users.

K. Kikuchi (✉) · T. Nakamura
Graduate School of Engineering, Osaka University, Suita City, Osaka, Japan
e-mail: kkikuchi@mls.eng.osaka-u.ac.jp

Y. Toyama et al. (eds.), *Make Life Visible*,
https://doi.org/10.1007/978-981-13-7908-6_7

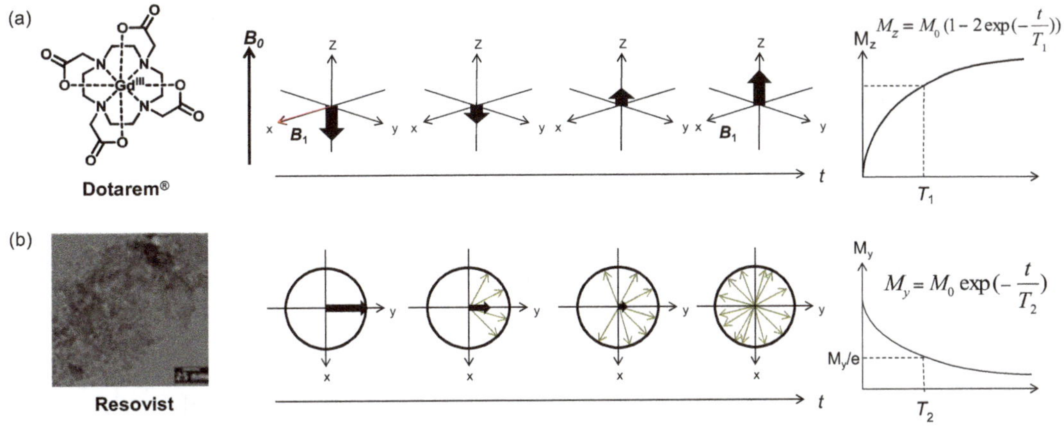

Fig. 7.1 (**a**) Clinically utilized T_1 contrast agent, Dotarem®, and T_1 relaxation. (**b**) Clinically utilized T_2 contrast agent, Resovist, and T_2 relaxation

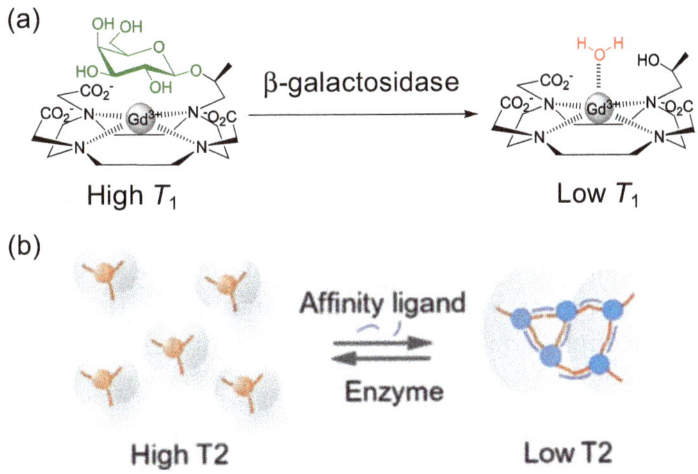

Fig. 7.2 The switching OFF/ON type probes based on (**a**) Gd^{3+} complexes and (**b**) SPIO

Table 7.1 NMR observable nucleus and the sensitivity

Nuclei	Resonant frequency ($MHz \cdot T^{-1}$)	Relative sensitivity	Natural abundance (%)	NMR sensitivity
^{1}H	42.58	1	99.985	1
^{13}C	10.71	1.59×10^{-2}	1.108	1.76×10^{-4}
^{15}N	4.31	1.04×10^{-3}	0.37	3.85×10^{-6}
^{19}F	40.05	8.33×10^{-1}	100	8.33×10^{-1}
^{29}Si	8.46	7.84×10^{-3}	4.70	3.69×10^{-4}
^{31}P	17.24	6.63×10^{-2}	100	6.63×10^{-2}
^{129}Xe	11.78	2.12×10^{-2}	26.4	5.60×10^{-3}

Toward this ends, ^{19}F MRI contrast agents (always ON type probes) have been utilized in visualization of foci, and cell tracker (Ahrens et al. 2005; Thurecht et al. 2010; Srinivas et al. 2007). In particular, perfluorocarbon (PFC) encapsulated nanoemulsions have attracted significant attention as highly sensitive ^{19}F MRI contrast agents (Srinivas et al. 2010), and have been utilized as a cell tracker, and oxygen delivery. Recently, several activatable ^{19}F MRI probes (switching OFF/ON type probes) have also been developed. However, there are only a few examples of in vivo applications owing to the low sensitivity of such probes.

7.2 Perfluorocarbon Encapsulated in Silica Nanoparticle (FLAME)

In the author's research group, novel unique shape nanomaterials, which are perfluoro-15-crown-5 ether (PFCE)-encapsulated silica nanoparticles, FLAMEs (**FL**uorine **A**ccumulated silica nanoparticle for **MRI** contrast **E**nhancement), were developed (Fig. 7.3) (Matsushita et al. 2014). FLAMEs are composed of a liquid PFCE, which shows the high molecular mobility to achieve the long T_2, and a silica shell, which can be easily surface-modified for various functionalization. Although Ahrens et al. reported lipid-based PFCE nanoemulsions as ^{19}F MRI contrast agents for immune cell tracking (Ahrens et al. 2005; Srinivas et al. 2007), the chemical modification of the lipid emulsion surface is limited due to the unstablity in organic solvents. In contrast, the silica shell fulfills the many demands such as high hydrophilicity, high stability in both aqueous and organic solutions, and chemically surface-modifiable property. In fact, various surface functionalization of FLAMEs was achieved and the functionalized FLAMEs were useful for monitoring a reporter protein expression in living cells and in vivo detection of a tumor. These biological applications represent only a fraction of the forthcoming applications.

7.3 Paramagnetic Relaxation Enhancement (PRE) Effect

There are three types of paramagnetic effects: paramagnetic relaxation enhancement (PRE) effect, pseudocontact shifts (PCSs), and residual dipolar couplings (RDCs) (Clore and Iwahara 2009). Since PCSs and RDCs are observed only in anisotropic electron systems, only PRE is effective in the case of SPIO and Gd^{3+}

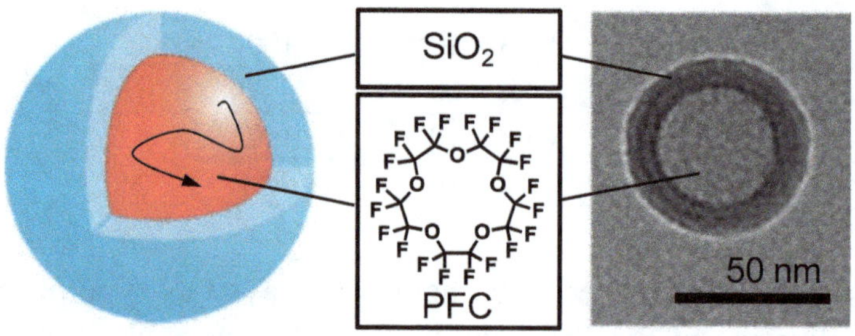

Fig. 7.3 Illustration and transmission electron microscope image of FLAME. The molecular motion of PFC is highly retained and thus the sensitivity of the nanoparticles is high sensitive

complexes (Keizer et al. 2007). The PRE decreases the spin-spin relaxation time (T_2) and results in the broadening of the NMR signals and the decrease of the MRI signals. There are two types of the relaxation mechanism of PRE effect. One is PRE through dipole-dipole interaction and the other is PRE through Curie-spin relaxation. The PRE effect of Gd^{3+} complexes is occurred through dipole-dipole interaction. The transverse (Γ_2) PRE rates of Gd^{3+} are described by the Solomon–Bloembergen (SB) equations (Solomon 1955; Bloembergen and Morgan 1961; Lipari and Szabo 1982):

$$\Gamma_2 = \frac{1}{15}\left(\frac{\mu_0}{4\pi}\right)^2 \gamma_I^2 g^2 \mu_B^2 S(S+1)\left\{4J_{SB}(0) + 3J_{SB}(\omega_I)\right\}$$

where μ_0 is the permeability of free space, μ_B is the magnetic moment of the free electron, γ_I the fluorine gyromagnetic ratio, g is the electron g-factor, S is the electron spin quantum number, and $\omega_I/2\pi$ is the Larmor frequency of the fluorine compound. $J_{SB}(\omega)$ is the spectral density function;

$$J_{SB}(\omega) = r^{-6}\frac{\tau_C}{1+(\omega\tau_C)^2}$$

τ_C is the correlation time, defined as $(\tau_r^{-1} + \tau_s^{-1})^{-1}$. τ_r is the rotational correlation time of the molecule, and τ_s is the effective electron relaxation time.

In contrast, Curie-spin relaxation arises from dipole-dipole interaction between a observable nuclide and the magnetization of the electron. The PRE effect of SPIOs is governed by Curie-spin relaxations owing to their high magnetic susceptibility. The Γ_2 PRE rates of Curie-spin relaxation are given by (Bertinin et al. 2002):

$$\Gamma_2 = \frac{1}{5}\left(\frac{\mu_0}{4\pi}\right)^2 \frac{\omega_I g^4 \mu_B^4 S^2 (S+1)^2}{(3k_B T)^2 r^6}\left(4\tau_r + \frac{3\tau_r}{1+\omega_I^2\tau_r^2}\right)$$

where k_B is the Boltzmann constant, T is temperature.

In both cases, PRE effect is effective over short distance due to its r^{-6} dependency, where r is the distance between NMR-observable nuclei and a paramagnetic center. When the T_2 relaxivity of SPIO is compared with that of Gd^{3+} complexes, SPIOs have higher T_2 relaxivity than Gd^{3+} complexes (Table 7.2). Thus, SPIO is efficient for decreasing the ^{19}F NMR/MRI signals of PFCE near the FLAME core compared with Gd^{3+} complexes.

Table 7.2 Relaxivities ($mM^{-1}\ s^{-1}$) of paramagnetic contrast agents in H_2O at 37 °C (Rohrer et al. 2005)

	0.47 T			1.5 T			3.0 T			4.7 T		
	r_1	r_2	r_2/r_1	r_1	r_2	r_2/r_1	r_1	r_2	r_2/r_1	r_1	r_2	r_2/r_1
Gd^{3+} complex												
Magnevist	3.4	4.0	1.18	3.3	3.9	1.18	3.1	3.7	1.19	3.2	4.0	1.25
Gadovist	3.7	5.1	1.38	3.3	3.9	1.18	3.2	3.9	1.22	3.2	3.9	1.22
ProHance	3.1	3.7	1.19	2.9	3.2	1.10	2.8	3.4	1.21	2.8	3.7	1.32
MultiHance	4.2	4.8	1.14	4.0	4.3	1.08	4.0	4.7	1.18	4.0	5.0	1.25
Dotarem	3.4	4.1	1.21	2.9	3.2	1.10	2.8	3.3	1.18	2.8	3.7	1.32
OmniScan	3.5	3.8	1.09	3.3	3.6	1.09	3.2	3.8	1.19	3.3	4.1	1.24
Teslascan	1.9	2.1	1.11	1.6	2.1	1.31	1.5	2.3	1.53	1.6	2.7	1.69
Optimark	4.2	5.2	1.24	3.8	4.2	1.11	3.6	4.5	1.25	3.8	4.7	1.24
SPIO												
Resovist	20.6	86	4.17	8.7	61	7.01	4.6	143	31.1	2.8	176	62.9
Feridex	27	152	5.63	4.7	41	8.72	4.1	93	22.7	2.3	105	45.7

7.4 Gadolinium Based-19F MRI Nanoprobe for Monitoring Reducing Environment

PRE effect is effective over short distance due to its r^{-6} dependency, where r is the distance between NMR-observable nuclei and a paramagnetic center (Clore and Iwahara 2009; Iwahara and Clore 2006). The author's research group has employed PRE effect to develop activatable ^{19}F MRI small molecule probes for detection of enzyme activity (Mizukami et al. 2008). The probes consist of fluorine compound, enzyme substrate, and Gd^{3+} complex. Gd^{3+} complex was conjugated with fluorine compounds through enzyme substrate. The distance between fluorine compound and Gd^{3+} complex was approximately 2.2 nm, determined by molecular mechanic method. Since PRE effect is effective at such close distance, ^{19}F NMR/MRI signal of the probes were decreased. Upon addition of enzyme, Gd^{3+} complexes were away from fluorine compounds, which results in high ^{19}F NMR/MRI signal enhancements.

In the case of FLAME, most of PFCE compounds are more than 50 Å away from the surface-modified Gd^{3+} complexes due to the thickness of the silica shell. Thus, it was assumed that the PRE effect might not sufficiently attenuate the ^{19}F NMR/MRI signals of FLAME.

The authors first confirmed whether the PRE of the Gd^{3+} complexes on the FLAME surface was effective. Different concentration of Gd^{3+} diethylenetriamine-pentaacetate (DTPA) complexes were attached to FLAME to yield FLAME-

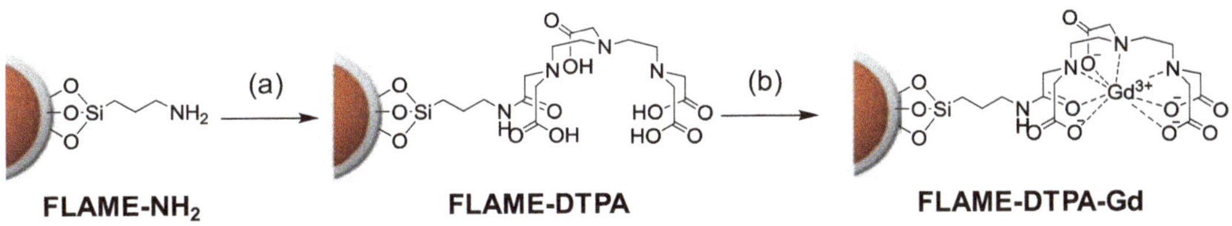

Scheme 7.1 Preparation of FLAME-DTPA-Gd. (**a**) diethylenetriaminepentaacetic acid dianhydride, TEA, DMF; (**b**) $GdCl_3{\cdot}6H_2O$, methanol

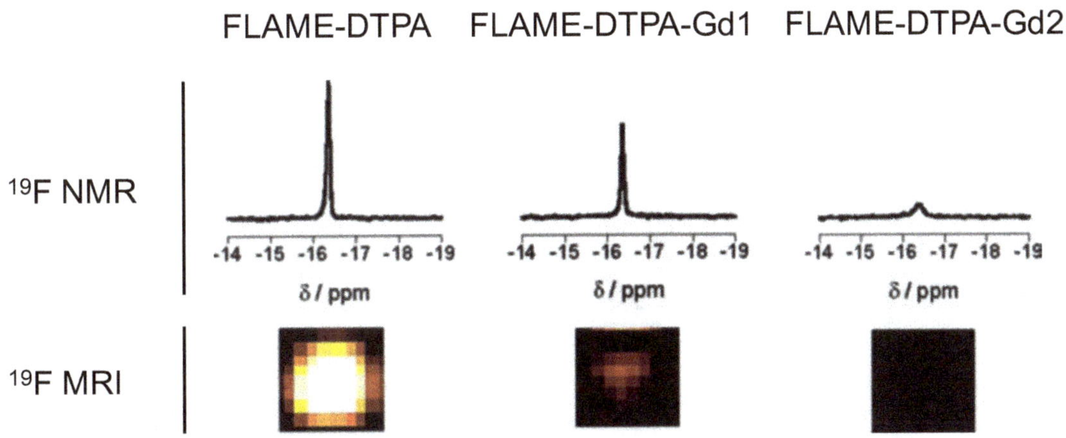

Fig. 7.4 ^{19}F NMR spectra and ^{19}F MRI phantom images of FLAME-DTPA and FLAME-DTPA-Gd. For ^{19}F NMR, C_{PFCE} = 0.6 mM, and the accumulation time was 1 min 22 s. For ^{19}F MRI (Rapid Acquisition with the Refocused Echoes (RARE) method): T_R was 3000 ms. $T_{E,eff}$ was 12 ms. The NEX was 64. The acquisition time was 12 min 48 s

DTPA-Gd1–2 (Scheme 7.1). The ^{19}F NMR spectrum of FLAME-DTPA without Gd^{3+} exhibited a sharp, single peak (T_2 = 420 ms). Meanwhile, that of FLAME-DTPA-Gd became a broader peak as Gd^{3+} concentration increased (Fig. 7.4a). The T_2 of FLAME-DTPA-Gds decreased in Gd^{3+} concentration dependent manner (T_2 = 68, 40 ms for FLAME-DTPA-Gd1, 2 respectively). Although the ^{19}F MRI signal of FLAME-DTPA were observed due to the long T_2, that of FLAME-DTPA-Gd was decreased with Gd^{3+} concentration increasing (Fig. 7.4b). These results indicated that the ^{19}F NMR/MRI signals of PFCE in FLAME were affected by the PRE from the surface-modified Gd^{3+} complexes. Therefore, the author expected that activatable ^{19}F MRI probes with high ^{19}F MRI signal enhancement would be achieved by introducing a cleavable linker between FLAME and the surface-modified Gd^{3+} complexes.

This result was explained by the molecular mobility on the NMR/MRI measurement time scale. Iwahara et al. reported that the PRE effect was efficient in spite of the long average distance, when NMR-observable nuclei can occasionally enter the effective range of the PRE effect (Lee et al. 2008). The long T_2 indicates that the PFCE in FLAME maintains high molecular mobility even in the nanoparticle structure (Matsushita et al. 2014). Although the PFCE at the center of the FLAME core is about 250 Å away from the surface Gd^{3+} complexes (where PRE is not efficient),

Fig. 7.5 Proposed relaxation mechanism of fluorine compounds in FLAME

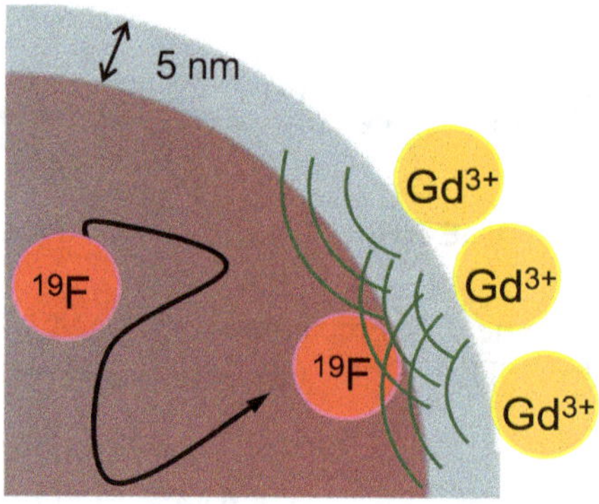

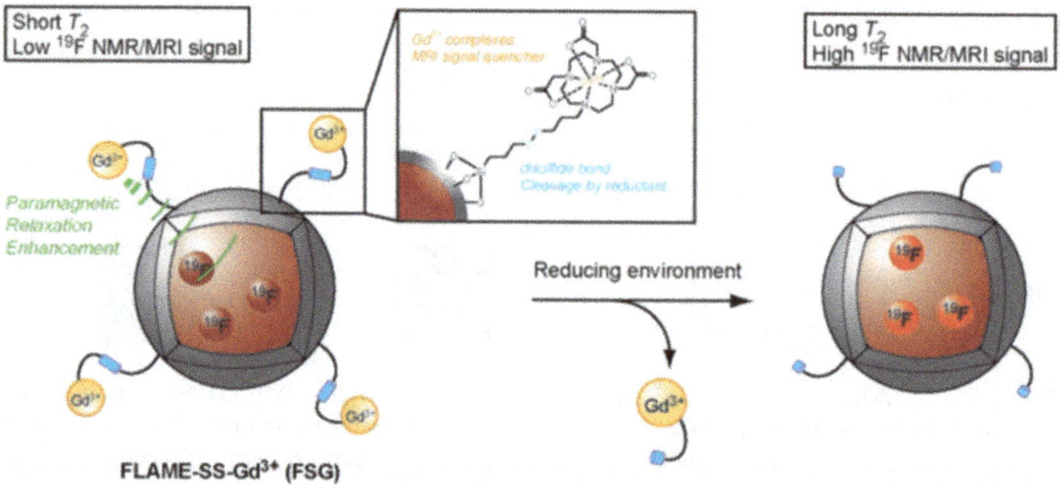

Fig. 7.6 Design of activatable FLAME, FLAME-SS-Gd^{3+} (FSG)

the fluorine compounds can access the inner shell of FLAME on the measurement time scale. Near the inner shell, although the contribution of one Gd^{3+} complex to the PRE effect is small, the PRE effect from multiple surface Gd^{3+} complexes is combined, and thus the T_2 of PFCE is efficiently decreased (Fig. 7.5). Although Grüll et al. observed the PRE of PFCE in Gd^{3+}-modified nanoemulsions, where the distance between the Gd^{3+} complexes and the fluorine core was less than 22 Å (De Vries et al. 2014), we confirmed that the PRE was effective as such distance for the first time.

Next, the authors designed activatable FLAMEs, FLAME-SS-Gd^{3+} (FSG), to image reducing environments. Gd^{3+} complexes were attached to the FLAME surface via disulfide linkers to reduce the T_2 of the fluorine compounds by the PRE effect, which attenuates the ^{19}F NMR/MRI signals (Fig. 7.6). When the disulfide of FSG was reduced, the Gd^{3+} complexes were cleaved from the FLAME surface. Then, the T_2 of the encapsulated PFCE would be elongated and the ^{19}F NMR/MRI signal intensity would increase.

To optimize the amount of Gd^{3+} complexes on the surface of FLAMEs, three types of FSGs with different concentrations of Gd^{3+} were prepared (Scheme 7.2). The synthetic intermediate FLAME-Py was prepared by the reaction of FLAME

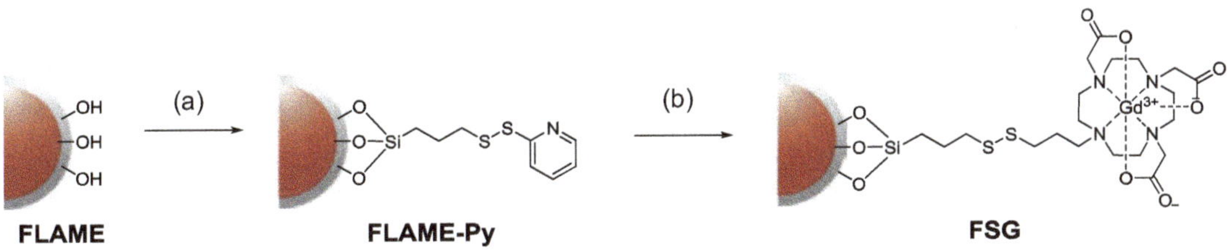

Scheme 7.2 Preparation of FLAME-SS-Gd^{3+} (FSG). (**a**) 2-((3-(trimethoxysilyl)propyl) dithio) pyridine, isopropanol; (**b**) Gd-DOTA-SH, MeOH

Table 7.3 Physical properties of FLAME and FSGs

	ς-potential/mV	$\boldsymbol{n}_{19F}$[a]	$\boldsymbol{n}_{Gd}$[a]	$\boldsymbol{n}_{19F}/\boldsymbol{n}_{Gd}$[a]	$T_{2,\,TCEP-}$/ms	$T_{2,\,TCEP+}$/ms
FLAME	−24.8 ± 1.7	1.7×10^6	0	–	420	–[b]
FSG1	−12.6 ± 2.4	1.7×10^6	9.1×10^2	1.8×10^3	120	383
FSG2	3.9 ± 1.4	1.7×10^6	2.1×10^3	7.7×10^2	66	365
FSG3	5.7 ± 1.5	1.7×10^6	3.1×10^3	5.3×10^2	27	371

$\boldsymbol{n}_{19F}$: the number of ^{19}F atoms in one nanoparticle, $\boldsymbol{n}_{Gd}$ the number of Gd^{3+} atoms in one nanoparticle

[a]These values were predicted assuming that FSG has a single size of 53.4 nm (diameter)

[b]Not measured

with different amounts of 2-((3-(trimethoxysilyl)propyl)dithio)pyridine (1 eq. for FSG1, 10 eq. for FSG2, and 100 eq. for FSG3). Then, 1 eq., 10 eq., or 100 eq. of Gd^{3+} complexes were conjugated to the FLAMEs via a thiol-disulfide exchange reaction to afford FSG1–3, respectively.

Next, the number of fluorine atoms and Gd^{3+} ions per nanoparticle were calculated as $\boldsymbol{n}_{19F}$ and $\boldsymbol{n}_{Gd}$, respectively (Table 7.3). The quantity of attached Gd^{3+} ions was measured by inductively coupled plasma atomic emission spectrometry (ICP-AES), and the amount of the fluorine atoms was quantified by ^{19}F NMR in comparison with that of an internal standard, sodium trifluoroacetate. The average diameter of FLAME was 53.4 nm with a 5 nm-thick silica shell, as measured by transmission electron microscopy. If FLAME has a single size of 53.4 nm, the mole of PFCE per one nanoparticle (m_{PFCE}) could be calculated as follows:

$$m_{\mathrm{PFCE}} = \frac{w_{\mathrm{PFCE}}}{MW_{\mathrm{PFCE}}} = \frac{d_{\mathrm{PFCE}} \times V_{\mathrm{core}}}{MW_{\mathrm{PFCE}}} = \frac{d_{\mathrm{PFCE}} \times \frac{4}{3}\pi r_{\mathrm{core}}^{3}}{MW_{\mathrm{PFCE}}} \approx 1.4 \times 10^{-19}\left(\mathrm{mol/particle}\right)$$

where w_{PFCE} is the weight of PFCE in FLAME, MW_{PFCE} is the molecular weight of PFCE, d_{PFCE} is the density of PFCE (1.86 g/cm^3), V_{core} is the volume of PFCE in FLAME, and r_{core} is the radius of the FLAME core (21.7 nm). Thus, the number of fluorine atoms per one nanoparticle ($\boldsymbol{n}_{19F}$) was calculated as:

$$n_{^{19}\mathrm{F}} = m_{\mathrm{PFCE}} \times 20 \times N_{\mathrm{A}} \approx 1.7 \times 10^{6}\left({}^{19}\mathrm{F\,atom/particle}\right)$$

where N_A is Avogadro's constant. Since the amount of the Gd^{3+} ions was measured by ICP-AES, the molar ratio of the Gd^{3+} ions to PFCE for FSG1, FSG2, and FSG3 was calculated to be 0.011, 0.026, and 0.038, respectively. Therefore, the number of Gd^{3+} ions per nanoparticle ($\boldsymbol{n}_{Gd}$) was calculated as:

$$\text{FSG1}: m_{\text{Gd}^{3+}} / m_{\text{PFCE}} = 0.011$$

$$n_{Gd} = m_{\text{Gd}^{3+}} \times N_{\text{A}} = 0.011 \times m_{\text{PFCE}} \times N_{\text{A}} \approx 9.1 \times 10^2 \left(\text{particle}^{-1}\right)$$

$$\text{FSG2}: m_{\text{Gd}^{3+}} / m_{\text{PFCE}} = 0.026$$

$$n_{Gd} = m_{\text{Gd}^{3+}} \times N_{\text{A}} = 0.026 \times m_{\text{PFCE}} \times N_{\text{A}} \approx 2.1 \times 10^3 \left(\text{particle}^{-1}\right)$$

$$\text{FSG3}: m_{\text{Gd}^{3+}} / m_{\text{PFCE}} = 0.038$$

$$n_{\text{Gd}} = m_{\text{Gd}^{3+}} \times N_{\text{A}} = 0.038 \times m_{\text{PFCE}} \times N_{\text{A}} \approx 3.1 \times 10^3 \left(\text{particle}^{-1}\right)$$

The ς-potentials of FSGs gradually shifted towards the positive direction with increasing amounts of surface Gd^{3+} ions (Table 7.3). This was because the slightly electronegative silanol groups on the FLAME surface were decreased owing to the coupling with 2-((3-(trimethoxysilyl)propyl)dithio)pyridine. The $\boldsymbol{n}_{Gd}$ and ς-potential data indicated that different concentrations of Gd^{3+} complexes were successfully introduced on the FLAME surface.

The ^{19}F NMR spectrum of FLAME without paramagnetic ions exhibited a sharp peak. In contrast, the ^{19}F NMR peaks of FSGs were decreased and more broad according to the concentration of surface Gd^{3+} on account of the PRE effect (Fig. 7.7a). Although the ^{19}F NMR of FSG1 exhibited a sharp peak, the T_2 of FSG1 (120 ms) was shorter than that of FLAME (420 ms) (Table 7.3). The T_2 of FSG2 and FSG3 was 66 ms, 27 ms, respectively. As such, the PRE effect was observed in all FSGs.

^{19}F NMR spectra and T_2 of FSGs were measured after treatment with a reducing agent, tris(2-carboxyethyl)phosphine (TCEP) (Fig. 7.7). Addition of TCEP made the ^{19}F NMR peaks of all FSGs sharper and taller as compared to those before the addition. The T_2 values of FSG1–3 were significantly increased upon addition of TCEP within 2 h, and were comparable to that of FLAME. All Gd^{3+} complexes were cleaved upon addition of more than 2 mM TCEP (Fig. 7.7b). The highest ^{19}F NMR SNR of FSG1–3 was obtained at 2 mM TCEP, and the values were 16.2 for FSG1, 19.5 for FSG2, and 17.9 for FSG3. The signal enhancement factors in response to the reductant were 3.1, 9.7, and 12.7 for FSG1–3, respectively. Thus, FSG3 was the most sensitive ^{19}F NMR probe in the detection of the reducing environment.

The ^{19}F NMR signals of the FSGs increased upon addition of other reducing agents such as glutathione, cysteine, and dithiothreitol (Fig. 7.8). In particular, addition of glutathione induced the greatest ^{19}F NMR signal enhancement. Although there are some concerns about the stability of reduction-triggered nanoparticles in normal tissues, rational optimization of the disulfide linkage will lead to practical in vivo applications.

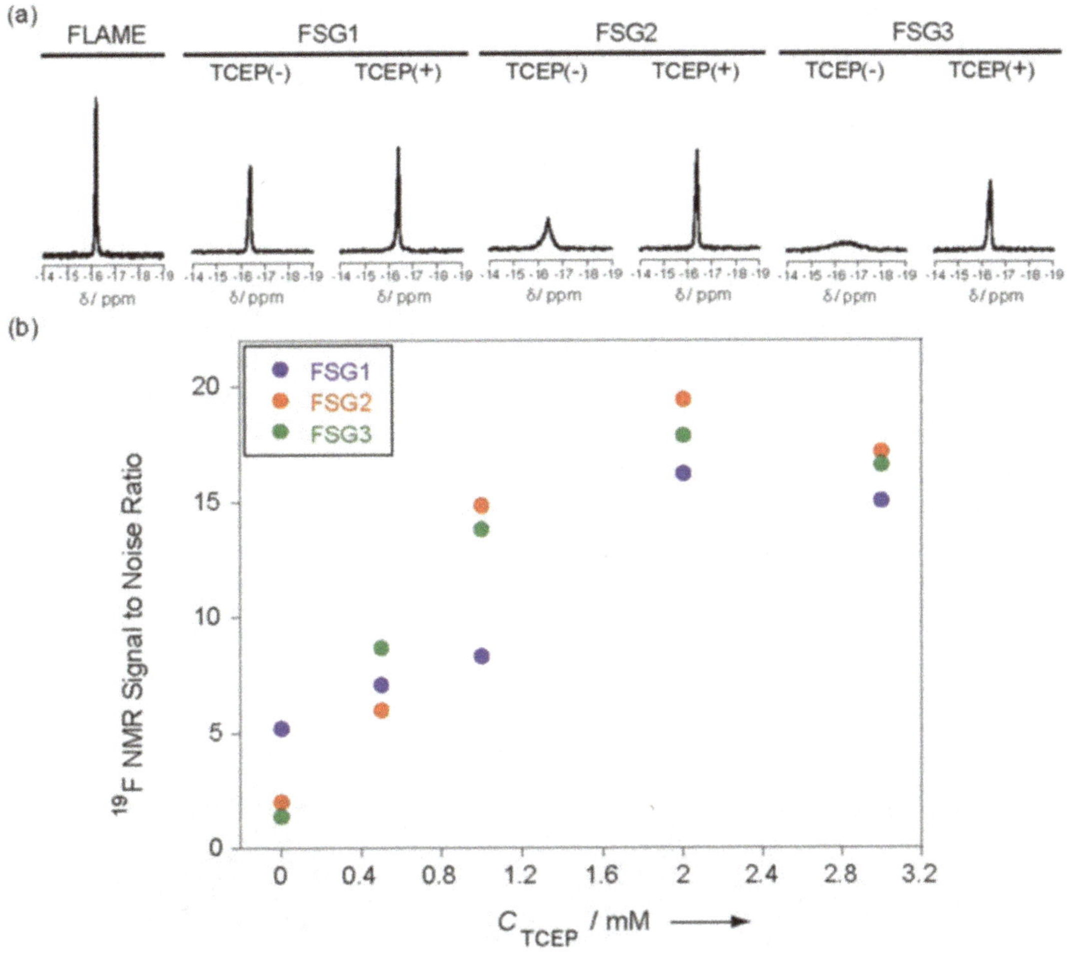

Fig. 7.7 (**a**) ^{19}F NMR spectra of FSGs incubated with or without TCEP. C_{PFCE}: 0.6 mM, C_{TCEP}: 1.0 mM, incubation time: 4 h, accumulation time: 10 min 55 s. (**b**) ^{19}F NMR signal to noise ratio of FSGs in the presence of TCEP (Blue: FSG1, Red: FSG2, Green: FSG3). C_{PFCE}: 0.15 mM

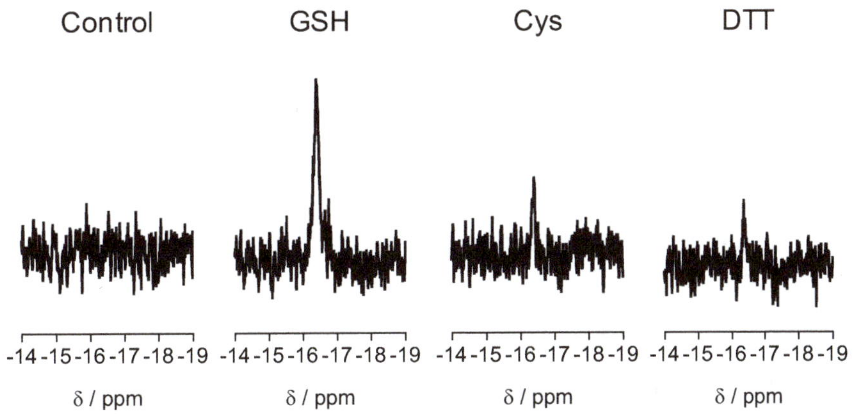

Fig. 7.8 ^{19}F NMR spectra of FSG2 (C_{PFCE} = 0.15 mM) incubated with several thiol-based reducing agents (3 mM). Left to right, control (without reductant), glutathione (GSH), cysteine (Cys), 1,4-dithiothreitol (DTT). The accumulation time was 1 min 22 s. Incubation time was 4 h

Finally, ^{19}F MR phantom images of FSGs solutions with or without TCEP were obtained by varying $T_{E,eff}$. In general, the MRI signal of the long T_2 component is well observed at both short and long $T_{E,eff}$. In contrast, the MRI signal of samples with moderately short T_2 is only visible at short $T_{E,eff}$, and that of the extremely short T_2 component is not observed even at short $T_{E,eff}$. As expected from the ^{19}F NMR results, almost no ^{19}F MRI signals of FSG2 and FSG3 were detected without TCEP at any $T_{E,eff}$ due to the strong PRE effect (Fig. 7.9a, b). In contrast, the ^{19}F MRI signals of FSG1 were observed at $T_{E,eff} \leq 84$ ms because of the moderately short T_2. However, the measurement of FSG1 without TCEP at $T_{E,eff} \geq 108$ ms extinguished the undesired ^{19}F MRI signals. Reductive reactions induced a noticeable ^{19}F MRI signal enhancement in FSG1–3 at any $T_{E,eff}$ (filled circles). At $T_{E,eff} = 12$ ms, approximately 60- and 40-fold increases were observed in FSG2 and FSG3, respectively. Although the signal the enhancement of FSG1 was only two-fold at $T_{E,eff} = 12$ ms, a 50-fold increase was observed at $T_{E,eff} = 108$ ms. These results indicated that FSG2 was the most effective probe for detecting reducing environments. One of the advantages of FSGs is the high sensitivity, because the ^{19}F NMR/MRI signals of 1.7×10^6 fluorine atoms in the core were decreased by ca. 1.0×10^3 Gd^{3+} complexes on the

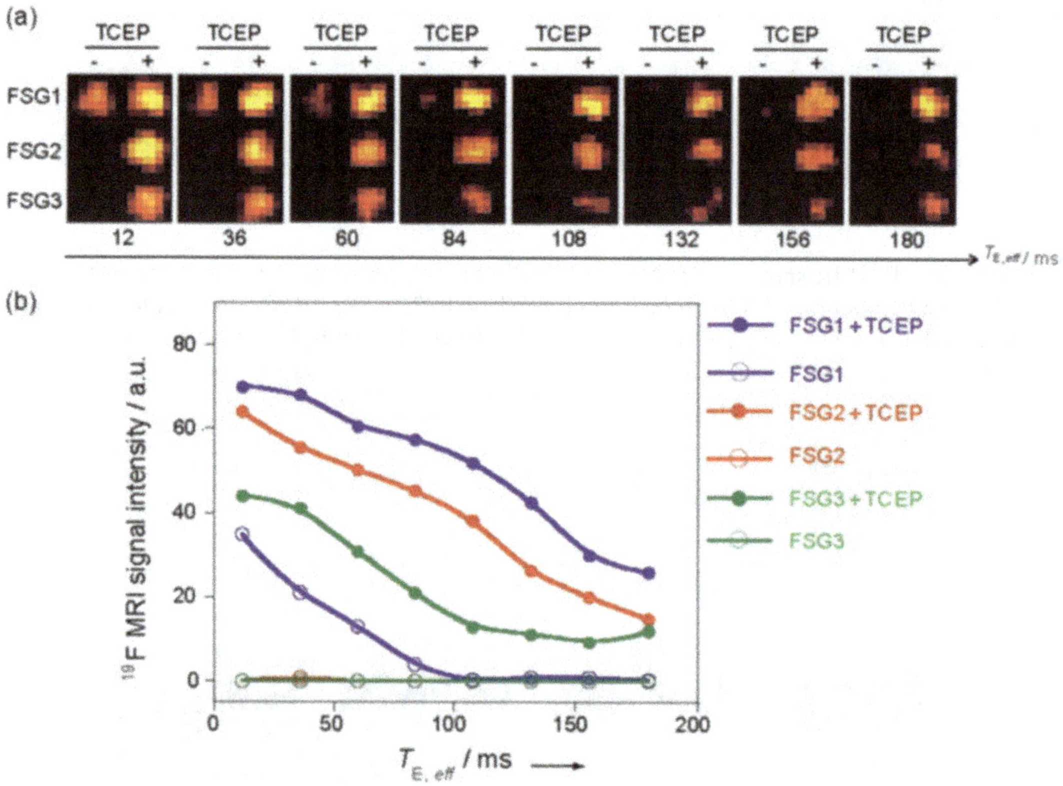

Fig. 7.9 ^{19}F MRI signal enhancement of FSGs by TCEP. (**a**) ^{19}F MRI phantom images of FSG1–3 with or without TCEP. (**b**) Plot of ^{19}F MRI signal intensity of FSG1–3 at different $T_{E,eff}$ with (filled circles) or without (open circles) TCEP. ^{19}F MRI RARE method: the matrix size was 128×64 and the slice thickness was 30 mm. T_R was 3000 ms. The NEX was 64. The acquisition time was 25 min 36 s

FLAME surface. The ratios of fluorine atoms to Gd^{3+} complexes (Table 7.1) are the highest among known PRE-based probes, of which the ratios were single digits. This high ratio led to the high signal amplification.

References

Ahrens ET, Flores R, Xu H, Morel PA (2005) In vivo imaging platform for tracking immunotherapeutic cells. Nat Biotechnol 23:983–987

Bertinin I, Luchinat C, Parigi G (2002) Magnetic susceptibility in paramagnetic NMR. Prog Nucl Mag Res Sp 40:249–273

Bloembergen N, Morgan LO (1961) Proton relaxation times in paramagnetic solutions. Effects of electron spin relaxation. J Chem Phys 34:842–850

Cassidy MC, Chan HR, Ross BD, Bhttacharya PK, Marcus CM (2013) In vivo magnetic resonance imaging of hyperpolarized silicon particles. Nat Nanotechnol 8:363–368

Clore GM, Iwahara J (2009) Theory, practice, and applications of paramagnetic relaxation enhancement for the characterization of transient low-population states of biological macromolecules and their complexes. Chem Rev 109:4108–4139

De Vries A, Moonen R, Yildirim M, Langereis S, Lamer-Ichs R, Pikkemaat JA, Baroni S, Terreno E, Nicolay K, Strijkers GJ, Grüll H (2014) Relaxometric studies of gadolinium-functionalized perfluorocarbon nanoparticles for MR imaging. Contrast Media Mol Imaging 9:83–91

Iwahara J, Clore GM (2006) Detecting transient intermediates in macromolecular binding by paramagnetic NMR. Nature 440:1227–1230

Keizer PHJ, Desreux JF, Overhand M, Ubbink M (2007) Increased paramagnetic effect of a lanthanide protein probe by two-point attachment. J Am Soc Chem 129:9292–9293

Lee H, Sun E, Ham D, Weissleder R (2008) Chip–NMR biosensor for detection and molecular analysis of cells. Nat Med 14:869–873

Lipari G, Szabo A (1982) Model-free approach to the interpretation of nuclear magnetic resonance relaxation in macromolecules. 1. Theory and range of validity. J Am Chem Soc 104:4546–4559

Louie AY, Hüber MM, Ahrens ET, Rothbächer U, Moats R, Jacobs RE, Fraser SE, Meade TJ (2000) In vivo visualization of gene expression using magnetic resonance imaging. Nat Biotechnol 18:321–325

Matsushita H, Mizukami S, Sugihara F, Nakanishi Y, Yoshioka Y, Kikuchi K (2014) Multifunctional core-shell silica nanoparticles for highly sensitive19F magnetic resonance imaging. Angew Chem Int Ed 53:1008–1011

Mizukami S, Takikawa R, Sugihara F, Hori Y, Tochio H, Wälchli M, Shirakawa M, Kikuchi K (2008) Paramagnetic relaxation-based 19F MRI probe to detect protease activity. J Am Chem Soc 130:794–795

Perez JM, Josephson L, O'Loughlin T, Högemann D, Weissleder R (2002) Magnetic relaxation switches capable of sensing molecular interactions. Nat Biotechnol 20:816–820

Rohrer M, Bauer H, Mintorovitch J, Requardt M, Weinmann H-J (2005) Comparison of magnetic properties of MRI contrast media solutions at different magnetic field strengths. Investig Radiol 40:715–724

Solomon I (1955) Relaxation processes in a system of two spins. Phys Rev 99:559–595

Srinivas M, Morel PA, Ernst LA, Laidlaw DH, Ahrens ET (2007) Fluorine-19 MRI for visualization and quantification of cell migration in a diabetes model. Mang Reson Med 58:725–734
Srinivas M, Cruz LJ, Bonetto F, Heerschap A, Figdor CG, de Vries IJM (2010) Customizable, multi-functional fluorocarbon nanoparticles for quantitative in vivo imaging using 19F MRI and optical imaging. Biomaterials 31:7070–7077
Thurecht KJ, Blakey I, Peng H, Squires O, Hsu S, Alexander C, Whittaker AK (2010) Functional hyperbranched polymers: toward targeted in Vivo19F magnetic resonance imaging using designed macromolecules. J Am Chem Soc 132:5336–5337

Chapter 8
Circuit-Dependent Striatal PKA and ERK Signaling Underlying Action Selection

Kazuo Funabiki

Cell-specific, time-lapsed changes in activities of dMSNs and iMSNs were examined by biosensors that allowed monitoring the active and inactive forms of PKA and ERK (Kamioka et al., *Cell Struct. Funct.* 2012). Four lines of transgenic mice were generated by crossing two lines of biosensor-expressing transgenic mice (floxed AKAR3EV for PKA and floxed EKAREV for ERK) with D1-Cre and D2-Cre BAC transgenic mice (Goto et al., *PNAS*, 2015, Fig. 8.1a). The D1-PKA and D1-ERK mice and the D2-PKA and D2-ERK mice exclusively expressed the respective FRET biosensors in the neural pathways of dMSNs and iMSNs, respectively. FRET imaging of the striatum of freely moving mice was achieved by developing fiber bundle-based micro-endoscope techniques (Fig. 8.1b). The pencil like-shaped tip of the optical fiber bundle was implanted into the mouse brain, and the flat end of the bundle was scanned with a confocal laser scanning microscope equipped with a 445-nm laser for excitation and a pair of band-path filters, 483 ± 16 nm for CFP and 542 ± 13 nm for FRET. Fluorescence excitation of the FRET biosensors was exclusively detected in the striatum of the transgenic mice. Upon quantitative analysis, *in vivo* administration of SP-8-Br-cAMPs (cAMP analog) through the cannula attached close to the endoscope caused a progressive increase in FRET responses (changes in FRET/CFP ratio) in both D1-PKA and D2-PKA mice (Fig. 8.1c), but not in PKA-neg mice. Conversely, the MEK inhibitor PD184352 gradually decreased FRET responses in both D1-ERK and D2-ERK mice (Fig. 8.1c). The FRET micro-endoscopy thus allowed us to monitor dynamic changes in activities of PKA and ERK specific for dMSNs and iMSNs.

Electronic Supplementary Material The online version of this chapter (https://doi.org/10.1007/978-981-13-7908-6_8) contains supplementary material, which is available to authorized users.

K. Funabiki (✉)
Institute of Biomedical Research and Innovation, Foundation for Biomedical Research and Innovation, Kobe, Japan
e-mail: funabiki@fbri.org; funabiki@ent.kuhp.kyoto-u.ac.jp

Y. Toyama et al. (eds.), *Make Life Visible*,
https://doi.org/10.1007/978-981-13-7908-6_8

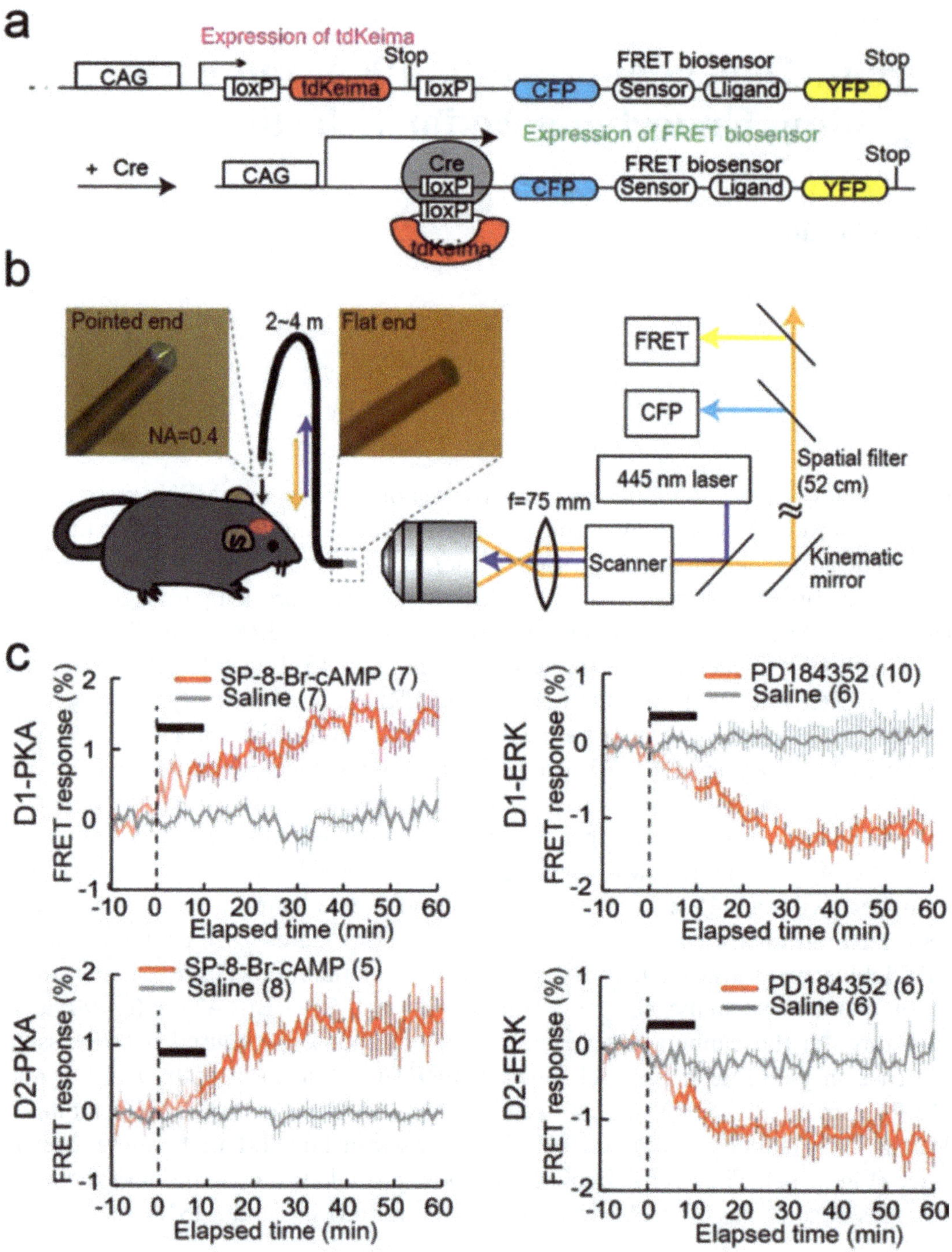

Fig. 8.1 Live monitoring of PKA and ERK activities in dMSNs and iMSNs of transgenic mice expressing FRET biosensors

(**a**) Construct for Cre-dependent expression of FRET biosensors

(**b**) Schema of the micro-endoscope system. Changes in FRET responses were monitored to measure the activity of PKA or ERK

(**c**) Local application of SP-8-Br-cAMP (2 mM) and PD184352 (10 μM) into the dorsal striatum of anesthetized transgenic mice (indicated by black bars) respectively increased FRET responses of D1-PKA and D2-PKA and decreased those of D1-ERK and D2-ERK

Exposure to cocaine causes a massive increase in the dopamine (DA) level in the striatum and results in activation of PKA and ERK in this brain region (Valjent et al., *J. Neurosci*, 2000; Bertran-Gonzales et al., *J. Neurosci*, 2008). Upon FRET micro-endoscopic analysis, administration of cocaine (25 mg/kg, i.p.), but not that of saline, rapidly and continuously increased the activities of both D1-PKA and D1-ERK with a concomitant increase in locomotor activity (Fig. 8.2a). This increase was in marked contrast to the response of iMSNs, in which the activities of both D2-PKA and D2-ERK were gradually decreased by the cocaine administration (Fig. 8.2a). Importantly, saline injection appreciably activated both D2-PKA and D2-ERK (Fig. 8.2a). Aversive stimuli transiently suppress tonic firings of most of DA neurons in the ventral tegmental area and disinhibit iMSNs via inactivation of Gi-coupled inhibitory D2 receptors (Gerfen and Surmeier, *Annu. Rev. Neurosci*, 2011; Ungless, *Science*, 2004). Because saline injection supposedly serves as an aversive stimulus, we more directly addressed how a strong aversive stimulus, i.e., an electric foot shock, would affect PKA and ERK in dMSNs and iMSNs. Both D2-PKA and D2-ERK were markedly activated in response to an electric foot shock (2 mA, 40 Hz for 2 sec) (Fig. 8.2b). Conversely, the activities of D1-PKA and D1-ERK were notably decreased in response to the electric shock (Fig. 8.2b). Thus, the activities of PKA and ERK are reciprocally controlled not only by rewarding and aversive stimuli but also between dMSNs and iMSNs. We further investigated involvement of D2-PKA and D2-ERK in the induction of aversive learning by pairing electric shocks with the sound of a bell (Fig. 8.2b). After habituation with repeated exposure to a bell sound, an additional bell sound never influenced the activities of PKA and ERK in either dMSNs or iMSNs and thus served as neutral information. Notably, both PKA and ERK were activated and inactivated in iMSNs and dMSNs, respectively, by the conditioned bell sound without electric shocks. Thus, the cell-specific regulation of PKA and ERK underlies the induction of both the acute aversive reaction and aversive learning behavior.

Naturally occurring rewarding stimuli such as food, drinking, and mating enhance DA release in the striatum and induce motivational reward-seeking behavior (Damsma et al., *Behav. Neurosci*, 1992; Salamone and Correa, *Neuron*, 2012). The role of striatal PKA and ERK in naturally occurring rewarding behavior was addressed by measuring the activities of PKA and ERK during the mating behavior of a male mouse after inclusion of a female mouse in the same chamber. The male mice showed a wide variety of mating reactions, including frequent sniffing, grooming, and mounting (Park 2011). We counted the percentages of time exhibiting mating behaviors (sniffing, grooming, mounting) every minutes during a 30-min period after inclusion of the female mouse (%PMR), and used it as an index to estimate the motivational strength for the male mice to the presented female mouse. When overall 30 min period (interaction with female) was averaged, a significant positive correlation was noted between the extent of the D1-PKA and D1-ERK activation and the percentage of positive mating reactions, and this correlation was inverted in the responses of D2-PKA and D2-ERK (Fig. 8.3a). When mating behaviors were arbitrarily divided into two groups exhibiting either frequent or infrequent mating reactions by values of 20% PMR (Fig. 8.3b), the D1-PKA and D1-ERK activities

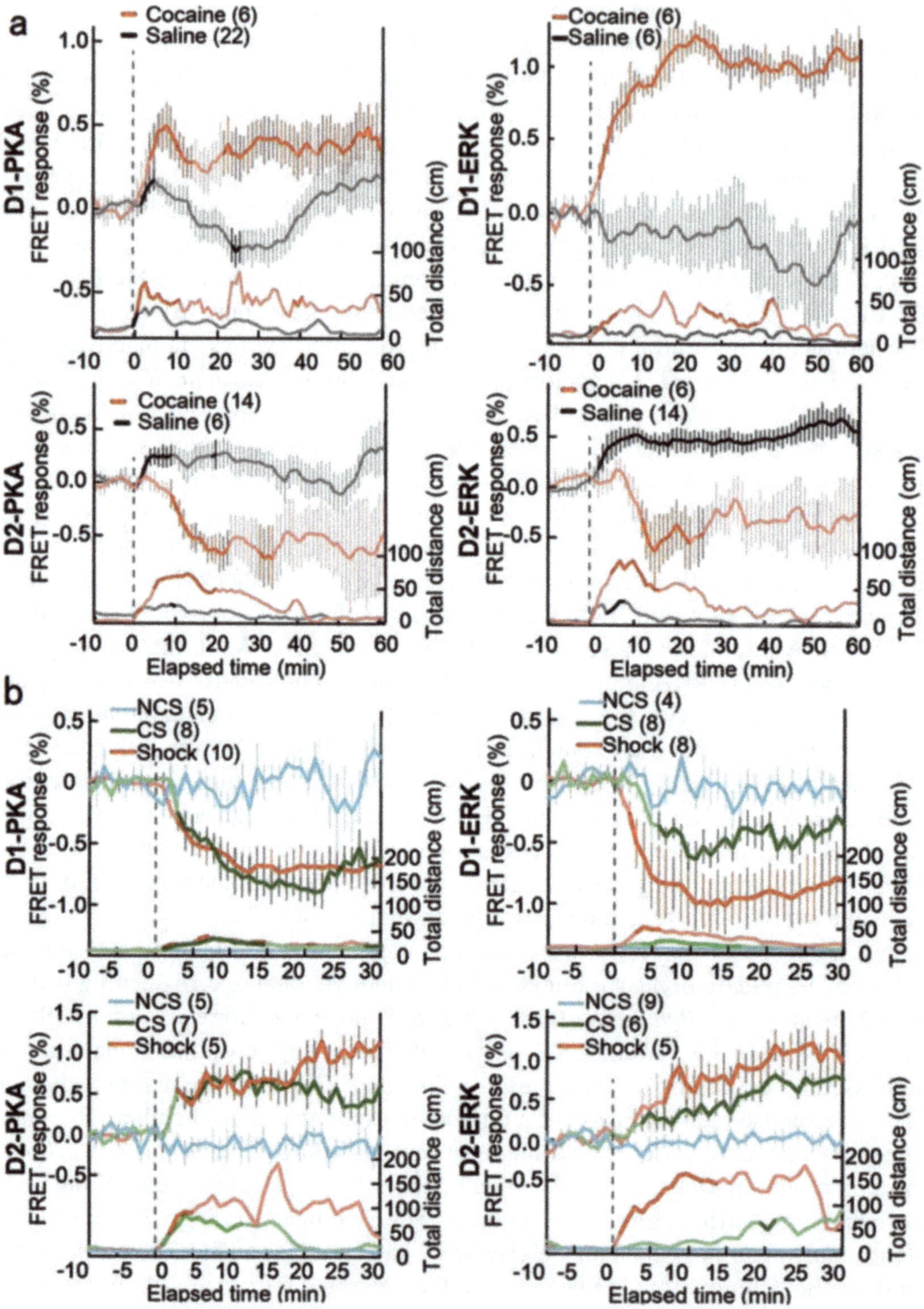

Fig. 8.2 Reciprocal regulation of PKA and ERK activities between dMSNs and iMSNs in response to cocaine administration and electric foot shocks

(**a**) PKA and ERK activities (upper traces) with SEM (vertical lines) and locomotor activities (lower traces) in response to cocaine or saline injection

(**b**) PKA and ERK activities in response to electric foot shocks (Shock), bell sound without unconditioned stimulus (NCS), and bell sound after conditioning with electric shocks (CS) significantly increased in frequently interacting mice, whereas the D2-PKA and D2-ERK activities were increased in the infrequently interacting ones (Fig. 8.3b). We noticed that the observed activity changes in frequently and infrequently interacting animals depended on whether these mice became successively motivated or indifferent to a female mouse during mating behaviors. Thus, the PKA and ERK activities of individual mice were pursued during the shift between the motivational phase and indifferent phase of mating behavior (defined as more than 50% PMR increase and decrease within 1–4 min, respectively) (Fig. 8.3c). This analysis revealed that the activities of D1-PKA and D1-ERK were elevated during the motivational phase of the mating reaction. In contrast, the activities of D2-PKA and D2-ERK were increased when a male mouse became indifferent to or escaped from a female mouse. Thus, the activities of both PKA and ERK (but more PKA) rapidly changed during mating behavior, and this rapid change reflected the shift between motivational and indifferent phases of the mating reaction. The above results suggest that activation of PKA and ERK in dMSNs and iMSNs underlies the induction and suppression of mating reactions, respectively. To substantiate this possibility, the ejaculation of a male mouse was facilitated by pairing the male mouse with a hormonally-primed female mouse (Ogawa et al., *Endocrinology*, 1998) and the activities of D1-PKA and D1-ERK were measured before and after ejaculation (Fig. 8.3e, f). The D1-PKA activity elevated during the mating reaction was rapidly reduced to lower levels within 4 min after ejaculation, whereas the D1-ERK activity continued to be elevated even after ejaculation, suggesting that PKA in the dMSNs was more relevantly associated with the rapid shift in the mating reaction.

To further address the causality of PKA activity in mating behavior, we artificially activated Gi or Gs by DREADDs (Designer Receptors exclusively Activated by a Designer Drug, Rogan & Roth, *Pharmacological reviews*, 2011) which were induced by adeno-associate virus in a Cre-dependent manner. CNO was injected 10 or 20 min after the female entry. Around 10 min after CNO injection, PKA activity was either decreased in AAV-hM4Di-mCherry injected mice, or increased in AAV-hDs-mCherry injected ones (Goto et al., *PNAS*, 2015). Concomitant to the increase or decrease in D1-PKA, male mouse exhibited increase or decrease in %PMR, respectively. Conversely, increase or decrease in D2-PKA either induced either decrease or increase in %PMR, respectively. These results indicate that the causal relationship between PKA activity of dMSNs and iMSNs in the dorsal striatum and the mating reactions in male mice.

Figure 8.4 summarizes differences in the amplitudes of the PKA and ERK responses in MSNs along different behavioral conditions. This summary explicitly demonstrates that PKA and ERK are coordinately stimulated or inhibited in both dMSNs and iMSN but oppositely regulated between these two cell types under different conditions. Animal behaviors can thus be orderly aligned from rewarding to aversive behaviors by taking into account the extents of activation and inactivation of PKA and ERK in individual behaviors. Intriguingly, highly interacting male mice with female mice exhibited higher PKA and ERK activities in dMSNs than those of cocaine-treated mice, suggesting that sexual behavior is highly emotional and motivational for male mice. Importantly, the motivational and indifferent phases of mat-

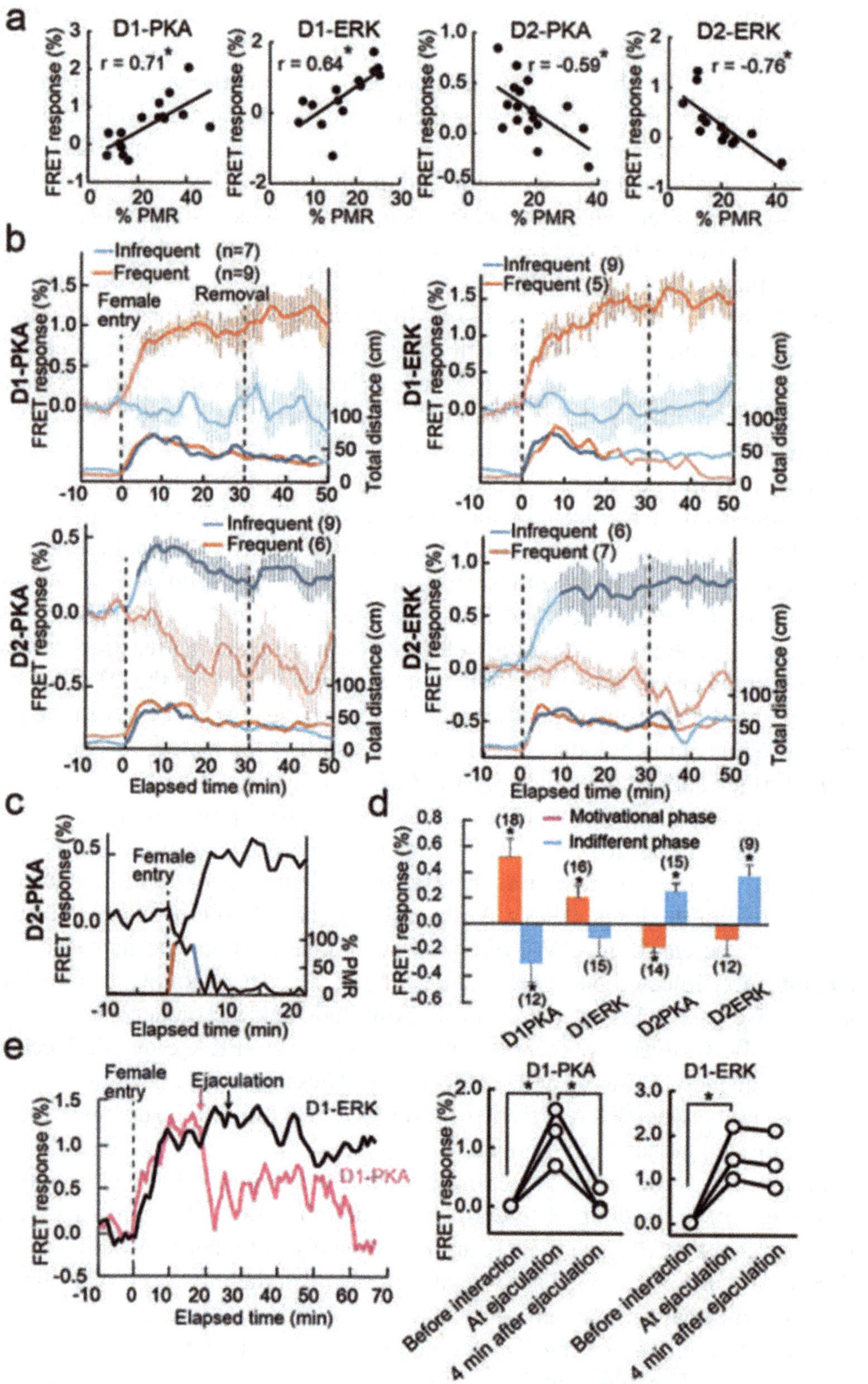

Fig. 8.3 PKA and ERK activities of dMSNs and iMSNs during sexual interaction
(**a**) A male mouse was exposed to an unfamiliar female mouse for 30 min and analyzed by the FRET micro-endoscopy. Percentages of PMR were measured, and average changes in activities of PKA and ERK of dMSNs and iMSNs during the 30-min period were plotted against % PMR

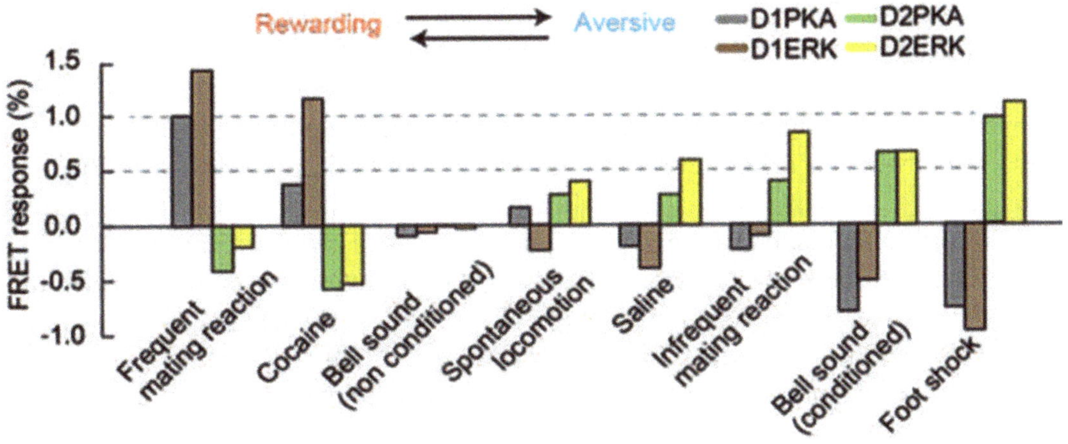

Fig. 8.4 Summary of PKA and ERK activities under rewarding and aversive/impassive conditions
Values of the PKA and ERK activities were calculated by averaging FRET responses during 5 min at the peak response under the different conditions. $***p < 0.001$, $**p < 0.01$, $*p < 0.05$, as compared with the non-conditioned bell sound (Mann-Whitney's U test). Reward-seeking and aversive/impassive animal behaviors can be orderly aligned according to the extents of activation and inactivation of PKA and ERK

ing reactions are tightly associated with the rapid shift in the activities of PKA and ERK in both dMSNs and iMSNs. Phosphorylation/dephosphorylation of PKA and ERK in these two types of MSNs could thus be a potential mechanism that controls this rapid shift between rewarding and aversive behaviors. Notably, the bell sound after conditioning with electric shocks induced profound effects on both dMSNs and iMSNs, indicating that robust and strong adaptive alterations in the striatal circuit are involved in the aversive learning behavior. Furthermore, saline injection, spontaneous locomotion, and indifference of male mice toward female mice caused up-regulation of the activities of PKA and ERK in iMSNs. This finding is consistent with the predominant expression of high-affinity (nM order) D2 receptors in iMSNs, which are capable of sensing subtle changes in synaptic DA concentrations in the

Fig. 8.3 (continued) (**b**) Changes in activities of PKA and ERK (upper traces) and locomotor activities (lower traces) of frequently or infrequently interacting male mice
(**c**, **d**) Up- and down-regulation of PKA and ERK activities at the active and indifferent phases of the mating reaction($*p < 0.05$, Mann-Whitney's U test). The numbers in parentheses indicate the sample numbers from 6 to 9 animals
(**e**), (left) Examples of changes in the PKA and ERK activities in dMSNs after ejaculation. Ejaculation is marked with the arrow in the D1-PKA (red) and D1-ERK (black) mouse
(right) Rapid inactivation of PKA in the D1-PKA mice after ejaculation ($*p < 0.05$, $n = 5$, Wilcoxon signed-rank test)

striatum (Gerfen & Surmeier, *Annu. Rev. Neurosci*, 2011). The iMSN transmission would thus greatly contribute to the innate tendency of animals to be more concerned about and to rapidly avoid uncomfortable environments and predators. Conversely, when animals encounter rewarding stimuli such as sexual interaction, these stimuli increase DA levels in the striatum and stimulate low-affinity (μM order) D1 receptors in dMSNs. Thus, the D1 and D2 receptors serve as key determinants to distinctly sense changes in synaptic DA transmission in a pathway-specific manner and to induce reward-directed and aversive behaviors via common PKA and ERK signaling cascades (Nakanishi et al., *Neuroscience*, 2014).

We also applied these techniques to measure the temporal dynamics of PKA response in the formation of aversive memory in the core part of nucleus accumbens (NAc). We found that PKA activities of iMSNs at NAc occurred not instantaneously after footshock but in a delayed and progressive manner (Yamaguchi et al., *PNAS*, 2015). We believe that the above methodologies allow us to study regulatory mechanisms of neural circuits involved in a wide range of animal behaviors.

References

Bertran-Gonzalez J et al (2008) Opposing patterns of signaling activation in dopamine D1 and D2 receptor-expressing striatal neurons in response to cocaine and haloperidol. J Neurosci 28:5671–5685

Bromberg-Martin ES, Matsumoto M, Hikosaka O (2010) Dopamine in motivational control: rewarding, aversive, and alerting. Neuron 68:815–834

Damsma G, Pfaus JG, Wenkstern D, Phillips AG, Fibiger HC (1992) Sexual behavior increases dopamine transmission in the nucleus accumbens and striatum of male rats: comparison with novelty and locomotion. Behav Neurosci 106:181–191

Gerfen CR, Surmeier DJ (2011) Modulation of striatal projection systems by dopamine. Annu Rev Neurosci 34:441–466

Gong S et al (2007) Targeting Cre recombinase to specific neuron populations with bacterial artificial chromosome constructs. J Neurosci 27:9817–9823

Goto A, Nakahara I, Yamaguchi T, Kamioka Y, Sumiyama K, Matsuda M, Nakanishi S, Funabiki K (2015) Circuit-dependent striatal PKA and ERK signaling underlies rapid behavioral shift in mating reaction of male mice. Proc Natl Acad Sci U S A 112(21):6718–6723

Graybiel AM (2008) Habits, rituals, and the evaluative brain. Annu Rev Neurosci 31:359–387

Kamioka Y et al (2012) Live imaging of protein kinase activities in transgenic mice expressing FRET biosensors. Cell Struct Funct 37:65–73

Luo Z, Volkow ND, Heintz N, Pan Y, Du C (2011) Acute cocaine induces fast activation of D1 receptor and progressive deactivation of D2 receptor striatal neurons: in vivo optical microprobe [Ca2+]i imaging. J Neurosci 31:13180–13190

Nakanishi S, Hikida T, Yawata S (2014) Distinct dopaminergic control of the direct and indirect pathways in reward-based and avoidance learning behaviors. Neuroscience 282:49–59

Ogawa S et al (1998) Modifications of testosterone-dependent behaviors by estrogen receptor-α gene disruption in male mice 1. Endocrinology 139:5058–5069

Park JH (2011) Assessment of male sexual behavior in mice. In: Mood and anxiety related phenotypes in mice, vol 63. Humana Press, New York, pp 357–373

Rogan SC, Roth BL (2011) Remote control of neuronal signaling. Pharmacol Rev 63(2):291–315

Salamone JD, Correa M (2012) The mysterious motivational functions of mesolimbic dopamine. Neuron 76:470–485

Ungless MA (2004) Uniform inhibition of dopamine neurons in the ventral tegmental area by aversive stimuli. Science 303:2040–2042

Valjent E et al (2000) Involvement of the extracellular signal-regulated kinase cascade for cocaine-rewarding properties. J Neurosci 20:8701–8709

Valjent E, Bertran-Gonzalez J, Hervé D, Fisone G, Girault J-A (2009) Looking BAC at striatal signaling: cell-specific analysis in new transgenic mice. Trends Neurosci 32:538–547

Yamaguchi T, Goto A, Nakahara I, Yawata S, Hikida T, Matsuda M, Funabiki K, Nakanishi S (2015) Role of PKA signaling in D2 receptor-expressing neurons in the core of the nucleus accumbens in aversive learning. Proc Natl Acad Sci U S A 112(36):11383–11388

Chapter 9
Making Life Visible: Fluorescent Indicators to Probe Membrane Potential

Parker E. Deal, Vincent Grenier, Rishikesh U. Kulkarni, Pei Liu, Alison S. Walker, and Evan W. Miller

9.1 Introduction

Cell membranes are central to all life on earth. The lipid bilayer composing cell membranes enables discrimination between the cell and its external environment. Far from a passive bystander, the lipid membrane plays an active role in sequestering and accumulating genetic material, proteins, nutrients and ions essential for life. Indeed, cells allocate a significant portion of their energy budget to maintain an unequal distribution of ions across the cell membrane. The unequal distribution of ions across the cell membrane results in an electrochemical potential, or voltage. Rapid changes in this membrane voltage drive the unique physiology of excitable cells like neurons and cardiomyocytes. Despite the central importance of voltage in the brain and body, the full contributions of voltage changes to both physiology and disease remain incompletely characterized due to a lack of methods that can report on membrane potential with high fidelity, high throughput, and minimal invasiveness.

Voltage imaging with fluorescent dyes offers a solution to this problem because it combines a direct readout of voltage changes, providing temporal resolution, with an imaging approach that offers spatial resolution. Attempts at voltage imaging with small molecules date back to the 1970s (Braubach et al. 2015; Loew 2015), and it is a measure of the difficulty of the task that voltage imaging has not yet become a wide-spread experimental approach. Rather, surrogates of voltage changes, notably Ca^{2+} ion fluxes have become the primary means of assessing neuronal and cellular activity. This is due, in part, to the fact that the experimental constraints on Ca^{2+} imaging are somewhat less stringent than voltage imaging in the context of neurobiology. First, transient fluctuations in intracellular Ca^{2+} concentration follow time-courses that are 10–100,000 times slower than neuronal action potentials. Second, an individual cell can accumulate >1000-fold more Ca^{2+} indicators relative to volt-

P. E. Deal · V. Grenier · R. U. Kulkarni · P. Liu · A. S. Walker · E. W. Miller (✉)
University of California, Berkeley, USA
e-mail: evanwmiller@berkeley.edu

Y. Toyama et al. (eds.), *Make Life Visible*,
https://doi.org/10.1007/978-981-13-7908-6_9

age indicators, owing to the requirement that voltage indicators must localize to the plasma membrane (which occupies ~0.1% the volume of the cytosol) in order to retain function. Finally, because the fluorescent signals from Ca^{2+} indicators emanate from the cytosol, it is relatively straightforward to segregate signals arising from distinct cells. For voltage indicators that localize to the plasma membrane, fluorescent signals from adjoining cells can overlap. These barriers, and others, have hindered the widespread adoption of voltage indicators because, compared to Ca^{2+} indicators, voltage indicators must do more with less (Kulkarni and Miller 2017).

To address these challenges, we have recently initiated a program to develop fluorescent sensors of membrane potential that circumvent previous limitations of speed, sensitivity and disruptive capacitive load. Our strategy uses small molecule fluorescent voltage sensors that employ photoinduced electron transfer (PeT) (De Silva et al. 1995; Li 2007) through a molecular wire as a voltage-sensing trigger. In the first generation of voltage-sensitive fluorophores, also known as VoltageFluors, or VF dyes, an electron-rich aniline donor is coupled to a fluorescent, fluorescein reporter via a phenylenevinylene molecular wire (Miller et al. 2012). Due to their amphipathic nature, VF dyes inserts into the plasma membrane with the chromophore protruding slightly above the phospholipid layer, on account of the anionic sulfonate. We hypothesized that, at resting membrane potential, which is slightly negative (approximately −60 mV in a typical mammalian neuron), the orientation of the electric field across the membrane accelerates PeT from the aniline donor to the excited chromophore, quenching fluorescence (Fig. 9.1). When a neuron fires an action potential, the membrane potential changes rapidly (<5 ms), depolarizing to approximately +40 mV. During this depolarization, the electric field across the membrane reverses, resulting in a reduction of the rate of PeT and subsequent fluorescence brightening. In this way, the membrane potential modulates PeT, (De Silva et al. 1995; Li 2007) which in turn alters the fluorescence, which can be read

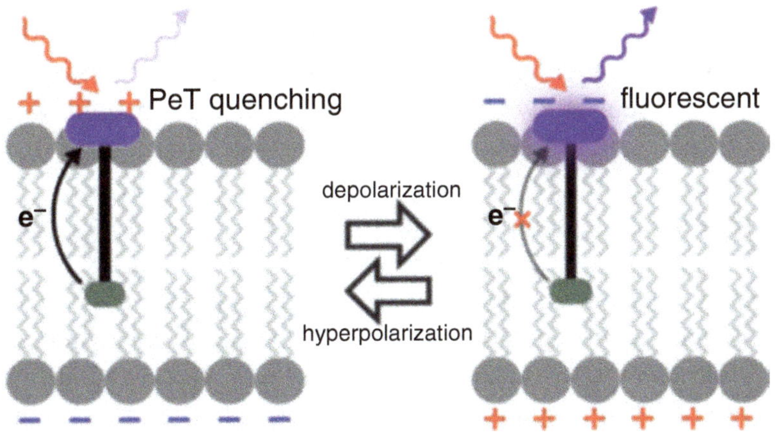

Fig. 9.1 General scheme for voltage sensing. At hyperpolarizing potentials, alignment between membrane potential and electron transfer accelerates electron transfer, quenching fluorescence. At depolarized potential, the rate of electron transfer is slowed, resulting in enhanced fluorescence. (Adapted with permission from Kulkarni and Miller, *Biochemistry* **2017**, *56*, 5171. Copyright 2017 American Chemical Society)

out optically using fluorescence microscopy. The first generation dye, VoltageFluor2.1.Cl, or VF2.1.Cl, possesses high voltage sensitivity (approximately 27% ΔF/F per 100 mV), linear and fast (sub-millisecond) fluorescence response to voltage changes, and no detectable increase in membrane capacitance (Miller et al. 2012). VF2.1.Cl (which has now been licensed by ThermoFisher and sold under the tradename "FluoVolt") has been utilized in a number of contexts, including leech ganglia (Fathiazar et al. 2016; Miller et al. 2012), cultured rat hippocampal neurons (Miller et al. 2012), mouse pancreatic tissue (Dolensek et al. 2013), cochlear tissues (Ceriani and Mammano 2013) and in cardiomyocytes (McKeithan et al. 2017). Below, we outline new chemical directions that have enabled improved sensitivity, voltage imaging in multiple colors, and targeting to defined cells.

9.2 Rational Design of VoltageFluor Dyes

While VF dyes have enabled voltage imaging in a variety of biological preparations, we hoped to increase the performance of VF dyes through tuning the redox properties of both the aniline donor and fluorescent reporter. The voltage sensitivity of VF dyes can be improved in this way, providing indicators with sensitivities approaching 50% ΔF/F per 100 mV (Woodford et al. 2015). Seeking a more general solution to improved performance, we also systematically investigated the orientation of VF dyes in cell membranes using a combination of computation and experiment (Kulkarni et al. 2017b). We hypothesized that a perfect perpendicular orientation of VF dyes with the plane of membrane should yield indicators with the maximum theoretical sensitivity. We used molecular dynamics (MD) simulations to calculate the tilt angle, or degree of displacement away from membrane normal and found that a typical VF dye containing a single sulfonate group shows significant variability and an approximate 35° departure from membrane normal (Fig. 9.2a and b). The calculations hinted at a structure—containing a symmetrical sulfonation pattern—that would resolve this rather large tilt angle, reducing it to 19°. Based on a theoretical model of voltage sensing, we hypothesized this change in angle would result in an approximate 16% increase in voltage sensitivity—a large improvement in a field where sensitivities typically fall below 20% ΔF/F per 100 mV.

We then confirmed this computational result by devising a new route to doubly sulfonated VF dyes. We synthesized nine new dyes, enabling six pairwise, experimental comparisons of monosulfoVF (msVF) and disulfoVF (dsVF) dyes in living cells to complement our computational study. In all cases, we saw increased voltage sensitivity for the dsVF dye variants relative to their msVF counterparts, with an average increase of 19%, which is in close agreement to the value predicted by MD simulation. This result not only validates our computational model of VF dyes in a lipid membrane, but has provided the most sensitive VF to date, dsVF2.2(OMe). Cl (Fig. 9.2c), with a voltage sensitivity of 63% ΔF/F per 100 mV. We showed that with this increased sensitivity, dsVF2.2(OMe). Cl can readily monitor spontaneous activity in mid-brain dopaminergic neurons derived from human pluripotent stem

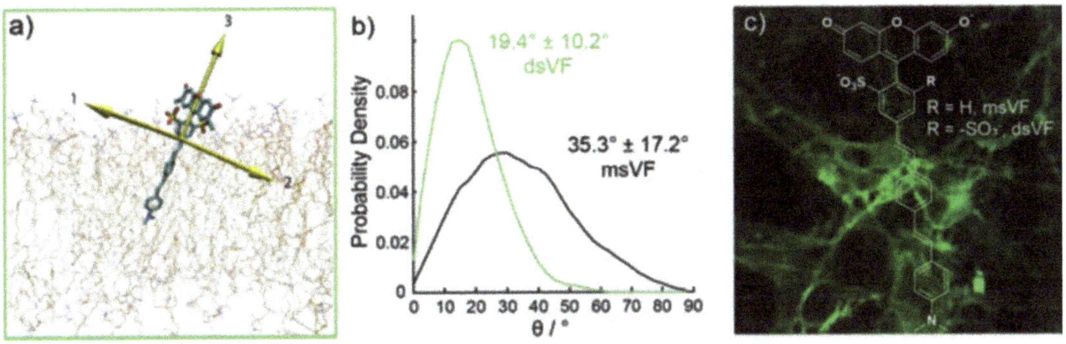

Fig. 9.2 Disulfonated VoltageFluors have better membrane orientation than monosulfonated VoltageFluors. (**a**) Molecular dynamics modeling of disulfoVoltageFluor in a POPC lipid bilayer demonstrated a slight deviation in angle from the normal. (**b**) DisulfoVF, or dsVF, has a small average angle of deviation as well as a smaller standard deviation, suggesting that it is more rigid in the membrane than msVF. (**c**) Confocal fluorescence image of dsVF in rat hippocampal neurons with structure of VF dyes overlaid. (Adapted with permission from Kulkarni, Yin, Pourmandi, James, Adil, Schaffer, Wang and Miller, *ACS Chem. Biol.* **2017**, *12*, 407. Copyright 2016 American Chemical Society)

cells. Over the course of differentiation, the stem cell-derived neurons began to demonstrate the characteristic pacemaker potential and activity of dopaminergic neurons (Rodrigues et al. 2017). Together, these results suggest that this particular modification – introduction of a second, complementary sulfonate – may be a general solution for improving the voltage sensitivity of VF-type dyes. More broadly, efforts to improve the orientation of the molecular wire voltage sensing domain with the electric field across the membrane represents a general strategy for improving voltage sensitivity.

9.3 Voltage Imaging with Red-Shifted Dyes

While synthetic modifications to fluorescein-based VFs have greatly improved their performance, they are inherently limited by their blue/green excitation and emission profiles, which overlap spectrally with optical tools such as GFP and ChannelRhodopsin2 (ChR2). VF dyes also rely on a synthetically challenging sulfonic acid for proper membrane targeting and orientation. With these limitations in mind, we aimed to develop a voltage sensing scaffold that would retain the high sensitivity of the VF dye series, expand the spectrum of colors available for voltage sensing, and circumvent the inclusion of the sulfonate that makes synthetic efforts challenging.

Toward this end we developed a new class of VF dyes based on tetramethylrhodamine (TMR), dubbed Rhodamine Voltage Reporters, or RhoVRs (Deal et al. 2016). RhoVRs were synthesized in isomerically pure form from 4′- and 5′-bromo TMRs. The bromo TMR derivatives were themselves generated from isomerically pure bromo phthalides, as we found separating the regioisomers at the phthalide stage (Mirabdolbaghi and Dudding 2012) much simpler than at the rhodamine stage.

Pd-catalyzed Heck couplings were used to attach aniline-substituted styrenes, generating the carboxy-functionalized TMR voltage reporters in good yields (41–55%). Initial studies with carboxy-functionalized RhoVRs revealed their tendency to localize to internal membranes of cells (Fig. 9.3b). We hypothesized this was due to the formation of a neutral spirocycle which could freely pass through the cell membrane. This problem was surmounted by the formation of an N-methylglycine-derived tertiary amide that both prevented spirolactonization and retained a negatively

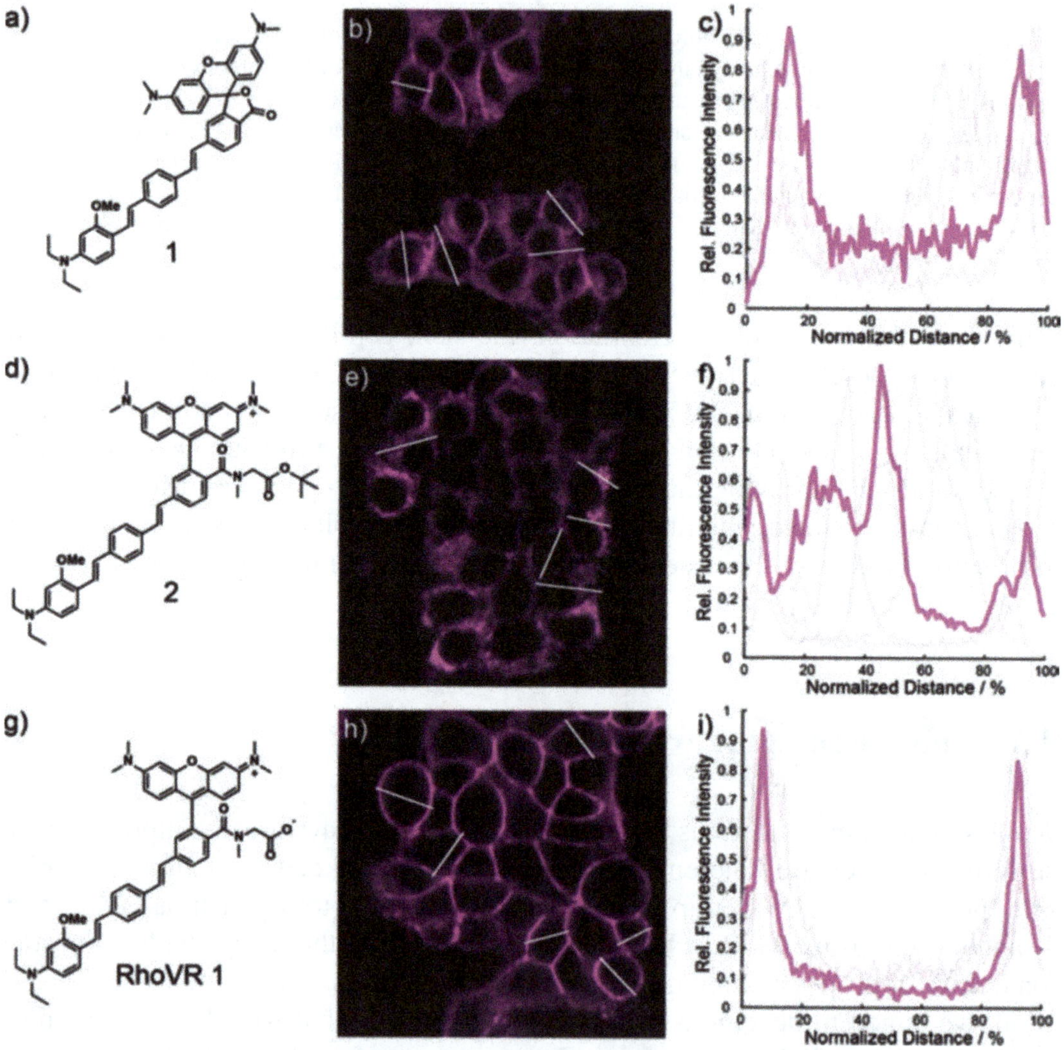

Fig. 9.3 Quantification of RhoVR 1 and rhodamine cellular localization. The fluorescence intensity of rhodamine signal was measured by measuring the pixel intensity across a line segment spanning individual HEK cells. Images are shown for RhoVR 1 (g-i), compound **1** (free carboxylate, no sarcosine, **a–c**), and compound **2**(*t*-Bu ester of RhoVR 1, **d–f**). Plots (**c**), (**f**), and (**i**) show the normalized fluorescence intensity for the rhodamine derivative (magenta) vs. the normalized widths of the white line segments in the fluorescence images on the left. Thick traces represent the average of five to six cells for each condition. Light traces represent individual intensity profiles. (Adapted with permission from Deal, Kulkarni, Al-Abdullatif, and Miller, *J. Am. Chem. Soc.* **2016**, *138*, 9085. Copyright 2016 American Chemical Society)

charged carboxylate group. Confocal microscopy confirmed that this strategy led to membrane staining identical to that seen with sulfonate-containing VFs (Fig. 9.3g–i).

Four RhoVR derivatives were synthesized to screen for maximal voltage sensitivity. All RhoVRs displayed absorption profiles centered at 564–565 nm ($\varepsilon = 70{,}000$ to 87,000 M^{-1} cm^{-1}) and emission profiles centered at 586–588 nm (Φ = 0.89–9.2%). The voltage sensitivity of each RhoVR was assessed in HEK cells using patch-clamp electrophysiology, which we found ranged from 3 to 47% ΔF/F per 100 mV. The most sensitive of the RhoVRs, which we called RhoVR 1, bore a 5′-methoxy substituted aniline (Fig. 9.4a–c). Interestingly, we found that RhoVRs derived from the 5′-substituted rhodamines were both more voltage-sensitive and brighter in cells than the 4′- equivalents. While we are still currently investigating the nature of this improvement. We speculate that the 5′ substitution pattern of RhoVR 1 improves orientation of the molecular wire with respect to the membrane, enhancing voltage sensitivity.

Given the high sensitivity and brightness of RhoVR 1 in HEK cells, we evaluated this dye in cultured rat hippocampal neurons. We found that bath-applying RhoVR 1 to neurons enabled the detection of spontaneously firing action potentials with an average ΔF/F of 15% with good SNR. We then showed that we could perform simultaneous two-color imaging using RhoVR 1 to record action potentials and GCaMP6s (a GFP-based Ca^{2+} indicator) to record the subsequent Ca^{2+} transients (Fig. 9.4d–g). From these experiments it was clear that monitoring V_m directly via RhoVR 1 enabled resolution and precise timing of spikes occurring in quick succession from multiple cells, a feat which would be impossible using traditional approaches such as Ca^{2+} imaging or single-cell electrophysiology.

In summary, we have developed a new class of voltage-sensitive dyes based on tetramethyl rhodamine. The best performing of these voltage indicators, RhoVR 1, displays an excitation and emission profile greater than 550 nm, good photostability and a voltage sensitivity of 47% ΔF/F per 100 mV. The development of RhoVRs revealed *ortho*-tertiary amides can be used in place of sulfonates to achieve membrane localization (Fig. 9.3), greatly simplifying the synthetic route to long-wavelength voltage sensors. We also revealed the importance of the substitution pattern of the molecular wire, with 5′- substituted RhoVRs outperforming the typical 4′- substitution pattern utilized in our previous voltage sensors and many other PeT-based analyte sensors. Current work with RhoVRs is now focused on utilizing the *ortho*-tertiary amide strategy to generate genetically targetable RhoVRs which will facilitate their use *in vivo*.

9.4 Far-Red Voltage Imaging for High Sensitivity

The biggest challenges in designing voltage-sensitive dyes (VSDs) for the measurement of neuronal action potentials (APs) are born from the fast timescale in which APs occur. Combining high speed imaging with the relatively small pool of dye molecules in the cell membrane leads to photon-starved conditions. To overcome

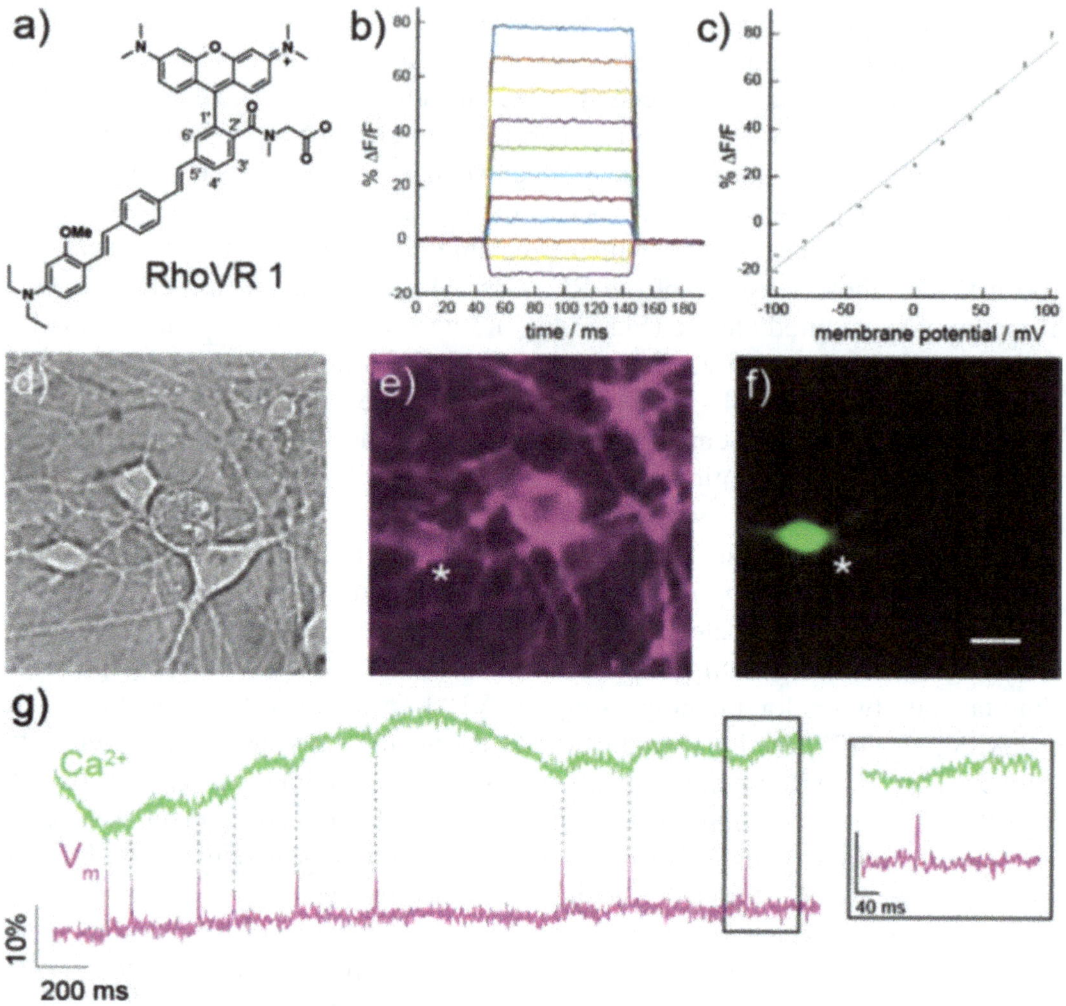

Fig. 9.4 RhoVR 1, a rhodamine-based voltage reporter. (**a**) Structure of RhoVR 1. (**b**) Plot of the fractional change in fluorescence vs time for 100 ms hyper- and depolarizing steps (±100 mV in 20 mV increments) from a holding potential of −60 mV for single HEK cells under whole-cell voltage-clamp mode. (**c**) Plot of % $\Delta F/F$ vs final membrane potential summarizing data from nine separate cells, revealing a voltage sensitivity of approximately 47% per 100 mV. Error bars are ±SEM. (**d–g**) Simultaneous two-color imaging of voltage and Ca^{2+} in hippocampal neurons using RhoVR 1 and GCaMP6s. (**d**) DIC image of neurons expressing GCaMP6s and stained with RhoVR 1. (**e**) Fluorescence image showing membrane localization of RhoVR 1 fluorescence from neurons in (**d**). (**f**) Fluorescence image of neurons in (**d**) showing GCaMP6s fluorescence. Scale bar is 20 μm. Simultaneous two-color imaging of voltage and Ca^{2+} in hippocampal neurons using RhoVR 1 and GCaMP6s. (**g**) The green trace shows the relative change in fluorescence from Ca^{2+}-sensitive GCaMP6s, while the magenta trace depicts relative fluorescence changes in RhoVR 1 fluorescence from neuron 1 in (**d**). (Adapted with permission from Deal, Kulkarni, Al-Abdullatif, and Miller, *J. Am. Chem. Soc.* **2016**, *138*, 9085. Copyright 2016 American Chemical Society)

these restrictions, a VF dye which generates signals with low noise and large changes in fluorescence would greatly improve AP detection. We hypothesized that signal-to-noise ratios (SNR) could be improved by red-shifting the VF fluorophore, where less overlap with blue/green spectrum cell autofluorescence should decrease baseline noise levels. Red-shifted VFs are also excited by longer wavelength light which causes less tissue damage and scatters less in tissue preparations. Furthermore, far-red sensors provide even larger spectral separation from useful green-spectrum optical tools and could therefore be used in conjunction with GFP, robust Ca^{2+} sensors like Oregon Green BAPTA or the GCaMP family, and optogenetic tools like ChannelRhodopsin2 (ChR2).

Silicon-rhodamines (Fu et al. 2008) are particularly desirable red-shifted fluorophores because they display photostable, far-red to NIR fluorescence that can be readily modulated by PeT (Koide et al. 2011). To synthesize a red-shifted VSD, a novel sulfonated silicon-rhodamine called Berkeley Red was first synthesized, which was combined with a phenylenevinylene molecular wire with electron-donating groups to generate Berkeley Red Sensor of Transmembrane potential 1 (BeRST 1, "burst"). As expected from the properties of Berkeley Red and other Si-Rhodamines, photophysical characterization of BeRST 1 showed excitation and emission profiles centered at 658 and 683 nm, respectively. BeRST 1 also showed excellent photostability, with a bleaching half-life of approximately 5 minutes under intense illumination conditions. By comparison, VF2.1.Cl had a bleaching half-life of <60 s under identical illumination intensities. Sensor photostability is highly advantageous, recommending the use of BeRST 1 for stable, relatively long-term imaging of neuronal activity (Huang et al. 2015).

The voltage sensitivity of BeRST 1 was tested after loading it into HEK cell membranes by applying voltage steps across the membrane via whole-cell patch-clamp electrophysiology. BeRST 1 has a voltage sensitivity of approximately 24% $\Delta F/F$ per 100 mV, comparable to VF2.1.Cl, and is linear over a physiologically relevant range spanning ±100 mV. Despite a relatively modest voltage sensitivity, BeRST 1 produced action potential traces during extracellular stimulation of dissociated neurons with very high signal-to-noise ratios (SNR; > 60:1). High SNR recordings permitted AP detection in single trials in dissociated hippocampal neurons, meaning that spontaneous neuronal activity could be recorded in multiple neurons simultaneously. By observing spontaneous AP patterns in neurons, it will be possible to study the nascent properties of neuronal firing and neuronal connectivity.

Finally, we showed that BeRST 1 is highly compatible for two-color functional imaging with GFP-based sensors. Using extracellular stimulation of dissociated hippocampal neurons, we could read-out separate BeRST 1 and GCaMP6s signals, examining the differences in the voltage and calcium readouts of AP firing at different frequencies. These experiments pave the way for investigations into interactions between voltage and calcium signaling under a variety of conditions. It was also possible to pair voltage recording with ChR2 where APs triggered by short pulses of cyan light could be detected in ChR2-expressing cells by reading out changes in BeRST 1 fluorescence (Fig. 9.5). This coupling shows the utility of BeRST 1 and ChR2 for non-invasive all-optical electrophysiological experiments.

In summary, BeRST 1 represents a new class of VSDs incorporating a far red/near infrared sulfonated Si-Rhodamine fluorophore. BeRST 1 is bright and highly photostable, making it ideal for imaging on longer timescales. BeRST 1 displays good voltage sensitivity and excellent signal-to-noise, making it advantageous for the detection of APs in single trials. Furthermore, BeRST 1 is ideally suited for

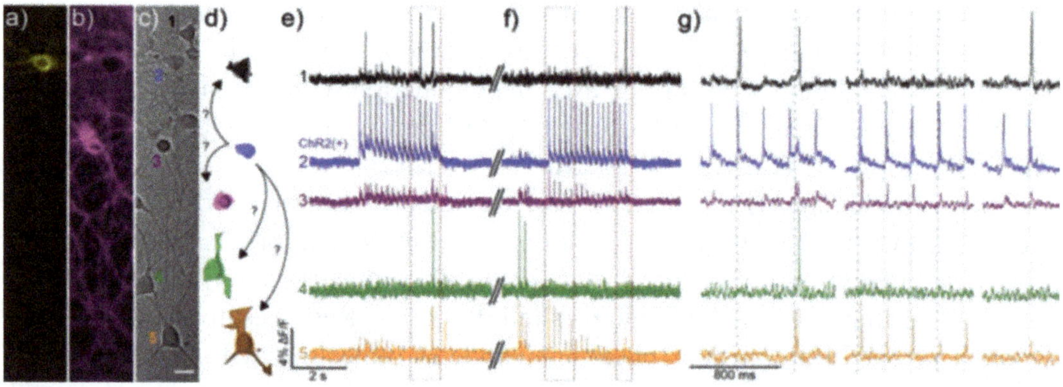

Fig. 9.5 Using BeRST 1 and ChR2 to perturb network activity. Cultured rat hippocampal (**c**) neurons transfected with (**a**) ChR2-YFP and stained with (**b**) BeRST 1 were stimulated with 475 nm light (80 mW/cm^2, 5 ms, 5 Hz, cyan bars) during two separate 3 s periods to evoke activity in the ChR2-YFP-expressing cell. Scale bar is 20 μm. (**d**) Schematic representation of neurons from DIC image in panel (**c**), color-coded to match the corresponding traces in (**e–g**). The blue ChR2(+) cell is depicted making possible connections to other neurons in the field of view. Optical records of BeRST 1 responses were acquired at 500 Hz with an sCMOS camera during (**e**) an optical recording session and (**f**) subsequent trial, separated by approximately 30 s (double hash). Numbers and colors of traces refer to specific neurons in panels (**a–d**). Red boxes indicate areas of the trace that have been magnified for clarity in panel (**g**). Dotted gray lines are provided in panel (**g**) to help visually estimate the spike timing of BeRST 1-stained neurons. (Reprinted with permission from Huang, Walker, and Miller, *J. Am. Chem. Soc.* **2015**, *137*, 10767)

multicolor imaging with GFP, Ca^{2+} indicators like GCaMP, as well as optogenetic tools like ChR2. Use of BeRST 1 alongside ChR2 permits non-invasive recording and control of AP firing.

9.5 Accessing Two-Photon Infrared Excitation for Imaging in Thick Brain Tissue

Observing neuronal activity in thick tissue preparations remains a challenge in part due to the relative lack of chromophores optimized for imaging under infrared excitation. The popularity of two-photon imaging for imaging intact brains and brain slices made a VoltageFluor optimized for two-photon absorption an attractive chemical target. Rhodols, a group of xanthene chromophores that are intermediates between fluoresceins and rhodamines (Whitaker et al. 1992), are well-suited for imaging applications (Dodani et al. 2014), due in part to their several-fold higher two-photon excitation cross sections than their fluorescein counterparts (Poronik et al. 2013). Rhodols are also relatively photostable compared to fluorescein-based dyes, potentially enabling long-term optical recordings of neurons in a variety of biological sample preparations. We hypothesized that rhodol-based VoltageFluors could serve as a complement to electrode-based techniques for monitoring voltage in neurons with two-photon imaging – facilitating recordings with high spatial resolution and the ability to record from several different neurons simultaneously. To this end, we designed and synthesized a rhodol-based voltage reporter optimized for two-photon microscopy and characterized its one- and two-photon photophysical properties (Kulkarni et al. 2017a).

Rhodol VoltageFluor-5, or RVF5, features a dichlororhodol xanthene chromophore, similar to the parent VF dye, VF2.1.Cl, but photobleaches four-fold more slowly and possess a four-fold higher two-photon excitation cross section relative to its parent dye. RVF5 demonstrates robust voltage sensitivity in HEK cells (28% $\Delta F/F$ per 100 mV) under one- and two-photon illumination. RVF5 can also be used to detect spontaneous and evoked activity in cultured neuron preparations (signal to noise = 10:1, $\Delta F/F = 11\%$ per action potential). Hippocampal neurons stained with RVF5 show no difference in action potential kinetics relative to neurons without RVF5, as measured by whole-cell patch-clamp electrophysiology. Additionally, action potentials recorded optically with RVF5 perfectly track with electrophysiologically recorded signals.

RVF5 enables dissection of epileptic-like activity in cultured neurons. We made optical recordings of RVF5 in neurons deficient in the protein tuberous sclerosis complex 1 (Tsc1). Fluorescence imaging revealed that these neurons exhibit increased spontaneous activity relative to wild-type neurons, consistent with multi-electrode array recording data (Bateup et al. 2013). Providing a powerful complement these electrode-based measures, the optical recordings showed that the proportion of active neurons in the network increased with the loss of Tsc1. RVF5 can also be used to characterize the firing activity of human stem-cell derived neurons as they mature. Finally, the high two-photon cross section of RVF5 enables imaging of neuronal voltage changes in acutely prepared mouse brain slices using two-photon microscopy. Bath applied RVF5 can be used to detect chemically evoked hippocampal spiking activity in mouse brain slices, validating RVF5 as a tool for performing voltage imaging in thick brain tissue samples (Fig. 9.6). Next generations of two-photon VoltageFluor dyes will be targeted towards imaging voltage changes in live animals to provide complementary information to classical extracellular electrode-based recordings.

9.6 Targeting VoltageFluor Dyes to Specific Cells

Amphipathic VoltageFluor dyes stain tissue indiscriminately (Fig. 9.6c), making it difficult to resolve signals from individual cells and placing important constraints on *in vivo* and *ex vivo* experiments, where it is often desirable to image from sparsely labeled neurons, or a genetically defined sub-population therein. To overcome these issues we designed a **s**mall-molecule, **p**hotoactivatable **o**ptical sensor of **t**ransmembrane potential, or SPOT2.1.Cl, a dimly fluorescent, caged derivative of VF2.1.Cl which could release the functional parent dye upon irradiation with near-UV light, permitting optical recording from arbitrarily defined cells of interest (Grenier et al. 2015).

SPOT2.1.Cl is accessible in a single step from VF2.1.Cl through alkylation of the phenolic oxygen with 2-nitro-4,5-dimethoxybenzyl bromide. The quantum yield of

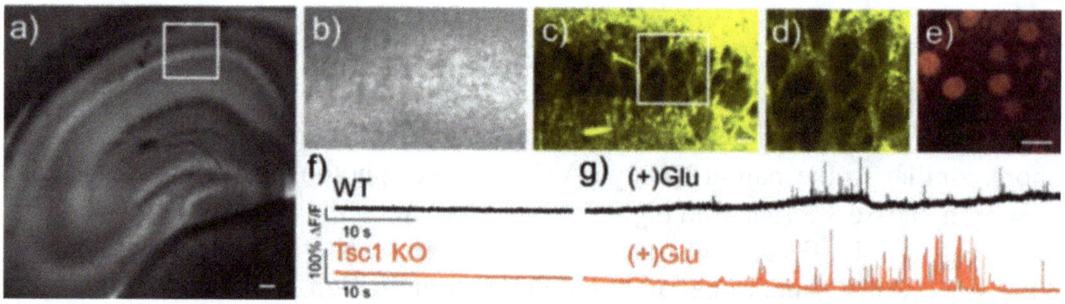

Fig. 9.6 Two-photon voltage imaging with RVF5 in mouse brain slices. Transmitted light images of mouse hippocampal brain slice stained with 10 μM RVF5 in oxygenated ACSF show (**a**) the entire hippocampus and (**b**) a zoomed region of CA1. (**c**) Fluorescence signals from RVF5 (10 μM, oxygenated ACSF) from the same region in panel (**b**) show membrane-localized staining. (**d**) and (**e**) A zoomed-in region from panel (**c**) shows RVF5 fluorescence primarily in cellular membranes and excluded from the cytosol and (**e**) nuclear-localized mCherry-Cre indicating Tsc1 KO neurons. Functional imaging was performed by creating a 8 × 64 pixel region over an area of CA1 and imaging at ~200 Hz for 20–40 s, first in the absence of glutamate (panel **f**) and then following addition of glutamate to the perfusate (panel **g** (+)Glu). Responses were recorded from neurons in the sham injected (control, "WT", black traces) and mCherry-Cre injected ("Tsc1 KO", red traces) hemispheres. Scale bars are 100 μm for panel a and 20 μm for panels (**b–e**). Fluorescence traces are single-trial ΔF/F values from single pixels and are uncorrected for photobleaching

SPOT2.1.Cl (Φ = 0.002) is 28 times lower than that of VF2.1.Cl (Φ = 0.057). Although the quantum yield of uncaging is low (Φ = 0.007) HPLC analysis of photolysis products indicated that VF2.1.Cl was cleanly released after irradiation. In HEK cells, we observed a maximal 12 ± 1.2 fold increase in fluorescence intensity after illumination at 390 nm. Fluorescence recordings indicated that voltage-sensitivity was maintained after triggered release of VF2.1.Cl – we measured a response of 17% ΔF/F per 100 mV, 77% of the response obtained from VF2.1.Cl under identical recording conditions. In cultured embryonic rat hippocampal neurons we measured a ΔF/F of 9 ± 0.2% in response to evoked action potentials, without a measurable change in action potential full width at half maximum. As an assessment of the effects on UV-irradiation and nitrobenzyl photochemistry on cell health we measured the electrophysiological parameters of HEK cells in whole-cell clamp before and after SPOT2.1.Cl uncaging and found no evidence that the membranes of target cells were compromised.

We next demonstrated our ability to uncage SPOT2.1.Cl with high spatial precision. Using either confocal microscopy or an iris diaphragm on a widefield microscope, we were able to release VF2.1.Cl with single cell precision in both HEK cells and cultured neurons. By illuminating over a small region of a single HEK cell we determined that released VF2.1.Cl diffuses laterally through cell membranes at an appreciable rate, gradually filling out the entire plasma membrane without a substantial increase in fluorescence in adjacent cells. To achieve our objective of selective recording from genetically defined populations of cells we envisioned using an expressed fluorescent protein as a fiduciary marker which could define regions for photoactivation. We sparsely transfected cultured neurons with a plasmid encoding

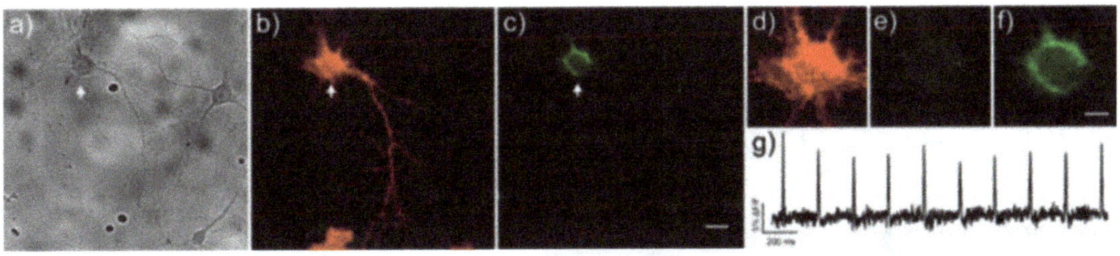

Fig. 9.7 SPOT2.1.Cl uncaging in single neurons. Dissociated, cultured rat neurons (**a**) were transiently transfected with CAAX-mCherry for use as a fiducial marker for illumination. Panels (**a**) and (**b**) show DIC and mCherry fluorescence images, respectively. Cells were loaded with 500 nM SPOT2.1.Cl and then photoactivated (390 nm, 10 s, 22.3 W/cm^2) over a region defined by the somatic staining of the mCherry signal (white arrow). (**c**) Following photoactivation, VF fluorescence appears to be membrane-localized. (**d–f**) EMCCD image of indicated cell, showing mCherry fluorescence. VF dye fluorescence from the mCherry-positive neuron, (**e**) prior to SPOT photoactivation and (**f**) immediately after. (**g**) Field stimulation of the SPOT-stained neuron at 5 Hz produced a train of optically recorded action potentials, which were captured at 500 Hz with an EMCCD camera. Scale bars are 20 μm for panels (**a–c**) and 10 μm for panels (**d–f**). (Reprinted with permission from Grenier, Walker, Miller, *J. Am. Chem. Soc.* **2015**, *137*, 10894. Copyright 2015 American Chemical Society)

mCherry, uncaged SPOT2.1.Cl in these cells, and recorded action potentials from target neurons (Fig. 9.7).

Retrograde tracers of neuronal connectivity have proven to be valuable tools for studying brain physiology. We envisioned that SPOT2.1.Cl could serve as a dual use, functional tracer. We first used a modified fluorescence recovery after photobleaching assay over a monolayer of HEK cells to determine that while VF2.1.Cl does have some ability to travel across cellular membranes, it does so at the same rate as the canonical tracer dye DiO. In a proof-of-principle experiment we next released VF2.1.Cl in the processes of cultured neurons, allowing the dye to back-fill the cell body of a neuron outside the illuminated region, and recorded optical action potentials from that cell. Further development of photoactivatable VoltageFluors will require the use of photocages with high 2-photon cross-sections to enable photoactivation with single-cell resolution in tissue slice.

Based on the success of the photoactivation approach for staining single cells, we envisioned a similar strategy could be employed for enzymatic activation of voltage-sensitive dye, providing contrast without the need for a separate photoactivation step (Liu et al. 2017). To achieve targeting, the parent VF dye is chemically modified to be minimally fluorescent and must be enzymatically activated prior to imaging (Fig. 9.8a). We appended a bulky methylcyclopropyl ester (Tian et al. 2012), a moiety cleaved only by pig liver esterase (PLE), to VF2.1.Cl to prepare two dyes VF-EX1 and VF-EX2. While VF-EX1 is masked only at the phenol, VF-EX2 is esterified at both phenol and sulfonic acid positions. Compared to the parent dye, both VF-EX1 and VF-EX2 showed diminished fluorescence, with 19- and 6.7-fold decreases in quantum yield, respectively. Robust fluorescence turn-on was observed upon enzyme treatment, confirming that both dyes are PLE substrates *in vitro*. Kinetic studies were also performed and revealed that VF-EX2 is a better substrate

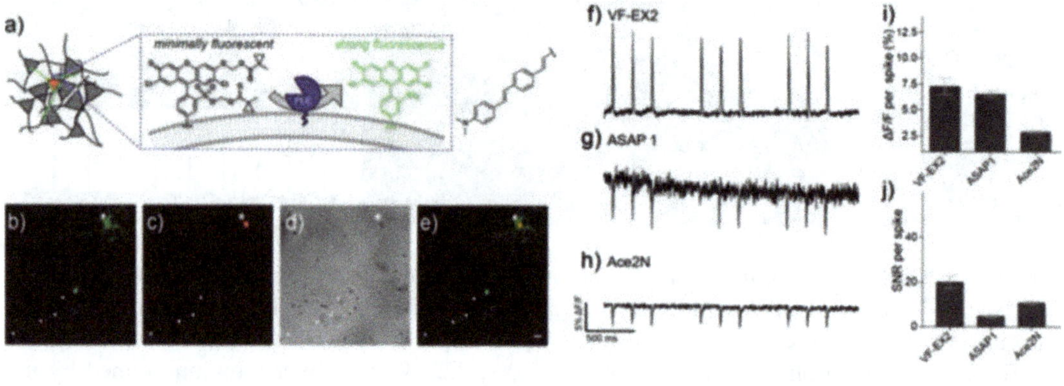

Fig. 9.8 VoltageFluor targeted by esterase expression (VF-EX), a fluorogenic voltage reporter targeted to cells of interest. (**a**) Scheme of neuron-specific targeting with ester/esterase pairs (components are not to scale). Widefield fluorescence microscopy of cultured hippocampal neurons (**b–e**) stained with VF-EX2 (1 μM) show membrane-associated fluorescence only in cells expressing cell-surface PLE. (**b**) Epifluorescence images showing VoltageFluor-associated fluorescence. (**c**) Fluorescence image of nuclear-localized mCherry indicating PLE expression. (**d**) Transmitted light image of neurons. (**e**) Merged imaging showing overlay of both VF and mCherry fluorescence. Scale bar is 20 μm. ΔF/F vs. time plots for action potentials evoked and optically recorded with either VF-EX2/PLE (**f**), ASAP 1 (**g**), or Ace2N (**h**). (**i–j**) Quantification of ΔF/F (**i**) and signal-to-noise (SNR, **j**). (Data are mean ± S.E.M Adapted with permission from Liu, Grenier, Hong, Muller, and Miller, *J. Am. Chem. Soc.* **2017**, *139*, 17334. Copyright 2017 American Chemical Society)

than VF-EX1, as evidenced by the larger k_{cat}/K_M value for VF-EX2 ($1.3 \times 10^6\ M^{-1}\ s^{-1}$) versus VF-EX1 ($2.1 \times 10^5\ M^{-1}\ s^{-1}$).

We next engineered a cell-surface PLE by removing a ER retention signal from the native sequence and adding a secretion signal derived from immunoglobulin K (IgK) and a membrane targeting sequence (a transmembrane domain from platelet-derived growth factor receptor) or a glycophosphatidyl inositol anchor signal). These modifications resulted in clear membrane localization of the enzyme on the cell surface in both HEK cells and neurons as determined by immunostaining. Bath application of the dyes exhibited selective staining in PLE-expressing HEK cells, with a 7- and 17-fold turn-on for VF-EX1 and VF-EX2 respectively. The activated dyes displayed high and linear voltage sensitivities around 20% ΔF/F per 100 mV, comparable to the value of 27% measured for VF2.1.Cl. By using neuron specific promoters, Synapsin (pan-neuronal) or CamKIIα (excitatory neuron), we expressed PLE selectively in neurons of interest. VF-EX dyes provided enhanced contrast in transfected neurons (Fig. 9.8b–e) and were able to record field-stimulation electrode-evoked action potentials as well as spontaneous spiking events in single trials. VF-EX2 was selected for further applications due to its greater brightness.

Our dye displays improved SNR in cultured neurons relative to purely genetically-encoded voltage indicators (GEVIs) including ASAP1 and Ace2N (Fig. 9.8f–j). This is due in part to the improved membrane localization of uncaged VF-EX dyes. Whereas a significant fraction of expressed fluorescent GEVIs remains in the cytosol and internal compartments, contributing to unresponsive background fluorescence, the genetically-encoded component PLE is non-fluorescent and the dye only localizes to, but does not cross, the cell membrane. By targeting VF-EX2 to excitatory neurons, we could interrogate the neuromodulatory effects of serotonin (5-HT), an important neuromodulator. Treatment of hippocampal cultures with 5-HT showed decreased spiking rates in excitatory neurons while washout of 5-HT resulted in a recovery of neuronal spiking. Using pharmacological blockade of 5-HT receptors, we identified 5-HT1A as the receptor responsible for the inhibitory effect of 5-HT on neuronal activity. Current work focuses on extending this fluorogenic approach to other VF dyes with different chromophores and improved sensitivity as well as applying these probes for *in vivo* and *ex vivo* imaging.

9.7 Conclusion/Summary

Voltage imaging remains an outstanding challenge. Methods that can faithfully report on changes in membrane potential in a non-invasive, high-throughput fashion will be critical in dissecting the roles that membrane potentials play in biology. Optical imaging of voltage, whether through small molecule fluorescent dye approaches described here, or through other creative solutions (Abdelfattah et al. 2016; Akemann et al. 2013; Gong et al. 2015; Hochbaum et al. 2014; Jin et al. 2012; Kralj et al. 2011a, b; Piatkevich et al. 2018), must address problems of low voltage sensitivity, low brightness, poor membrane localization, and/or poor localization to cells of interest (Kulkarni and Miller 2017). In a related fashion, new modalities to enable high-speed optical sampling (~kHz) from deep brain regions, with high spatial resolution (μm) across large regions (mm) are required to fully realize the potential of voltage imaging.

References

Abdelfattah AS et al (2016) A bright and fast red fluorescent protein voltage indicator that reports neuronal activity in organotypic brain slices. J Neurosci 36:2458–2472. https://doi.org/10.1523/JNEUROSCI.3484-15.2016

Akemann W, Sasaki M, Mutoh H, Imamura T, Honkura N, Knopfel T (2013) Two-photon voltage imaging using a genetically encoded voltage indicator. Sci Rep 3:2231. https://doi.org/10.1038/srep02231

Bateup HS, Johnson CA, Denefrio CL, Saulnier JL, Kornacker K, Sabatini BL (2013) Excitatory/inhibitory synaptic imbalance leads to hippocampal hyperexcitability in mouse models of tuberous sclerosis. Neuron 78:510–522. https://doi.org/10.1016/j.neuron.2013.03.017

Braubach O, Cohen LB, Choi Y (2015) Historical overview and general methods of membrane potential imaging. In: Canepari M, Zecevic D, Bernus O (eds) Membrane potential imaging in the nervous system and heart. Springer, Cham, pp 3–26. https://doi.org/10.1007/978-3-319-17641-3_1

Ceriani F, Mammano F (2013) A rapid and sensitive assay of intercellular coupling by voltage imaging of gap junction networks. Cell Commun Signal 11:78. https://doi.org/10.1186/1478-811X-11-78

De Silva AP, Gunaratne HQN, Habibjiwan JL, Mccoy CP, Rice TE, Soumillion JP (1995) New fluorescent model compounds for the study of photoinduced electron-transfer - the influence of a molecular electric-field in the excited-state. Angew Chem Int Edit 34:1728–1731. https://doi.org/10.1002/anie.199517281

Deal PE, Kulkarni RU, Al-Abdullatif SH, Miller EW (2016) Isomerically pure tetramethylrhodamine voltage reporters. J Am Chem Soc 138:9085–9088. https://doi.org/10.1021/jacs.6b05672

Dodani SC et al (2014) Copper is an endogenous modulator of neural circuit spontaneous activity. Proc Natl Acad Sci 111:16280–16285. https://doi.org/10.1073/pnas.1409796111

Dolensek J, Stozer A, Skelin Klemen M, Miller EW, Slak Rupnik M (2013) The relationship between membrane potential and calcium dynamics in glucose-stimulated beta cell syncytium in acute mouse pancreas tissue slices. PLoS One 8:e82374. https://doi.org/10.1371/journal.pone.0082374

Fathiazar E, Anemuller J, Kretzberg J (2016) Statistical identification of stimulus-activated network nodes in multi-neuron voltage-sensitive dye optical recordings. Conf Proc IEEE Eng Med Biol Soc 2016:3899–3903. https://doi.org/10.1109/EMBC.2016.7591580

Fu MY, Xiao Y, Qian XH, Zhao DF, Xu YF (2008) A design concept of long-wavelength fluorescent analogs of rhodamine dyes: replacement of oxygen with silicon atom. Chem Commun:1780–1782. https://doi.org/10.1039/B718544h

Gong Y, Huang C, Li JZ, Grewe BF, Zhang Y, Eismann S, Schnitzer MJ (2015) High-speed recording of neural spikes in awake mice and flies with a fluorescent voltage sensor. Science 350:1361–1366. https://doi.org/10.1126/science.aab0810

Grenier V, Walker AS, Miller EW (2015) A small-molecule photoactivatable optical sensor of transmembrane potential. J Am Chem Soc 137:10894–10897. https://doi.org/10.1021/jacs.5b05538

Hochbaum DR et al (2014) All-optical electrophysiology in mammalian neurons using engineered microbial rhodopsins. Nat Methods 11:825–833. https://doi.org/10.1038/nmeth.3000

Huang YL, Walker AS, Miller EW (2015) A photostable silicon rhodamine platform for optical voltage sensing. J Am Chem Soc 137:10767–10776. https://doi.org/10.1021/jacs.5b06644

Jin L, Han Z, Platisa J, Wooltorton JR, Cohen LB, Pieribone VA (2012) Single action potentials and subthreshold electrical events imaged in neurons with a fluorescent protein voltage probe. Neuron 75:779–785. https://doi.org/10.1016/j.neuron.2012.06.040

Koide Y, Urano Y, Hanaoka K, Terai T, Nagano T (2011) Evolution of group 14 rhodamines as platforms for near-infrared fluorescence probes utilizing photoinduced electron transfer. ACS Chem Biol 6:600–608. https://doi.org/10.1021/cb1002416

Kralj JM, Douglass AD, Hochbaum DR, Maclaurin D, Cohen AE (2011a) Optical recording of action potentials in mammalian neurons using a microbial rhodopsin. Nat Methods 9:90–95. https://doi.org/10.1038/nmeth.1782

Kralj JM, Hochbaum DR, Douglass AD, Cohen AE (2011b) Electrical spiking in Escherichia coli probed with a fluorescent voltage-indicating protein. Science 333:345–348. https://doi.org/10.1126/science.1204763

Kulkarni RU, Miller EW (2017) Voltage imaging: pitfalls and potential. Biochemistry 56:5171–5177. https://doi.org/10.1021/acs.biochem.7b00490

Kulkarni RU, Kramer DJ, Pourmandi N, Karbasi K, Bateup HS, Miller EW (2017a) Voltage-sensitive rhodol with enhanced two-photon brightness. Proc Natl Acad Sci U S A 114:2813–2818. https://doi.org/10.1073/pnas.1610791114

Kulkarni RU et al (2017b) A rationally designed, general strategy for membrane orientation of photoinduced electron transfer-based voltage-sensitive dyes. ACS Chem Biol 12:407–413. https://doi.org/10.1021/acschembio.6b00981

Li LS (2007) Fluorescence probes for membrane potentials based on mesoscopic electron transfer. Nano Lett 7:2981–2986. https://doi.org/10.1021/nl071163p

Liu P, Grenier V, Hong W, Muller VR, Miller EW (2017) Fluorogenic targeting of voltage-sensitive dyes to neurons. J Am Chem Soc 139:17334–17340. https://doi.org/10.1021/jacs.7b07047

Loew LM (2015) Design and use of organic voltage sensitive dyes. In: Canepari M, Zecevic D, Bernus O (eds) Membrane potential imaging in the nervous system and heart, Advances in experimental medicine and biology, vol 859. Springer, Berlin, pp 27–53. https://doi.org/10.1007/978-3-319-17641-3_2

McKeithan WL et al (2017) An automated platform for assessment of congenital and drug-induced arrhythmia with hiPSC-derived cardiomyocytes. Front Physiol 8:766. https://doi.org/10.3389/fphys.2017.00766

Miller EW, Lin JY, Frady EP, Steinbach PA, Kristan WB Jr, Tsien RY (2012) Optically monitoring voltage in neurons by photo-induced electron transfer through molecular wires. Proc Natl Acad Sci U S A 109:2114–2119. https://doi.org/10.1073/pnas.1120694109

Mirabdolbaghi R, Dudding T (2012) An indium-mediated allylative/transesterification DFT-directed approach to chiral C(3)-functionalized phthalides. Org Lett 14:3748–3751. https://doi.org/10.1021/ol301566f

Piatkevich KD et al (2018) A robotic multidimensional directed evolution approach applied to fluorescent voltage reporters. Nat Chem Biol. https://doi.org/10.1038/s41589-018-0004-9

Poronik YM, Clermont G, Blanchard-Desce M, Gryko DT (2013) Nonlinear optical chemosensor for sodium ion based on rhodol chromophore. J Org Chem 78:11721–11732. https://doi.org/10.1021/jo401653t

Rodrigues GMC et al (2017) Defined and scalable differentiation of human oligodendrocyte precursors from pluripotent stem cells in a 3D culture system. Stem Cell Rep 8:1770–1783. https://doi.org/10.1016/j.stemcr.2017.04.027

Tian L et al (2012) Selective esterase-ester pair for targeting small molecules with cellular specificity. Proc Natl Acad Sci U S A 109:4756–4761. https://doi.org/10.1073/pnas.1111943109

Whitaker JE, Haugland RP, Ryan D, Hewitt PC, Prendergast FG (1992) Fluorescent rhodol derivatives: versatile, photostable labels and tracers. Anal Biochem 207:267–279

Woodford CR et al (2015) Improved PeT molecules for optically sensing voltage in neurons. J Am Chem Soc 137:1817–1824. https://doi.org/10.1021/ja510602z

Chapter 10
Molecular Dynamics Revealed by Single-Molecule FRET Measurement

Tomohiro Shima and Sotaro Uemura

FRET techniques have been widely used for measuring the dynamics of biomolecules because of its high sensitivity as a nanoscale distance sensor. Between two closely located fluorescent molecules, energy in an excited donor fluorescent probe is resonantly transferred to an adjacent acceptor fluorescent probe, thereby decreasing the donor's fluorescence intensity and increasing the acceptor's fluorescence intensity. The efficiency of this energy transfer is inversely proportional to the sixth power of the distance between the two fluorescent molecules. Accordingly, FRET is an extremely sensitive measurement system for detecting changes in the distance between two fluorescent probes, particularly around what is called the Förster distance, namely, a distance that yields a FRET efficiency of 0.5 (4–7 nm for a pair of typical fluorescent probes) (Lakowicz 2006). As such, FRET measurement is ideally suited for detecting changes in the distance between domains or subunits within a protein or nucleic acids during conformational changes. Moreover, based on the ratio of fluorescence intensities of two fluorescent molecules, it can achieve high signal-to-noise ratio in measurements of binding and dissociation reactions compared with measurements involving a single fluorescent molecule. These advantages have made FRET an extensively used technique for researching the dynamics of biomolecules.

Conventional bulk FRET measurements, however, only yield mean measurement values of a large number of molecules. Therefore, these measurements are unable to extract information on the distribution of multiple molecules. The development of single-molecule imaging technologies, capable of distinguishing fluorescence intensities from individual molecules, has overcome this limitation. In combination with the single-molecule imaging techniques, FRET measurements are able to distinguish the state of each molecule in real time. This combination has

T. Shima · S. Uemura (✉)
The University of Tokyo, Tokyo, Japan
e-mail: uemura@bs.s.u-tokyo.ac.jp

Y. Toyama et al. (eds.), *Make Life Visible*,
https://doi.org/10.1007/978-981-13-7908-6_10

led to the discoveries of diversities in dynamics and states of biomolecules in the same conditions.

In this chapter, we first outlines the single-molecule imaging techniques, which provide the basis for establishing smFRET measurement, then presents examples of protein dynamics research employing smFRET, and finally introduces some state-of-the-art smFRET applications.

10.1 Single-Molecule Fluorescence Imaging

To detect single molecule fluorescent probes using optical microscopy, the techniques to reduce background light combined with an intense illumination and highly sensitive camera systems are required. By the late 1980s, illumination and imaging systems had already been refined to the point of theoretically being able to detect single molecules of fluorescent probes. Nevertheless, the influence of background light from non-observed fluorescent probes had stalled the development of a system capable of identifying fluorescence from a single molecule. In 1990, Shera et al. succeeded in distinguishing fluorescent signals emitted from a single fluorescent probe molecule using pulsed light to induce photoexcitation of a low-concentration fluorescent probe solution streaming through a flow cell (Shera et al. 1990). However, this technique is arguably more pertinent to classifying as flow cytometry rather than microscopic imaging. Later, in 1993, Betzig et al. paved the way for the technology of single-molecule fluorescence imaging by employing near-field scanning optical microscopy (Betzig and Chichester 1993). Their method took advantage of the phenomenon in which illuminating a small hole with a diameter less than the wavelength of the light results in the light emerging only in the immediate vicinity of the hole. By limiting the area of illumination to a minimum, that is, reducing the background light from fluorescent probes outside the observation area, they achieved single-molecule fluorescence imaging. Thereafter, total internal reflection fluorescence microscopy (TIRFM) also has realized single-molecule fluorescence imaging by employing a similar strategy (Funatsu et al. 1995). TIRFM uses evanescent waves that occur in the immediate vicinity (~200 nm) of the interfacial surface between glass and water. Thus, only fluorescent probes present within ~200 nm from the glass surface were illuminated under TIRFM (Axelrod 1981). Compared with the near-field scanning microscopy, TIRFM is easy to set up and eligible for high-speed imaging. TIRFM requires only a standard fluorescence laser microscope with the ability to adjust the incidence angle of excitation light. Moreover, unnecessity of the scanning process makes TIRFM capable to swiftly capture images of an extensive area in a single shot. These two advantages have contributed to the widespread usage of TIRFM in the single-molecule imaging field. Today, modified epifluorescence microscopy (Sase et al. 1995), confocal microscopy (Nie et al. 1994), oblique illumination microscopy (Tokunaga et al. 2008), and light sheet microscopy (Ritter et al. 2010), which have a deeper range of photoexcitation than TIRFM, can also be applied to single-molecule imaging. Furthermore, the availability of increasingly bright commercial light-emitting diodes means that laser lighting equipment is no longer a prerequisite. These technical advances provide many options for building up a single-molecule microscopy appropriate for each experiment.

Although the above-mentioned high-speed single-molecule imaging techniques incorporate methods to reduce background light, it is necessary to limit the concentrations of fluorescent probes in solution up to the nanomolar order to distinguish single molecules from each other. Any higher concentrations render it difficult to distinguish single molecules. However, most biomolecules have a dissociation constant within the micromolar range, necessitating measurement at concentrations approximately 1000 times higher than the maximum detection limit of TIRFM techniques. To address this issue, zero-mode waveguides (ZMWs) have been developed (Levene et al. 2003). A ZMW is an optical wave guide that uses a glass foundation onto which a metallic lamina with numerous pores with a diameter of less than 100 nm is attached through vapor deposition. In a ZMW, only fluorescent probes present very close to the glass surface, approximately 10–20 nm in depth, are photoexcited. Therefore, ZMWs method can distinguish single-molecule signals under far higher fluorescent probe concentrations compared with TIRFM (Fig. 10.1). Indeed, Uemura et al. succeeded in visualizing the dynamics of tRNA that binds and dissociates from single-molecule ribosomes in the presence of fluorescently labeled tRNA at a high concentration of 2 μM during translation, thereby resolving a long-standing mystery regarding the timing of tRNA binding and dissociation from the three tRNA binding sites (Uemura et al. 2010). In addition to the capability of single-molecule imaging in the presence of high concentration probes, high-throughput data acquisition ability makes ZMWs prominent among the

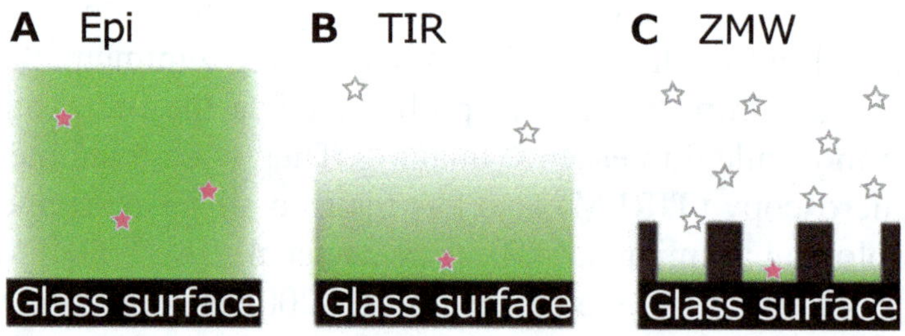

Fig. 10.1 Schematic diagrams of typical illumination systems using a fluorescence microscope
(a) Conventional epi-illumination. Fluorescent probes (magenta stars) that exist outside the focal plane are also photoexcited, making it difficult to eliminate background light
(b) Total internal reflection (TIR) illumination. Fluorescent probes that exist within the 100–200 nm distance from the glass surface are photoexcited. The fluorescent probes that exist outside of this range (white stars) do not interfere with observation
(c): Zero-mode waveguide illumination. An aluminum lamina with pores with a diameter of approximately 100 nm is attached to the glass surface through vapor deposition. Only the fluorescent probes that exist within the 10–20 nm distance from the glass surface are photoexcited. This trait gives this system the ability to measure single molecules under the presence of fluorescent probes at much higher concentrations compared with total internal reflection fluorescence microscopy

single-molecule imaging techniques. A large number of small pores in a ZMWs cell enables the simultaneous and parallel acquisition of single-molecule reaction data in huge quantities. Taking advantage of these high-throughput data acquisition capabilities, one of the third-generation sequencers now incorporate ZMWs. The single-molecule real-time sequencers of Pacific Biosciences, for instance, monitor and quantify hundreds of thousands of molecular reactions simultaneously, thus achieving a throughput that is one to ten million times faster than conventional Sanger sequencing (Perkel 2016). Therefore, using ZMWs, we can now acquire data of a large number of single molecules even in the presence of high concentration fluorescent probes.

10.2 Molecular Dynamics of Proteins Measured by smFRET

Advances in single-molecule fluorescent imaging technology have made it possible to perform smFRET measurements. smFRET measurements have revealed diversities in behavior of individual molecules in many types of bio-reactions, overturning the conventional view that molecules in same conditions show uniform reaction and dynamics. Inhibition of protein synthesis mediated by aminoglycoside antibiotics presents an example of such diversity among similar molecules revealed by smFRET. The three aminoglycoside antibiotics, apramycin, paromomycin and gentamycin, are known to inhibit protein synthesis by binding to the A site of the bacterial ribosomal small subunit. Until recently, it remained unclear which step of the ribosome-mediated protein translation process these antibiotics inhibit. Tsai et al. explored steps inhibited by these antibiotics by visualizing behavior of individual ribosomes with smFRET and ZMWs methods (Tsai et al. 2013). The major conformational changes in ribosomes (rotation of the large and small subunits) and tRNA selection processes at the A site were monitored by smFRET in ZMW cells. As a result, Tsai et al. found that apramycin inhibited the translocation of tRNA from the A site, but not affecting the major conformational change in ribosome that precedes the tRNA translocation. Meanwhile, paromomycin and gentamicin induced non-cognate tRNA binding and inhibited the ribosomal conformational change (Fig. 10.2). These results obtained from smFRET measurements clarify the detailed steps of protein synthesis, and reveal the diverse inhibition mechanisms of the antibiotics in the same type.

smFRET measurement is an exceptionally versatile technique, capable of tracking the dynamics of not only ribosomes but also many other molecules in real time. Next, we present some of the latest findings regarding the dynamics of the RNA-guided Cas9 endonuclease, which has been recognized as a powerful genome-editing tool. Cas9 protein binds to a single-stranded guide RNA (sgRNA) to form an sgRNA–Cas9 complex, which then binds to a double-stranded DNA with a specific base sequence (NGG for *S. pyogenes* Cas9), known as the protospacer adjacent

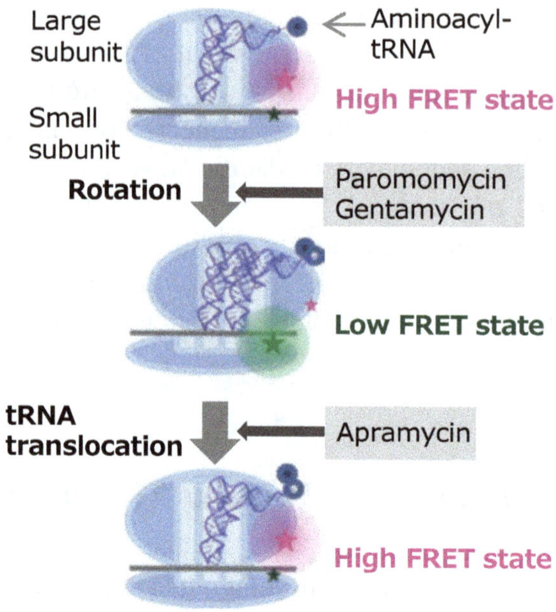

Fig. 10.2 Action mechanism of aminoglycoside antibiotics revealed by monomolecular FRET measurement
Normally, when a second aminoacyl tRNA binds to a ribosome, the large and small ribosomal subunits rotate. This is followed by the translocation of tRNA, with the ribosome returning to the original conformation. Fluorescently labeling of the two subunits visualizes this inter-subunit rotation. smFRET measurements have revealed that paromomycin and gentamicin inhibit the first rotation and apramycin inhibits the tRNA translocation and the second ribosomal rotation, which returns the ribosome to its original conformation (Tsai et al. 2013)

motif (PAM). When the DNA sequence preceding the PAM is same as that of the sgRNA, the Cas9 complex cleaves both DNA strands. Intriguingly, smFRET measurements revealed that DNA sequences scarcely affect the DNA binding rate with sgRNA-Cas9 (Singh et al. 2016). In contrast, the dissociation rate considerably increases on the introduction of mismatches proximal to the PAM sequence. This mechanism probably suppresses further reactions against off-target DNAs. Another smFRET analysis revealed heterogeneity in the behavior of the Cas9 molecules during the DNA cleavage process. In any crystal structures of the DNA-sgRNA-Cas9 ternary complex solved to date, the active site of the HNH nuclease domain in Cas9 does not attach to the DNA cleavage site (Nishimasu et al. 2014; Sternberg et al. 2015; Jiang et al. 2016). Thus, the ternary complex has been predicted to take additional temporal conformations beyond the solved crystal structures during DNA cleavage. Single-molecule measurements of intramolecular FRET between probes in the HNH domain and the domain proximal to the DNA cleavage site demonstrated that the ternary complex shows both static and fluctuating phases (Osuka et al. 2018). In the static phase, the HNH domain stays at the DNA-undocked position, which is 3-nm away from the DNA cleavage site, for an extended period.

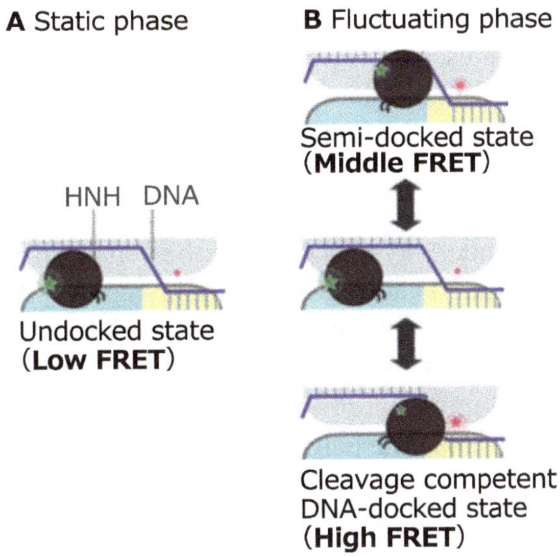

Fig. 10.3 Dynamics of the DNA cleavage domain of Cas9. (Reproduced from Osuka et al. 2018) smFRET measurements have revealed that HNH nuclease domain of Cas9 assumes two different phases: **(a)** a static phase in which the HNH domain remains stationary for an extended period (over 100 s) and **(b)** a fluctuating phase in which the domain moves frequently between multiple positions (Osuka et al. 2018). Only during the fluctuating phase, the Cas9 takes structure capable to cleave DNA strands. In addition, the measurement has also suggested that the HNH domain needs to temporarily translocate into the undocked position during transitions between the semi-docked and docked positions

Contrarily, in the fluctuating phase, the HNH domain frequently moves between DNA-undocked, semi-docked and cleavage competent docked positions. Because the complex cleaves DNA only when the HNH is in the docked position, mutations that unstabilize the other HNH positions may enhance the nuclease activity of the Cas9. The fact that smFRET detected this temporal cleavage competent conformation, which is not solved by crystal structures, demonstrates the usefulness of smFRET as an analytical tool for investigating polymorphisms and fluctuations in protein structures (Fig. 10.3).

10.3 Advances in smFRET Methods

The smFRET techniques presented in this chapter have been advancing further by incorporating other methodologies. For instance, attempts are being made to apply luminescent probes to observe single-molecule dynamics. Luminescent probes do not require illumination light, surmounting the obstacles of fluorescence imaging: autofluorescence, photo-damage to the samples and the strict limitations in the use of optogenetic tools. However, low brightness of the luminescent probes has limited the application of luminescent imaging. Recently, several bright and multicolor luminescent probes were developed by employing resonance energy transfer from luminescent probes to fluorescent proteins (Suzuki and Nagai 2017). The developed probes have greatly improved the sensitivity of luminescent imaging. In addition to the luminescent probes, various biosensors using FRET technique have been developed, enabling elucidation of the localization and dynamics of diverse intracellular molecules in single-molecule sensitivities.

Now, efforts are also underway to accelerate the smFRET measurement process. While conventional smFRET is able to detect the dynamics of biomolecules within 10–100 millisecond order, a recent study demonstrated that smFRET can track protein conformational changes at the microsecond level (Otosu et al. 2015). When FRET occurs, the donor fluorescent probe shows a decreased fluorescence intensity as well as a shortened cycle of time before returning to the ground state after photoexcitation (fluorescence lifetime). Compared with conventional intensity measurements, the lifetime measurements require fewer fluorescent photons to monitor FRET efficiency, and hence, can improve the temporal resolution of FRET measurements. The study using this method revealed the detailed process of conformational changes in cytochrome c protein at a sub-microsecond temporal resolution (Otosu et al. 2015).

Although the FRET techniques presented above are premised on the labeling of samples with two (or more) probes in different colors, smFRET can be measured using a fluorescent probe. Using non-fluorescent quenchers allows experimenters to perform an analysis similar to two-colored FRET measurement simply by measuring the fluorescence intensity of one fluorescent probe. When the donor fluorescent probe approaches a quencher, the fluorescence intensity decreases due to resonance energy transfer from the donor to the quencher. Therefore, one can observe conformational changes, bindings, and dissociations of labeled biomolecules simply by measuring the change in fluorescence intensity of the donor probe (Chen et al. 2012). Moreover, not only between heterologous molecules, FRET between homologous probes (referred to as homo-FRET) can be measurable. When illuminated by polarized light, only fluorescent probes in specific orientation are photoexcited and emit polarized fluorescence. If two identical fluorescent probes locate close together, because of FRET between the probes, the probes not in the photo-excitable orientation also emit fluorescence light polarized differently than that from the photoexcited donor probe, resulting in decreased anisotropy of the fluorescence. Therefore, distance changes between identical probes can be monitored by measuring the polarization components of fluorescence. This homo-FRET technique expands the application of FRET measurement in the studies of dynamics of biomolecules which can be labeled with only one-type of fluorescent probe, such as oligomerization processes of an endogenous protein (Bader et al. 2011). These advanced optical techniques have further sophisticated the smFRET method, so that we can elucidate more detailed behaviors of wider range of biomolecules.

10.4 Conclusion

smFRET is a particularly useful technique for investigating the behavior of individual biomolecules. Its applications have been steadily expanding by incorporating various other optical technologies. The strength of smFRET lies in its ability to track dynamic conformational changes and bindings/dissociations of ligands under near physiological conditions in real-time. Although smFRET measurements only detect distances and angles between a few positions labeled with FRET probes, this drawback can be complemented by X-ray crystal structure and electron microscopic analyses that visualize entire structures at high resolution. The appropriate combinations of technologies will further deepen our understanding of the molecular basis of biological phenomena.

References

Axelrod D (1981) Cell-substrate contacts illuminated by total internal reflection fluorescence. J Cell Biol 89(1):141–145

Bader AN, Hoetzl S, Hofman EG, Voortman J, van Bergen en Henegouwen PM, van Meer G et al (2011) Homo-FRET imaging as a tool to quantify protein and lipid clustering. ChemPhysChem 12(3):475–483

Betzig E, Chichester RJ (1993) Single molecules observed by near-field scanning optical microscopy. Science 262(5138):1422–1425

Chen J, Tsai A, Petrov A, Puglisi JD (2012) Nonfluorescent quenchers to correlate single-molecule conformational and compositional dynamics. J Am Chem Soc 134(13):5734–5737

Funatsu T, Harada Y, Tokunaga M, Saito K, Yanagida T (1995) Imaging of single fluorescent molecules and individual ATP turnovers by single myosin molecules in aqueous solution. Nature 374(6522):555

Jiang F, Taylor DW, Chen JS, Kornfeld JE, Zhou K, Thompson AJ et al (2016) Structures of a CRISPR-Cas9 R-loop complex primed for DNA cleavage. Science 351(6275):867–871

Lakowicz JR (2006) Principles of fluorescence spectroscopy. Springer, New York

Levene MJ, Korlach J, Turner SW, Foquet M, Craighead HG, Webb WW (2003) Zero-mode waveguides for single-molecule analysis at high concentrations. Science 299(5607):682–686

Nie S, Chiu DT, Zare RN (1994) Probing individual molecules with confocal fluorescence microscopy. Science 266(5187):1018–1021

Nishimasu H, Ran FA, Hsu PD, Konermann S, Shehata SI, Dohmae N et al (2014) Crystal structure of Cas9 in complex with guide RNA and target DNA. Cell 156(5):935–949

Osuka S, Isomura K, Kajimoto S, Komori T, Nishimasu H, Shima T et al (2018, in press) Real-time observation of flexible domain movements in Cas9. EMBO J 37(10):e96941

Otosu T, Ishii K, Tahara T (2015) Microsecond protein dynamics observed at the single-molecule level. Nat Commun 6:7685

Perkel J (2016) Elaine Mardis and Richard Wilson, directors of the McDonnell Genome Institute at Washington University, in front of an Illumina HiSeq 2000 sequencer. BioTechniques 60(2):56–60

Ritter JG, Veith R, Veenendaal A, Siebrasse JP, Kubitscheck U (2010) Light sheet microscopy for single molecule tracking in living tissue. PLoS One 5(7):e11639

Sase I, Miyata H, Corrie J, Craik JS, Kinosita K Jr (1995) Real time imaging of single fluorophores on moving actin with an epifluorescence microscope. Biophys J 69(2):323–328

Shera EB, Seitzinger NK, Davis LM, Keller RA, Soper SA (1990) Detection of single fluorescent molecules. Chem Phys Lett 174(6):553–557

Singh D, Sternberg SH, Fei J, Doudna JA, Ha T (2016) Real-time observation of DNA recognition and rejection by the RNA-guided endonuclease Cas9. Nat Commun 7:12778

Sternberg SH, LaFrance B, Kaplan M, Doudna JA (2015) Conformational control of DNA target cleavage by CRISPR–Cas9. Nature 527(7576):110

Suzuki K, Nagai T (2017) Recent progress in expanding the chemiluminescent toolbox for bioimaging. Curr Opin Biotechnol 48:135–141

Tokunaga M, Imamoto N, Sakata-Sogawa K (2008) Highly inclined thin illumination enables clear single-molecule imaging in cells. Nat Methods 5(2):159

Tsai A, Uemura S, Johansson M, Puglisi EV, Marshall RA, Aitken CE et al (2013) The impact of aminoglycosides on the dynamics of translation elongation. Cell Rep 3(2):497–508

Uemura S, Aitken CE, Korlach J, Flusberg BA, Turner SW, Puglisi JD (2010) Real-time tRNA transit on single translating ribosomes at codon resolution. Nature 464(7291):1012

Chapter 11
Comprehensive Approaches Using Luminescence to Studies of Cellular Functions

Atsushi Miyawaki and Hiroko Sakurai

In 1962, Dr. Osamu Shimomura discovered and purified green fluorescent protein (GFP) from the jellyfish *Aequorea victoria*. In 1992, the jellyfish GFP gene was cloned, causing a revolution in fluorescent labeling technology in cell biology. The use of genetic engineering techniques made the fluorescent labeling of cells, subcellular organelles and biomolecules possible. In 1999, new fluorescent proteins (FPs) were cloned from coral animals. At the turn of the century, genome structures of various life forms were clarified, with the players in cell workings (biomolecules) gathering together. With the demand for visualization of how biomolecules behave in live cells, expectations are high for innovations in fluorescent imaging technology and the spread of such technology. The dynamic behavior of biomolecules is crucial to understanding the mechanisms of cell proliferation, differentiation, and canceration, and the field itself has attracted the attention of the drug discovery industry, in particular. Here I describe several novel probes for cell functions that we developed in the last decade, including Fluoppi, Fucci, GEPRA, and UnaG.

11.1 <Fluoppi>

Protein-protein interactions (PPIs) play fundamental roles in cellular functions and disease development and are considered to be important targets for drug discovery. Current fluorescence-based technologies to detect PPIs, including fluorescence

Electronic Supplementary Material The online version of this chapter (https://doi.org/10.1007/978-981-13-7908-6_11) contains supplementary material, which is available to authorized users.

A. Miyawaki (✉) · H. Sakurai
RIKEN Brain Science Institute, Wako, Japan
e-mail: atsushi.miyawaki@riken.jp; hiroko.sakurai@riken.jp

Y. Toyama et al. (eds.), *Make Life Visible*,
https://doi.org/10.1007/978-981-13-7908-6_11

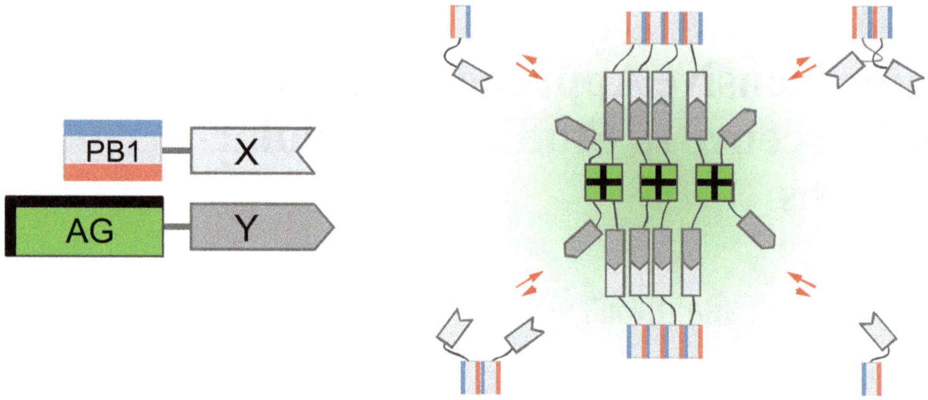

Fig. 11.1 Design and validation of Fluoppi, a PPI detection system using PB1/AG tags
Left, Homo-oligomerization of the p62 PB1 domain and the green-emitting fluorescent protein AG (Azami-Green). PB1 self-associates in an equilibrium in a front-to-back topology to form a high-molecular-weight homo-oligomer. The conserved acidic/hydrophobic and lysine/arginine residues of PB1 are indicated by red and blue bars, respectively. AG forms an obligate tetramer complex to become fluorescent (green). The hydrophobic interfaces between AG subunits are indicated by thick bars on two adjacent sides. Right, Schematic representation of PPI-dependent formation of fluorescent puncta. Due to the interaction between X and Y, PB1-X and AG-Y build crosslinks, resulting in the concentration of AG fluorescence (green shading)

resonance energy transfer (FRET), bimolecular fluorescence complementation (BiFC), and translocation/aggregation-based methods, have limited dynamic range to perform robust, reversible, scalable quantitative measurements. We harnessed liquid phase transitions to develop a genetic method for optical monitoring of PPIs at the single cell level (Watanabe et al. 2017). We employed two protein modules that homo-oligomerize with PPI-dependent association to drive phase separation and condensation of crosslinked products into liquid droplets (Fig. 11.1). One module is the PB1 domain, whose concatemerizing property is crucial for phase separations. The second module is a coral-derived FP, which forms a tetrameric complex. With this system, PPI-dependent formation of liquid-phase droplets can be detected as fluorescent puncta in live cells. The method, called Fluoppi, is amenable to FP technologies and applicable to many different PPI monitoring systems that utilize high content assay (HCA) and high-throughput screening (HTS) approaches. Fluoppi is superior to other PPI-monitoring methods in contrast, sensitivity, speed, reversibility, and simplicity.

Dynamic phase transitions of proteins in condensed liquid compartments are emerging as a ubiquitous process in biology that underlies intracellular fluidic organization. An increasing number of membrane-less intracellular structures are known to behave like liquid-droplet phases of the cytoplasm/nucleoplasm. While many of the structures are ribonucleoprotein (RNP) granules, such as P granules and nucleoli, it was demonstrated that multivalent binding of signaling proteins is capable of assembling liquid phase droplets. Our proof-of-concept experiments revealed the rapid appearance and disappearance of cytoplasmic liquid-phase droplets in a PPI-dependent fashion (Fig. 11.2), and the stable propagation of droplets across cell division (Fig. 11.3).

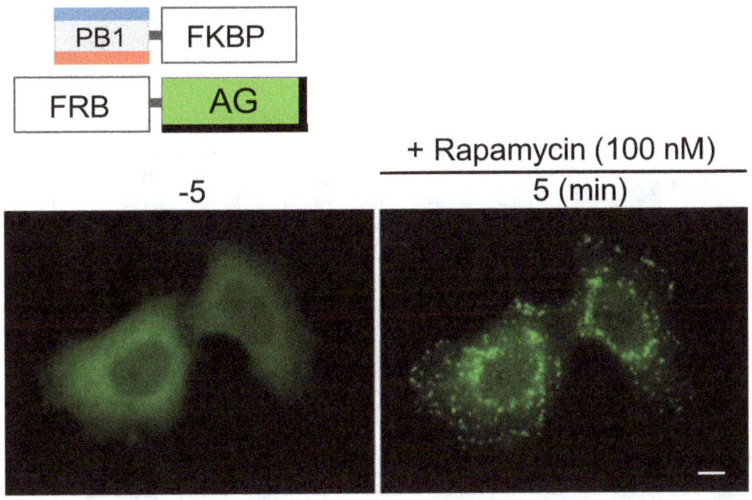

Fig. 11.2 Visualization of Rapamycin-induced association between FRB and FKBP in HeLa cells co-expressing PB1-FKBP and FRB-AG

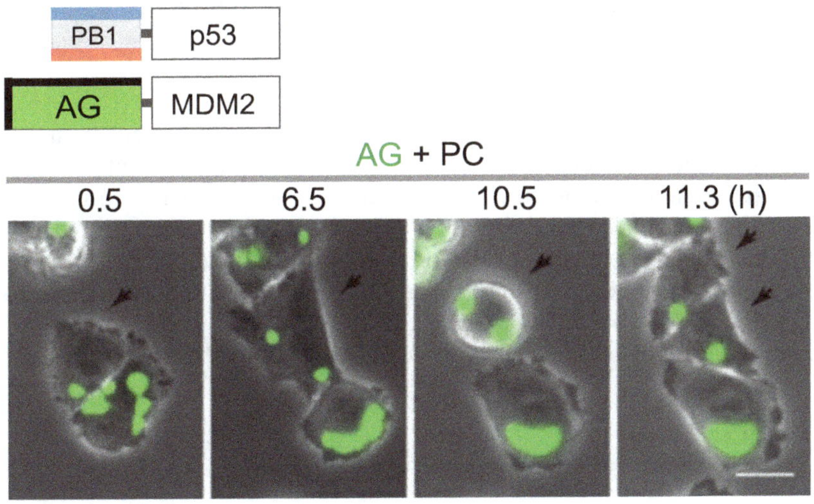

Fig. 11.3 Liquid-like state inside Fluoppi punctate structures in CHO-K1 cells stably co-expressing PB1-p53 and AG-MDM2. Cells were time-lapse imaged. PC, phase-contrast images. AG + PC, fluorescence images merged with phase-contrast images. One cell-division event is marked by black arrows. Most large puncta (> 10 μm) were irregular in shape

We used the Fluoppi method to visualize, for the first time, ERK2-dimer formation in single living cells stimulated with EGF. Although the ERK2-dimer was originally solved by a crystal structure of phosphorylated ERK2, its *in vivo* existence has been debatable. Our Fluoppi method revealed not only functional *in vivo* dimerization but that this PPI occurs in a cell-specific wave-like manner (Fig. 11.4). Because this novel wave behavior is not synchronized among cells, our findings provide a novel caution to researchers who conventionally harvest cells for *in vitro* biochemical detection of ERK2-dimer formation. These discoveries could only be obtained with Fluoppi technology, which provides rapid, reversible, and quantitative PPI readouts, thus introducing a general method for discovery of novel PPIs and modulators of established PPIs.

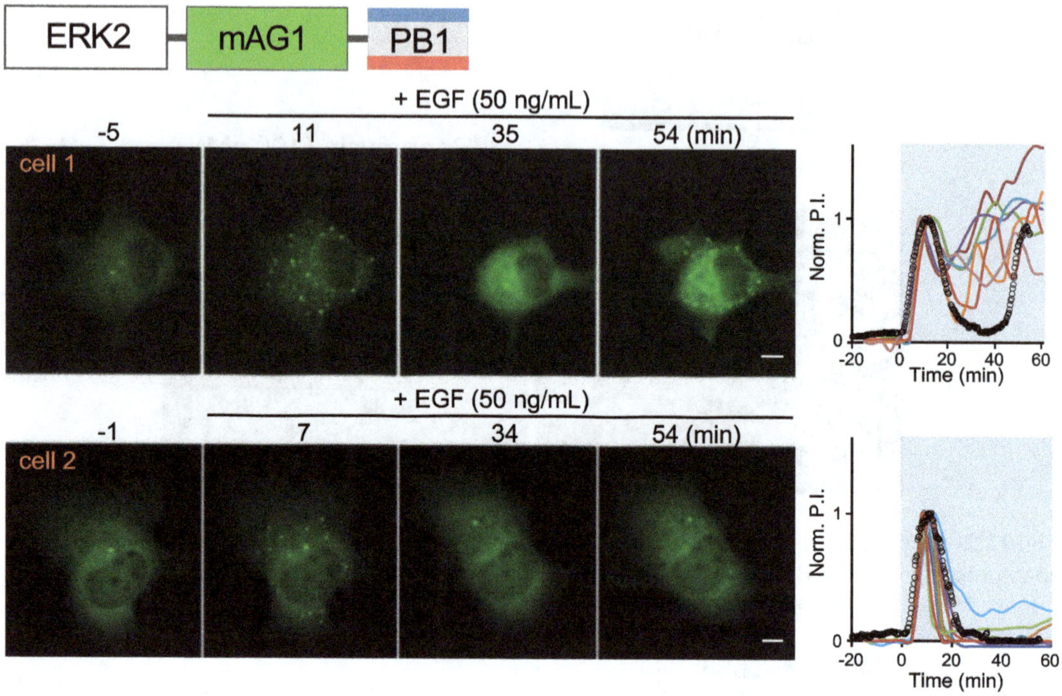

Fig. 11.4 HomoFluoppi using mAG1-PB1 tag for visualizing homo-dimerization
EGF-evoked homo-dimerization of ERK2 monitored in Cos-7 cells transiently expressing ERK2-mAG1-PB1. ERK2 homo-dimerization was quantified in 21 cells. Punctum formation was oscillatory in 9 cells and transient in 12 cells as represented by cell 1 (upper) and cell 2 (lower), respectively. Time points of image acquisition were counted after the addition of 50 ng/mL EGF. Despite heterogeneity of the temporal profile, initial punctum formation was observed 5–10 min after the addition of EGF. The time courses of P.I. normalized to the initial peak are shown (rightmost). Data points from cell 1 and cell 2 are indicated by black open circles

11.2 <Fucci>

Although considerable progress has been made towards understanding the mechanisms regulating cell cycle progression in single cells, little is known about the pathways coordinating the cell cycle with differentiation, morphogenesis, and cell death within multi-cellular tissues and organisms. Cell division is tightly regulated, and cells maintain tight control over the expression levels of proteins involved in the cell cycle. For example, Cdt1 and Geminin have opposite effects on DNA replication, and the amount of these proteins within cells is temporally controlled through the targeted destruction of unwanted protein. We exploited this tightly regulated process to develop a precise visual indicator of cell cycle status in living cells (Sakaue-Sawano et al. 2008). In our technique, which we call "Fucci (*f*luorescent *u*biquitination-based *c*ell *c*ycle *i*ndicator)", cells are genetically modified to express the G_1 marker Cdt1 and the S/G_2/M marker Geminin fused to red and green fluorescent tags, respectively. As a result, actively replicating cell nuclei in S/G_2/M phases exhibit green fluorescence, while nuclei that are in G_1 and not yet actively dividing fluoresce red (Fig. 11.5). Using Fucci technology, we directly observed active tumor

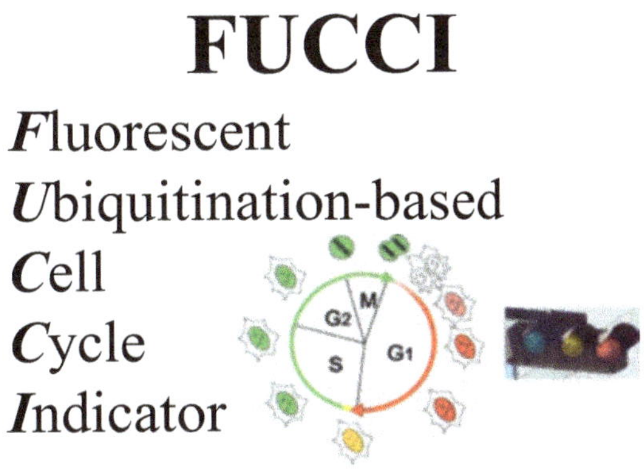

Fig. 11.5 Fucci probe labels individual G1 phase nuclei in red and S/G2/M phase nuclei green

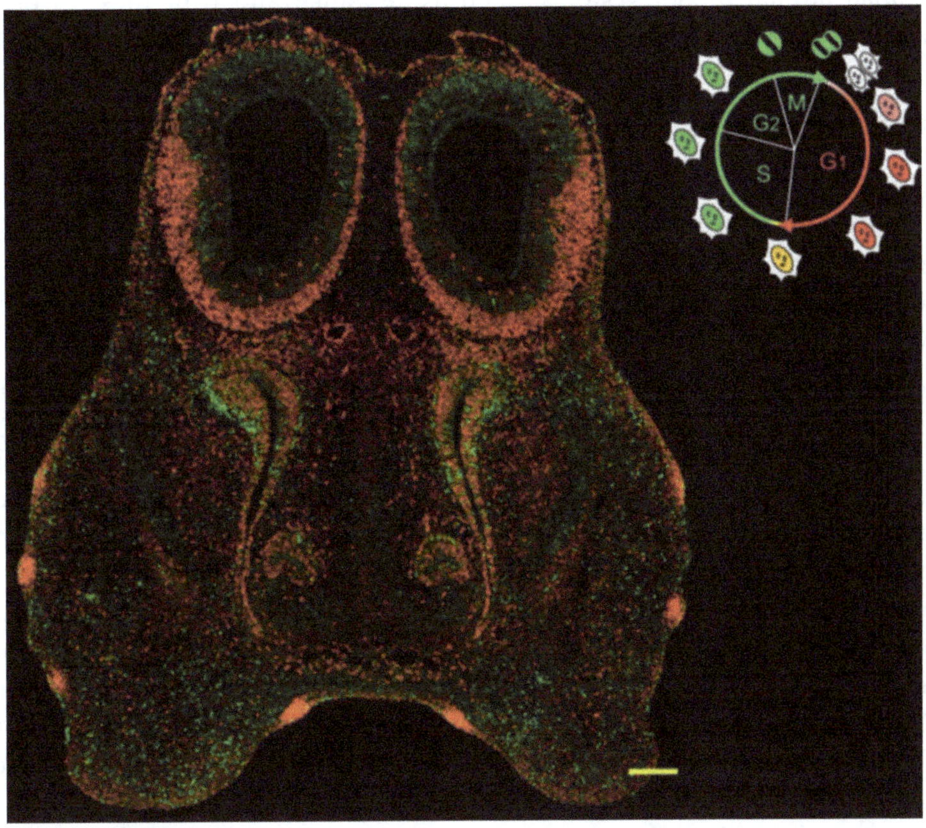

Fig. 11.6 A coronal section of an E13 Fucci transgenic embryo, containing the bran, olfactory system, and vomeronasal system. Red and green fluorescence signals are merged. Scale bar, 0.1 mm

cell growth in living animals over the course of a month. We also generated transgenic Fucci-expressing mice (Fig. 11.6), and we used these animals to perform detailed analyses of cell cycle profiles in various regions of the developing brain.

While our original paper represented a significant step forward in the understanding of cell cycle regulation, many challenges remain, and foremost among these is the development of a reliable and multifaceted screening technique for the discovery and characterization of novel anticancer drugs. We identify several significant variations in the cell cycle that cells exposed to chemotherapeutic agents can undergo. The variations would be missed by conventional cytometry analysis that only quantifies dye-incorporation to examine DNA content. By combining cytometry analysis with the Fucci probe, we have developed a novel assay that fully integrates the complexity of cell cycle regulation into drug discovery screens (Sakaue-Sawano et al. 2011). We believe that this assay system represents a powerful drug-discovery tool for the development of the next generation of anti-cancer therapies.

Since 2008, we have received many requests for Fucci-related products, including cDNAs, cell lines, and transgenic mouse lines. Importantly, quite a few people have also contacted us with inquiries about the performance of Fucci in non-mammalian animal model systems, such as zebrafish and fruit flies. In order to compile dynamic profiles of cell proliferation in the whole embryo, we turned to zebrafish, a powerful vertebrate model whose external embryonic development and transparency provide good access to almost all stages of embryogenesis for *in vivo* imaging. Thus, we examined whether the original Fucci based on human Cdt1 and Geminin operates effectively in fish cells. Unfortunately, we found that the original Fucci does not fully function in fish cells because the ubiquitin-mediated degradation of Cdt1 differs between mammals and fish. In 2009, however, we reported the development of zebrafish Fucci (zFucci), a time- and work-intensive project that involved the generation of DNA constructs using the zebrafish homologs of Cdt1 and Geminin, the characterization of these constructs using cultured fish cells, and the construction of transgenic zebrafish, Cecyil (Cell cycle illuminated) (Sugiyama et al. 2009). The transgenic lines, Cecyil and Cecyil2, which express zFucci and zFucci-S/G2/M(NC), respectively, exhibit normal development, confirming that the indicators do not affect normal cell cycle progression of fish cells. As the developers of this tool, we were privileged to be the first to use fish embryos to reveal the intricate and dynamic patterns of cell cycle progression in several parts of the body. Two organs were highlighted for their cell-cycle related morphogenesis. One was the retina, which has already been very well characterized, and the other was the notochord, which is a less explored embryonic structure in vertebrates in terms of cell proliferation/differentiation. Remarkably, we discovered two waves of cell-cycle transitions traveling from the anterior to the posterior of the notochord (Fig. 11.7) (Sugiyama et al. 2014).

11.3 <GEPRA>

Owing to the combined efforts of molecular biologists and geneticists in the last half century, our understanding of the spatiotemporal regulation of embryonic development has greatly advanced, particularly by the discovery of morphogens, diffusible molecules that impart positional information to cells within the embryo. Nevertheless, it remains unclear how a morphogen is spatially distributed along various axes of the body. Even though a source-sink model of morphogen dynamics

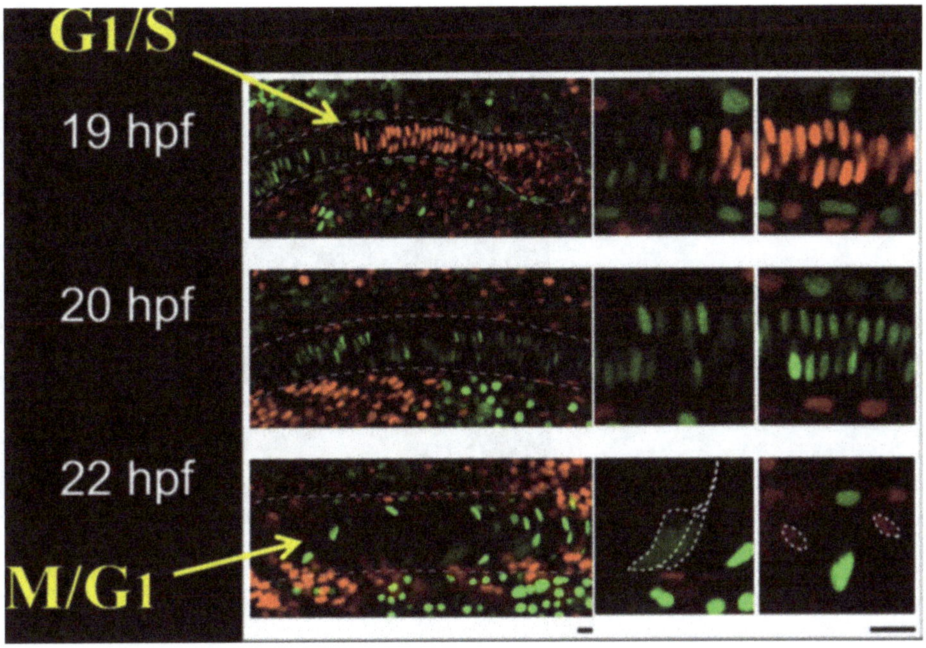

Fig. 11.7 Cell-cycle transition waves in the differentiating notochord. Confocal images of the posterior region of the notochord at 19, 20, and 21 hpf (hours post-fertilization)

was proposed by Francis Crick in 1970 predicting that a local source and a local sink can generate a linear concentration gradient of a morphogen based on simple diffusion, no one had yet succeeded in real-time monitoring of endogenous morphogen concentrations in a live embryo. Generally, morphogen gradients are surmised based on data that map the regions of enzymes that synthesize or degrade morphogen molecules in fixed samples. This is also the case with retinoic acid (RA). Despite the importance of RA in vertebrate development, the presence of its gradient in the zone flanked by synthesis (raldh2 enzyme) and degradation (cyp26 enzyme) regions is still controversial. Some researchers think that there is no RA gradient but a uniform or rectangular distribution. Moreover, assuming that a RA gradient exists, it is unknown whether it is linear or not. Due to its non-peptidic nature it is not possible to obtain even static images of RA distribution.

We developed three genetically encoded probes for RA (GEPRAs) with different binding affinities, for quantitative real-time imaging of the intracellular concentration of RA ($[RA]_i$) in live zebrafish embryos (Fig. 11.8) (Shimozono et al. 2013). By imaging both $[RA]_i$ and morphology over an extended period and combining the imaging with pharmacological and genetic manipulations, we were able to gain a comprehensive understanding of $[RA]_i$ dynamics along the anterior-posterior axis in relation to hindbrain formation and somitogenesis. The $[RA]_i$ distribution was demonstrated to be linear which definitively resolves the historical controversy.

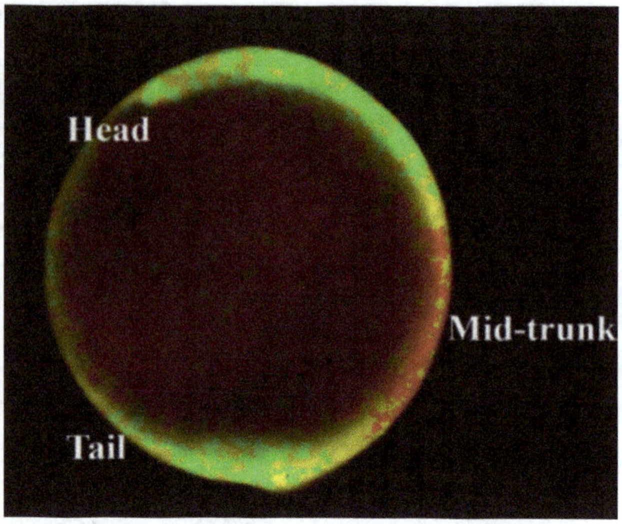

Fig. 11.8 A ratiometric $[RA]_i$ image in a bud-stage embryo expressing GEPRA

11.4 <UnaG>

The discovery and utilization of FPs has catalyzed rapid advances in many fields of biomedical research. While new variants continue to be genetically-engineered, nature remains the best source of novel fluorescent sensors. In 2009, researchers at Kagoshima University in Japan described a green fluorescence in the muscle of the Japanese eel (Hayashi and Toda 2009), a traditional part of Japanese cuisine but suffering from population decline. In 2013, we reported a comprehensive characterization of the protein that is responsible for the fluorescence, named 'UnaG,' including its molecular cloning, mechanism, structure and clinical use (Kumagai et al. 2013).

The mechanism of UnaG fluorescence is unexpected: we found that it binds non-covalently to the heme catabolite molecule bilirubin that serves as a fluorogenic chromophore. This is in marked contrast to the autocatalytic but oxygen-dependent chromophore formation of GFP and GFP-like proteins. The binding of bilirubin to UnaG is strong (K_d = 98 pM) and highly specific to the lipophilic bilirubin species of medical importance. We resolved the crystal structure of holoUnaG at considerably high resolution (1.2 Å), and defined the binding pocket as co-planar non-covalent interactions (Fig. 11.9). All of known bilin (linear tetrapyrrole)-binding proteins found in the plant/protozoan kingdom and their derivatives contain covalently bound bilin chromophores (Miyawaki 2016). However, UnaG is the first bilin-inducible FP, the first bilin-binding FP that belongs to the fatty-acid binding protein (FABP) family, and the first FP from the vertebrate subphylum. In many respects, therefore, UnaG can be regarded as a novel FP.

The accumulation of bilirubin in the human body causes the diseases jaundice and kernicterus, and bilirubin itself is a global health indicator of liver function. Until our molecular cloning of UnaG, however, humankind had not obtained a

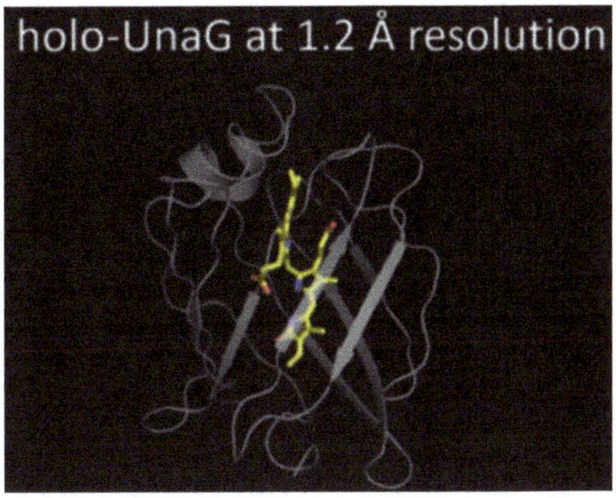

Fig. 11.9 A crystal structure of holo-UnaG (complex with bilirubin). The bilirubin chromophore is shown as a stick representation with atoms colored (carbon, green; oxygen, red; nitrogen, blue)

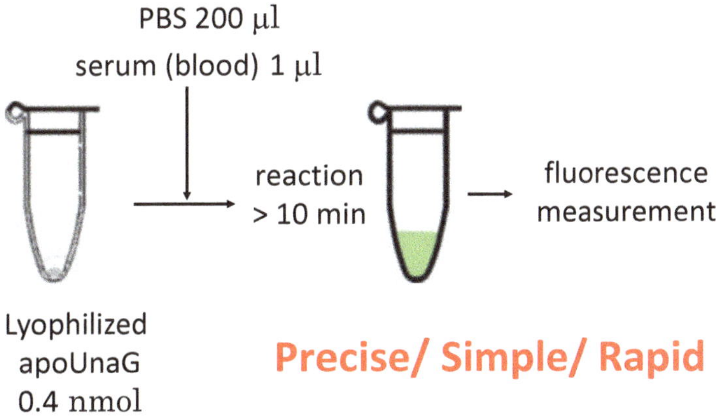

Fig. 11.10 A schematic showing the simple procedure for bilirubin level determination in a sample using lyophilized apoUnaG

direct sensor for this substance. On the whole, there have been significant problems related to current measurements of bilirubin in clinical laboratories. One of the problems stems from the principle of bilirubin detection that uses light absorption; absorptiometric methods are insensitive and affected by many factors. With UnaG, in contrast, we have developed a much superior fluorescence measurement assay that will revolutionize the ability to monitor bilirubin in human samples (Fig. 11.10). Our study also provides new insight on the role of a fluorescent protein system in the muscle of migratory eels.

References

Hayashi S, Toda Y (2009) A novel fluorescent protein purified from eel muscle. Fish Sci 75(6):1461–1469

Kumagai A, Ando R, Miyatake H, Greimel P, Kobayashi T, Hirabayashi Y, Shimogori T, Miyawaki A (2013) A bilirubin-inducible fluorescent protein from eel muscle. Cell 153(7):1602–1611

Miyawaki A (2016) Exploiting the cyanobacterial light-harvesting machinery for developing fluorescent probes. Nat Methods 13(9):729–730

Sakaue-Sawano A, Kurokawa H, Morimura T, Hanyu A, Hama H, Osawa H, Kashiwagi S, Fukami K, Miyata T, Miyoshi H, Imamura T, Ogawa M, Masai H, Miyawaki A (2008) Visualizing spatiotemporal dynamics of multicellular cell cycle progression. Cell 132(3):487–498

Sakaue-Sawano A, Kobayashi T, Ohtawa K, Miyawaki A (2011) Drug-induced cell cycle modulation leading to cell-cycle arrest, nuclear mis-segregation, or endoreplication. BMC Cell Biol 12:2

Shimozono S, Iimura T, Kitaguchi T, Higashijima SI, Miyawaki A (2013) Visualization of an endogenous retinoic acid gradient across embryonic development. Nature 496(7445):363–366

Sugiyama M, Sakaue-Sawano A, Iimura T, Fukami K, Kitaguchi T, Kawakami K, Okamoto H, Higashijima S, Miyawaki A (2009) Illuminating cell-cycle progression in the developing zebrafish embryo. Proc Natl Acad Sci U S A 106(49):20812–20817

Sugiyama M, Saitou T, Kurokawa H, Sakaue-Sawano A, Imamura T, Miyawaki A, Iimura T (2014) Live imaging-based model selection reveals periodic regulation of the stochastic g1/s phase transition in vertebrate axial development. PLoS Comput Biol 10(12):e1003957

Watanabe T, Seki T, Fukano T, Sakaue-Sawano A, Karasawa S, Kubota M, Kurokawa H, Inoue K, Akatsuka J, Miyawaki A (2017) Genetic visualization of protein interactions harnessing liquid phase transitions. Sci Rep 7:46380

Part II
Imaging Disease Mechanisms

Chapter 12
Making Chronic Pain Visible: Risks, Mechanisms, Consequences

A. Vania Apkarian

12.1 Summary Abstract for Presentation Delivered at Uehara Meeting, June 2017

By drawing an analogy between color perception (in the visual system) and pain perception, I highlight the fact that pain states must be considered conscious conditions, and in this sense ultimately our understanding of mechanisms of pain requires elucidation of fundamentals of consciousness. Thus, until we gain such understanding, we need to remember that current knowledge about pain mechanisms remain brain/behavioral correlates for subjectivity (SLIDE 2).

SLIDE 3: The current lecture deals primarily with mechanisms of chronic pain, and we need to differentiate between acute and chronic pain. Acute pain is necessary for avoiding damage based on conscious negative affectively colored states, which give rise to appropriate behaviors, such as avoidance. In contrast, chronic pain is a persistent state of negative affect where appropriate behaviors are no longer available. It is a state of conscious pain perception once the healing process of the initial injury has subsided. Current estimates are that >20% of world population suffers from chronic, proper treatments are missing, and its management imparts a very high cost to society.

SLIDE 4: Descartes' drawing in 1644, illustrates the basic elements that constitute any given sensory system, illustrated specifically for pain. The figure shows transduction, transmission, and cortical representation, which have become the main organizational concepts for each of the sensory systems; and the constituent

---

Electronic Supplementary Material The online version of this chapter (https://doi.org/10.1007/978-981-13-7908-6_12) contains supplementary material, which is available to authorized users.

A. V. Apkarian (✉)
Northwestern University Feinberg School of Medicine, Chicago, IL, USA
e-mail: a-apkarian@northwestern.edu

Y. Toyama et al. (eds.), *Make Life Visible*,
https://doi.org/10.1007/978-981-13-7908-6_12

cellular/molecular elements remain a main research direction in all senses. There is now ample evidence that persistence of pain, or transition from acute to chronic pain, is associated with peripheral, spinal cord, and cortical changes in functional and even in anatomical properties.

SLIDE 5: Within this context, this lecture deals with recent advances in our understanding mechanisms of chronic pain. The lecture emphasizes: (1) acute and chronic pain are distinct brain states; (2) recent studies show that we can derive a brain signature for chronic pain; (3) human and rodent-model longitudinal studies show that the limbic brain is critically and causally involved in the transition to chronic pain.

SLIDE 6: The general viewpoint for chronic pain is simply that it must be comprised of four distinct elements: (1) predisposition: necessary as only a minority of subjects with similar injuries develop chronic pain; (2) an injury: often the inciting event is clearly identifiable, but in many cases it may not be; (3) transition: recent evidence shows that both humans and rodent respond differently with treatments and show distinct perceptual properties early after an inciting event, in contrast to later stages of chronic pain. Mechanisms of the transition is a main emphasis of this lecture. (4) The maintenance stage is when the pain persists for long periods (usually years), a stage where treatments are also least effective. The specific mechanisms of maintenance of chronic pain remain minimally understood. The traditional (nociceptive) view has been that all these stages are embedded and thus need to be understood within the properties of the nociceptive circuitry, emphasizing the role of afferent fibers and spinal cord mechanisms of sensitization. Our viewpoint, based on recent advances in the topic instead posit that: (1) Limbic brain properties define risk; (2) the interaction between injury and emotional-learning processes underlie transition to chronic pain; and (3) chronic pain state is a new brain anatomical and functional condition carved during the transition to chronic pain.

SLIDES 7–11: If we compare brain properties between chronic pain patients and healthy controls, then we identify the components that make up the maintenance state of chronic pain. We observe anatomical distortions, and brain activity that seem to uniquely correlate with chronic pain perception.

SLIDE 12: There is also some evidence that when chronic pain is properly treated at least some of the brain anatomy renormalizes to correspond to the healthy brain state.

SLIDES 13–14: Illustrates brain oscillations, recorded in resting state fMRI, in a single subject. These oscillations reflect learning, memory and myriad other properties. Here we use it to derive a signature for the presence of chronic pain.

SLIDE 15: The overall approach is to use brain oscillations to construct an undirected graph of connectivity, and reduce this information to nodal links (degree): the number of nodes (degree, link) any given node communicates with.

SLIDE 16: Healthy subjects group average map for degree is shown. This is a map of the amount of information sharing any given brain location performs with the rest of the brain. If we calculate such a map for a single chronic pain patient, and plot, voxel by voxel, the one subject versus control degree map we can then calculate a distortion index kd.

SLIDE 17: kd provides a whole-brain unitary measure of extent of information sharing distortion a given patient or a group of patients exhibit. We see the index is present in 3 chronic pain conditions, and in all cases individual kd correlate with patients' magnitude of chronic pain. SLIDE 18 shows that we can used kd in a validation data set to predict individual subjects' magnitude of chronic pain, which we can do at an accuracy of about 60–70% correct.

SLIDES 19–28 summarize results from a longitudinal study, where we tracked brain properties of back pain patients, over a 3-year period. These patients entered the study within a few weeks of onset of their back pain (sub-acute stage) and were followed with repeated brain scanning while they transitioned either to recovery or to chronic pain. SLIDE 19 illustrates the general concept of the study, sub-acute back pain patients in time transition into recovering or persistence (based on the level of back pain), and properties that predict long-term outcome identify predispositions, while properties that change in time create the chronic pain state.

SLIDE 20: Brain activity maps are plotted related to the spontaneous fluctuations of back pain, in the recovering group (SBPr), and persistent group (SBPp), over time. We observe that both groups initially show similar brain activity, that matches activity for acute pain, but in time the respective maps diverge. The SBPr brain activity disappears while the SBPp activity moves away from sensory regions and instead engages limbic circuits. Thus, brain activity for back pain shifts in brain location as a function of time.

SLIDES 21–23: Summarize the main functional connectivity that predicts the long-term outcome, namely extent of information sharing between medial prefrontal cortex and nucleus accumbens (mPFC-NAc), which we interpret as a signal of the brain becoming addicted to nociceptive inputs. We suggest that the value of nociceptive afferents is modulated by these connections, which increase their importance to the individual, thus interpreting event small nociceptive inputs as pain.

SLIDES 24–28 summarize our approach to build a comprehensive model for factors that determine risk for chronic pain. SLIDE 24 shows that pain intensity and pain disability begin at equivalent levels but diverge in time between SBPp and SBPr. Thus we try to identify factors that predict these outcomes.

SLIDE 25: We create a brain anatomical network (based on white matter tracks derived from diffusion tensor imaging brain scans, DTI) for the limbic brain, defined as to be composed of amygdala, hippocampus, accumbens, and medial prefrontal cortex. This network was segregated into 3 sub-networks (based on within and across connectivity), one of which (green) had properties predictive of long-term back pain outcomes. This network anatomically and functionally could differentiate between groups, up to 1 year, but only anatomically at 3 years.

SLIDE 26: The volume of the hippocampus (as well as of the amygdala, data not shown) were also distinct between groups and constant over time.

SLIDE 27: The structured approach used to build the model predictive of chronic pain is illustrated. Only parameters that differentiated between the SBPp and SBPr groups were entered into the model.

SLIDE 28: Resultant model is shown. We also performed a limited gene analysis, and identified a single gene mediating contribution of amygdala volume to the model. The model shows three independent parameters all significantly contributing to the prediction of chronic pain, including limbic brain functional properties, anatomy of its connectivity, and the volume of the amygdala (or hippocampus). This result then shows that the limbic brain properties play a critical role in humans transitioning to chronic pain.

SLIDES 29–36 present correlates of the human studies in rodent models for chronic neuropathic pain. SLIDE 29 emphasizes the fact that rodent models provide the opportunity to study injury effects, transition and maintenance of chronic pain, but not predisposition, as these models always exhibit transition to chronic pain. The rest of the slides show the evidence that limbic brain in the rat also undergoes time dependent reorganization, as in the humans. Also, physiological and anatomical reorganization of accumbens indirect pathway is involved in transition to chronic pain.

SLIDE 30: In rats where we perform a neuropathic injury (spared nerve injury model, SNI), resting state fRMI scans show that the brain connectivity remains unchanged at 5 days, but it is reorganized at 28 days after injury. Note the animals show pain-like behavior (data not shown) at both time points. Moreover, the functional connectivity changes are mainly between limbic and somatosensory brain regions.

SLIDE 31: In the same animals as in slide 30, when we specifically examine functional connectivity for nucleus accumbens, again we only observe changes at 28 days, across many brain regions and for different parts of the nucleus.

SLIDE 32: In the same animals as in slide 30, when we examine nucleus accumbens levels of protein expression for various receptors, we observe dopamine receptor type 1 and 2 and kappa opioid receptor levels decreasing in time, which become significant at 28 days after injury.

SLIDE 33: In the same animals as in slide 30, when we examine functional connectivity for 2 sub-regions of the accumbens, we observe that functional connectivity, protein expression for dopamine receptor 2 and pain-like behavior (tactile allodynia) are all inter-related at day 28 after injury.

SLIDES 34–36 are patch recordings from accumbens shell dopamine neurons in mice genetically modified to express dopamine cells with d1 receptor with red and with d2 receptor with green fluorescence. SLIDE 34 shows that 5 days after neuropathic injury, excitability of d2 neurons (but not d1 neurons, data not shown) are increased, their dendritic expanse is shrunk, and afferent inputs are decreased. Moreover, extracellular dopamine levels are decreases and firing frequency of ventral tegmental neurons (the primary source of dopamine to nucleus accumbens) are decreased. Thus, we see both anatomical and functional reorganization of specific cell type in the shell of accumbens, just days after a peripheral neuropathic injury.

SLIDE 35 show that if such animals are treated twice a day either by a combination of L-dopa and naproxen or with pramipexole their tactile allodynia can be decreased together with renormalization of physiology and anatomy of accumbens shell d2 neurons.

SLIDE 36 demonstrates that chemogenetically controlling excitability of accumbens shell d2 neurons can upregulate and downregulate neuropathic pain-like behavior (tactile allodynia). The 5HT3 virus inserts sodium channels, while GLYR virus inserts chloride channels in infected cells. When these proteins are activated with a promoter (PSEM) they increase/decrease d2 neuron excitability and control tactile allodynia. Therefore, the level of excitability of d2 accumbens shell neurons causally controls neuropathic pain.

SLIDES 37–39 summarize the concepts presented in this lecture. SLIDE 37 highlights the circuitry associated with the 4 phases of chronic pain. SLIDE 38 demonstrates the interaction between nociception, limbic circuits and neocortex, pointing the role of limbic modulation of the neocortex to define the chronic pain state.

SLIDE 40 states the main conclusions of the lecture.

SLIDE 41 shows the contribution of Apkarian lab members to our ongoing research, and the 5 NIH institutes that have funded and continue to fund our studies.

Chapter 13
Visualization of the Pathological Changes After Spinal Cord Injury (*-From Bench to Bed Side-*)

Masaya Nakamura

Spinal cord injury (SCI) results in devastating loss of function, because spinal cord of human beings never regenerates after injury. However, there is an emerging hope for regeneration-based therapy of the damaged spinal cord due to the progress of neuroscience and regenerative medicine including stem cell biology. Stimulated by the 2012 Nobel Prize in Physiology or Medicine awarded for Shinya Yamanaka and Sir John Gurdon, there is an increasing interest in the iPS cells and reprogramming technologies in medical science. There is no doubt that iPS cells are expected to open new era providing enormous opportunities in the biomedical sciences in terms of cell therapies for regenerative medicine.

We previously established a reproducible spinal cord injury model (SCI) in adult common marmosets and demonstrated that transplantation of human iPS derived neural stem/progenitor cells (NSPC) into the injured spinal cord promoted functional recovery (Kobayashi et al. 2012). There are several potential mechanisms of the functional recovery after iPS-NSPC transplantation including axonal regrowth, re-myelination and trophic support (Fig. 13.1). We confirmed these findings through the histological examinations such as immunostaining for GAP43, which is a marker for regenerating axons and Luxol fast blue (LFB) myelin sheath staining. The question is how to evaluate these findings in patients with SCI. We have to replace these histological examinations as imaging examinations in clinical setting. We sought to replace them as diffusion tensor tractography (DTT) and Myelin map. Furthermore, central re-organization could also occur after cell therapy and neuro-rehabilitation in SCI patients. In the previous animal study, we confirmed it with

Electronic Supplementary Material The online version of this chapter (https://doi.org/10.1007/978-981-13-7908-6_13) contains supplementary material, which is available to authorized users.

M. Nakamura (✉)
Department of Orthopaedic Surgery, Keio University, School of Medicine, Shinjuku, Tokyo, Japan
e-mail: masa@keio.jp

Y. Toyama et al. (eds.), *Make Life Visible*,
https://doi.org/10.1007/978-981-13-7908-6_13

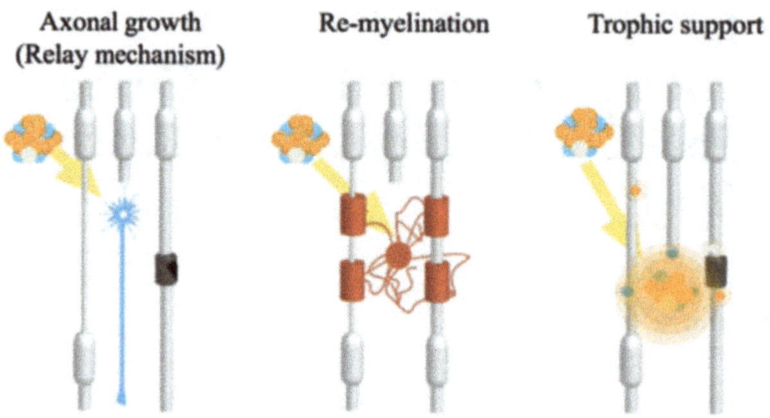

Fig. 13.1 Potential mechanisms of functional recovery after iPS-NSPC transplantation for SCI

tracer experiment to examine the changes in connectivity among the specific sites in brain. We also sought to replace them as connectivity analysis based on resting-state functional MRI.

13.1 Diffusion Tensor Tractography

13.1.1 Basic Research

Although the evaluation of axonal fibers is essential to assess the severity of SCI and efficacy of any treatment protocol, conventional methods such as tracer injection in brain parenchyma are highly invasive and technically demanding. Furthermore, since histological examinations are required to evaluate tracer studies, it has been impossible to evaluate axonal fibers in vivo and follow the sequential growth of axonal fibers in the same animal. We therefore sought to establish a non-invasive method to evaluate axonal fibers *in vivo* using DTT, a new MRI technique that makes *in vivo* tracing of axonal fibers possible. The properties and clinical applications of DTT in the brain have been reported, but technical difficulties have limited DTT studies of the spinal cord. Previously, we examined the effectiveness of DTT to visualize both intact and surgically disrupted spinal long tracts in adult common marmosets (Fujiyoshi et al. 2007). We induced a hemisection SCI at the 5th cervical vertebral (C5) level in adult common marmosets, and the spinal cord was imaged in a 7.0 Tesla MRI (Bruker Biospin) at several different time-points after injury. Furthermore, histological examination using Hematoxylin-Eosin, LFB and calmodulin dependent protein kinase to detect the corticospinal tract was conducted and confirmed the DTT findings in these animals.

We found that DTT clearly illustrated spinal projections such as the corticospinal tract and afferent fibers in control animals and depicted the severed long tracts in the injured animals. Furthermore, we succeed in demonstrating the pyramidal decussation of the marmoset. Histology of the spinal cords in both control and injured groups were consistent with DTT findings, verifying the accuracy of DTT. We also conducted DTT after contusion SCI in live marmosets and demonstrated that DTT can be performed in live animals to reveal *in vivo* nerve fiber tracing images, providing an essential tool to evaluate axonal conditions in the injured spinal cord (Konomi et al. 2012). Taken together, these findings demonstrate the feasibility of applying DTT to preclinical and clinical studies of spinal cord injury. DTT of the spinal cord is a powerful tool with tremendous potential if its properties and limitations are fully understood and correctly applied.

13.1.2 Clinical Significance of DTT

Based on our previous findings of DTT in adult common marmosets, we moved on to the study of DTT for cervical spondylotic myelopathy (CSM) to determine the clinical significance of DTT. The aims of this study were to (1) compare DTT of the cervical spinal cord in patients suffering from CSM with their clinical assessment, (2) compare DTT with the signal intensity of the spinal cord achieved with conventional MRI sequences and (3) determine whether postoperative changes in DTT have prognostic significance of patients with CSM after decompression surgery (Nakamura et al. 2012).

In twenty-one patients with CSM, T2-weighted imaging and DTI were performed before and 1 year after the decompression surgery. The value of fractional anisotropy was analyzed and fiber tracking was performed and analyzed using VOLUME-ONE software. Fiber tracts were generated by placing the region of interest (ROI) at the second cervical vertebral (C2) level (normal spinal cord) or at the most compressed level with reference to the sagittal MR images. The tract fiber (TF) ratio was calculated using a following formula: (Number of the tract fibers at the most compressed level) / (Number of the tract fibers at C2 level) × 100%. Japanese Orthopaedic association (JOA) scoring system of CSM was used to determine pre- and postoperative functional status and recovery rate was calculated by Hirabayashi method. We performed statistical analyses to determine the differences in preoperative JOA score, preoperative TF ratio and recovery rate between the patients with and without high signal intensity on T2-weighted image: T2HSI (+) and (−) groups. We also performed Nonparametric correlation analysis to determine the relationship between pre- and post-operative JOA scores and pre- and post-operative TF ratio respectively and also preoperative TF ratio and recovery rate.

We found that there was a significant difference in preoperative JOA scores between T2HSI (+) and (−) groups, whereas no significant difference in the recovery ratio was observed between them. There was also no significant correlation between the preoperative JOA score and the preoperative TF ratio, suggesting that the preoperative TF ratio did not reflect the severity of neurological deficit before the surgery. In contrast, there was a significant correlation between the preoperative TF ratio and the recovery rate. It was noteworthy that we can anticipate a poor prognosis (recovery ratio < 40%) of patients with CSM, whose preoperative TF ratio is

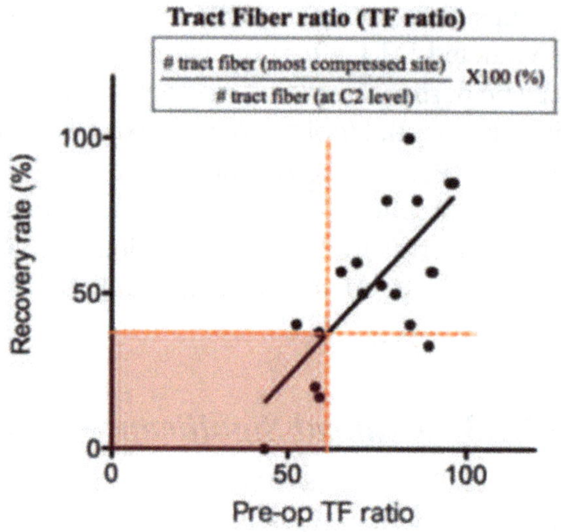

Fig. 13.2 Clinical application of DTT to Cervical Spondylotic Myelopathy **A poor outcome (recovery rate <40%) could be anticipated for CSM patients with preoperative tract fiber ratios below 60%**

below 60% (Fig. 13.2). Taken together, preoperative TF ratio was significantly correlated with CSM patients' recovery rate, suggesting that preoperative DTT could become a new prognostic predictor of CSM patient after decompression surgery.

13.2 Myelin Map

13.2.1 Basic Research

To assess the severity of SCI and efficacy of its treatment, it is essential to evaluate the histopathological state of myelin sheaths in the injured spinal cord. Therefore, the development of a new method for non-invasively evaluating myelin sheath was desired. We developed a novel technique, called the Myelin map, which uses pulsed gradient spin-echo MRI to visualize myelin *in vivo*, by focusing on the non-Gaussian diffusion distribution of water molecules confined by myelin sheaths (Fujiyoshi et al. 2016).

First, to validate the accuracy of this technique *in vivo*, we obtained Myelin maps of the spinal cords of postmortem myelin-deficient *shiverer* and *jimpy* mice as well as wild-type littermates, and compared them with histological findings of the same tissues. We found that there were almost no myelin sheathes in the spinal cords of myelin-deficient mice, which were closely associated with the findings of Myelin map, but not the other images such as T2-weighted image and FA map.

Second, we induced chemical SCI by injecting lysophosphatidylcholine into the posterior funiculus as well as contusive SCI at the C5 level using a modified NYU device in adult common marmosets. Furthermore, we performed transplantation of NSPC into the contused spinal cord of adult common marmosets. We took myelin map using a 7.0 Tesla MRI at the several different time-points. Myelin maps accurately depicted the demyelination/remyelination in marmoset chemical SCI, as well as the remyelination after allogeneic NS/PC transplantation in common marmosets. Immuno-EM analysis revealed that the transplanted NSPCs actively re-myelinated the de-myelinated axons in the injured spinal cords of common marmosets.

Taken together, we succeeded in developing a straightforward way to image the myelination of the spinal cord that should allow clinicians to evaluate the normal and pathological state of myelination more easily than with current methods. Using Myelin map, we also succeeded in obtaining strong evidence that the remyelination brought by transplanted NSPCs is a key mechanism for functional recovery. Myelin maps have an unparalleled ability to non-invasively visualize both normal myelin and its pathological state, and therefore this technique promises to be a powerful tool for researchers and clinicians examining diseases of the central nervous system. Furthermore, this method uses equipment that is already widely available, and so has the potential for immediate clinical application.

13.2.2 Clinical Significance of Myelin Map

Based on the findings of our basic research about Myelin map, we moved onto the clinical application of Myelin map. Brain MRI of neuromyelitis opticaspectrum disorders (NMOSD) patients often reveals multiple T2 high signal lesions, for which patients may be misdiagnosed as multiple sclerosis (MS) and treated with MSmodifying drugs potentially harmful to NMOSD. It is well known that distinct pathologies exist in NMOSD and MS, however the correct diagnosis is often jeopardized by the non specific nature of T2 signals. We sought to determine whether Myelin map enable us to differentiate NMOSD from MS.

A 54yearold female patient with newly diagnosed NMOSD with positive anti-aquaporin 4 antibody serostatus and a 30yearold female patient with 7month history of relapsingremitting MS were included in the study. Both patients experienced acute exacerbation explainable by Gadolinium (Gd)enhancing T2 lesion and they were treated with intravenous methylprednisolone therapy (IVMP). 3 T MRI studies with conventional modalities (T1 and T2weighted images, with Gd enhancement) and myelin map were repeated before and after IVMP with 3month intervals (Tanikawa et al. 2017).

In both NMOSD and MS patients, T2 lesions surrounded Gdenhancing inflammatory rims, however Myelin map supported demyelination existed outside the rim in NMOSD whereas it was localized inside the rim in MS. After the IVMP, Gdenhancing rims disappeared in both cases, albeit T1 hypointense cavity was left behind only in NMOSD. T2 lesion remained around the cavity in NMOSD or inside the diminished rim in MS, but neither of them were indicative of persistent demyelination. Myelin map supported remyelination was fast and extensive, already near complete at 3 months post IVMP in NMOSD, whereas remyelination slowly progressed inward from the rim, but remained incomplete even at 6 months postIVMP in MS. In conclusions, Non-myelin specific nature of T2 signals were confirmed in both NMOSD and MS. Distinct patterns in relative location of demyelination to inflammatory core may suggest differential pathogenesis underlying these diseases. Our cases also suggest a possible difference in remyelination capacity in NMOSD and MS, however a larger clinical study is required to draw a final conclusion.

13.3 Resting-State Functional MRI

It is recently reported that after SCI, neuronal connectivity changes occur not only in the spinal cord, but also in the brain. However, there has been no report investigating the changes of the neuronal functional communication among the several regions of the cerebral cortex after SCI.Therefore, we examined the changes in neuronal functional connectivity of the brain after SCI by taking the resting state-functional MRI (rs-fMRI) (Matsubayashi et al. 2018).

Adult mice were subjected to rs-fMRI without anesthesia. After careful acclimation to environmental stress in taking MRI, rs-fMRI was performed and the data of different mice brain were standardized with the stereotaxic MRI brain template. By classifying the regions of the brain based on the Allen mouse brain atlas, the neuronal functional connectivity was analyzed among the specific regions. Next, complete transection or contusion SCI was induced at the 10th thoracic vertebral level in these mice. rs-fMRI was taken at the several time-points after injury and the changes in neuronal functional connectivity of their brain were visualized using SPM12 software and CONN toolbox, and these data were analyzed using graph theory.

We succeeded in detecting the normal neuronal functional connectivity in the brain of the awake mice through rs-fMRI. In the comparative analyses before and after the transection SCI, the changes in functional connectivity was observed between the primary and secondary motor cortex. Moreover, by analyzing the brain connectivity after the contusion SCI, we detected the changes in the neuronal functional connectivity in accordance with the motor function recovery. Based on the graph theory, quantitative analyses of the whole brain structural community revealed the decrease in the density of the whole brain network and the changes in the pattern of the components of the specific brain community structure after SCI. In the current study, we demonstrated the feasibility to examine neuronal functional connectivity in the brain of awake mice using rs-fMRI. We also showed the relative changes in the neuronal functional connectivity in the brain after SCI and identified the regions that were strongly related to the functional recovery after SCI. In addition, we detected that the networks changed in the brain after SCI by the analyses using a graph theory. These networks were divided into small communities and the density of these networks decreases immediately after SCI, then individual regions change the importance of their network, suggesting that brain networks were reorganized and changed the efficiency of the entire network after SCI.

References

Fujiyoshi K, Hikishima K, Nakahara J, Tsuji O, Hata J, Konomi T, Nagai T, Shibata S, Kaneko S, Iwanami A, Momoshima S, Takahashi S, Jinzaki M, Suzuki N, Toyama Y, Nakamura M, Okano H (2016) Application of q-space diffusion MRI for the visualization of white matter. J Neurosci 36(9):2796–2808

Fujiyoshi K, Yamada M, Nakamura M, Yamane J, Katoh H, Kitamura K, Kawai K, Okada S, Momoshima S, Toyama Y, Okano H (2007) In vivo tracing of neural tracts in the intact and injured spinal cord of marmosets by diffusion tensor tractography. J Neurosci 27(44):11991–11998

Kobayashi Y, Okada Y, Itakura G, Iwai H, Nishimura S, Yasuda A, Nori S, Hikishima K, Konomi T, Fujiyoshi K, Tsuji O, Toyama Y, Yamanaka S, Nakamura M, Okano H (2012) Pre-evaluated safe human iPSC-derived neural stem cells promote functional recovery after spinal cord injury in common marmoset without tumorigenicity. PLoS One 7(12):e52787

Konomi T, Fujiyoshi K, Hikishima K, Komaki Y, Tsuji O, Okano HJ, Toyama Y, Okano H, Nakamura M (2012) Conditions for quantitative evaluation of injured spinal cord by in vivo diffusion tensor imaging and tractography: preclinical longitudinal study in common marmosets. NeuroImage 63(4):1841–1853

Matsubayashi K, Nagoshi N, Komaki Y, Kojima K, Shinozaki M, Tsuji O, Iwanami A, Ishihara R, Takata N, Matsumoto M, Mimura M, Okano H, Nakamura M (2018) Assessing cortical plasticity after spinal cord injury by using resting-state functional magnetic resonance imaging in awake adult mice. Sci Rep 8(1):14406

Nakamura M, Fujiyoshi K, Tsuji O, Konomi T, Hosogane N, Watanabe K, Tsuji T, Ishii K, Momoshima S, Toyama Y, Chiba K, Matsumoto M (2012) Clinical significance of diffusion tensor tractography as a predictor of functional recovery after laminoplasty in patients with cervical compressive myelopathy. J Neurosurg Spine 17(2):147–152

Tanikawa M, Nakahara J, Hata J, Suzuki S, Fujiyoshi K, Fujiwara H, Momoshima S, Jinzaki M, Nakamura M, Okano H, Takahashi S, Suzuki N (2017) q-Space Myelin Map imaging for longitudinal analysis of demyelination and remyelination in multiple sclerosis patients treated with fingolimod: a preliminary study. J Neurol Sci 373:352–357

Chapter 14
Multimodal Label-Free Imaging to Assess Compositional and Morphological Changes in Cells During Immune Activation

Nicholas Isaac Smith

First I would like to acknowledge the support of the Uehara Foundation, who supported the research discussed here. Aside from financial support, which is crucial, members of the foundation also expressed their interest in developing new ways to visualize and measure cellular processes. Other recipients of Uehara support also were enthusiastic and provided useful feedback and support of this research. It has been an honor to be a part of this program. I would also like to thank the members of my lab, especially Dr. Nicolas Pavillon and Dr. Alison Hobro, without whom this work would not have been what it is. Also my colleagues and collaborators, particularly in Raman imaging at Osaka university, and in immunology at our institute have been very supportive.

Since joining the IFReC immunology institute, our lab research has been aimed at creating new optical tools to understand some of the less clear aspects of the immune response, especially on the single-cell level. Most of the tools used by researchers to study the cell response involve tagging specific target molecules and seeing how they are expressed in different cell types, and determining how that expression changes during dynamic processes such as the stimulation of different immune pathways. There are a large number of pathways, signaling ions, expression levels of different proteins, RNA, and more that can be targeted (Spiller et al. 2010) and this number continually grows as researchers unlock new information on how the cell is built, and how it responds. The growing number of known pathways means that at any given time, we have had, and continue to have, only a partial view of the basic mechanisms of the cell. This is where the developments in this project can play a role: using label-free optical methods to interrogate the cell, we are able to analyze changes in molecular content and morphology which can correlate with how the cell is responding to immune stimulation. This approach does not give the same level of specificity as using fluorescent markers, PCR, or other analytical

N. I. Smith (✉)
Immunology Frontier Research Center, Osaka University, Suita, Japan
e-mail: nsmith@ap.eng.osaka-u.ac.jp

Y. Toyama et al. (eds.), *Make Life Visible*,
https://doi.org/10.1007/978-981-13-7908-6_14

chemistry-based techniques, but instead allows the generation of quantitative data which corresponds to the entire cellular composition and shape, which in turn, can be correlated with cell type, cell state, or other features of interest. It also allows mining the data to look for emergent patterns, correlations with other measurements, or to look for new features or indicators of cellular reactions which may not have been observed with other measurements.

A main technique we use is based on measuring how light is scattered from the sample, and by spectrally resolving the scattered light, we see the shifts, known as Raman shifts, in the light where the wavelength of scattered light is shifted due to the molecular vibrations in the sample. Rather than just elastically scattering the incident light, the sample molecules appropriate some of the photon energy, so that the scattered photons are red-shifted. The degree of energy absorbed, and therefore the wavelength shift, depends on vibrational modes in the sample molecules. Using this process, Raman imaging then gives us an image where the contrast, color, or both are determined by the molecules that make up the sample. This can then be exploited to visualize some of the basic activities of the cell such as cell division (Hamada et al. 2008), apoptosis (Okada et al. 2012), and can be expanded to take advantage of emerging high-resolution techniques (Watanabe et al. 2015). Taking the Raman spectra from a cell provides a signature of the cell's chemical makeup. Not surprisingly, most cells have a roughly similar composition and therefore Raman spectra look similar between different cells. The slight differences, however, in Raman spectral features either within cells, between cells, or from different time-points, can have enough statistical weight to discriminate cellular behavior or type that can be difficult to distinguish using any other methods, except by breaking the cell apart for analysis or by introducing a specific exogenous material to probe the cell states (Fig. 14.1).

Raman imaging produces large amounts of highly useful data, and when performed with conservative laser excitation powers, does not harm or modify the cell. However, it is possible to simultaneously multiplex Raman imaging with other label-free modes (Pavillon et al. 2014) and thereby gain complementary data from the sample. The only downside to this approach is complexity of the optical setup, which once solved, allows simultaneous multimodal quantitative label-free imaging and analysis. To this end we also use quantitative phase imaging, which works by measuring the differences in optical path length across the cells, and provides a spatially resolved map of the sample morphology. From a collimated beam of laser light, a partial mirror splits the beam, sending half of the light through the sample, while the other beam acts as a reference and does not pass through the sample. Both beams are then combined and interfered on a detector. This gives a spatially resolved map of the optical path length and attenuation characteristics of the sample. The technique we use, known as digital holographic microscopy (DHM), provides quantitative morphological data that has been shown to be highly useful, for example demonstrating the ability to predict cell death at an early stage by detecting the changes in cellular ionic homeostasis (Pavillon et al. 2012)

Combining these two optical measurement approaches, see Fig. 14.2, allows us to use either or both sets of complementary information. Of particular note is the

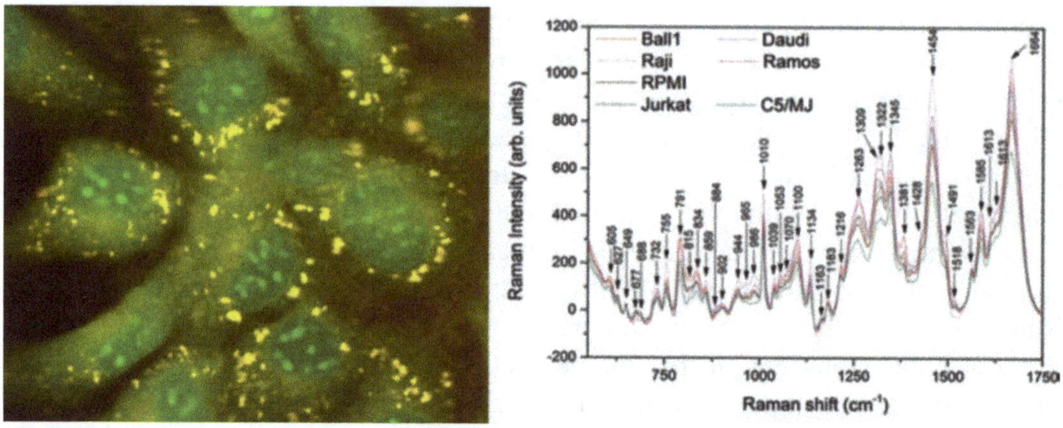

Fig. 14.1 (Left panel) Label-free Raman image of mouse embryonic fibroblast cells, cultured on a quartz substrate. Cells were excited by 532 nm laser, in a line-scan configuration, with spectrometer and cooled CCD detector. The green channel is a summation of Raman shifts between 2930–2940 cm^{-1} (shared by protein and lipid) and the red channel is between 2848–2856 cm^{-1} (predominantly lipid). Even with some overlap between the channels, nuclear features appear in saturated green, while lipid droplets appear as strong yellow. It is possible to further separate channels by processing if required. (Right panel) Average Raman spectra for different lymphocyte cell lines showing overall similarity, but statistically significant differences between ratios of peaks allows the discrimination of cell type by spectra. (See Hobro et al. 2016 for details)

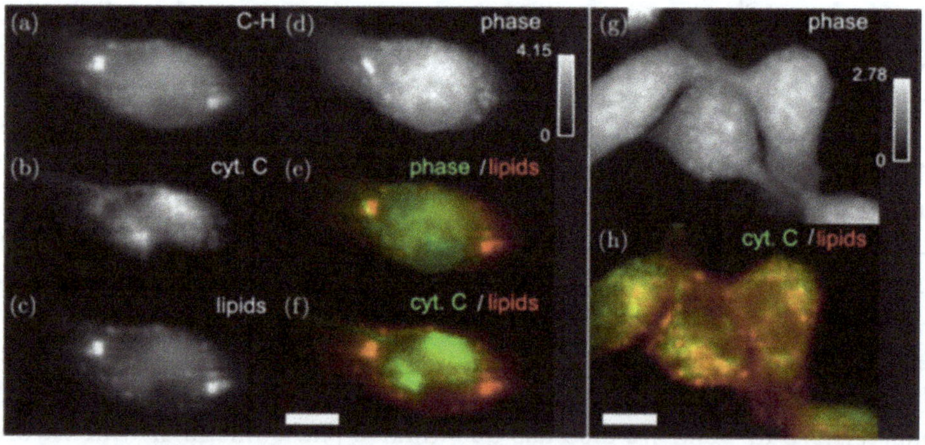

Fig. 14.2 Simultaneous label-free quantitative phase imaging (DHM) and Raman imaging of MH-S macrophages (**a**)–(**f**) and HeLa (**g**) and (**h**) cells. The image contrast is as labelled for each panel in (**a**)–(**f**), from (**a**) the C-H stretching band (2935–2955 cm^{-1}), (**b**) the cytochrome C band (740–780 cm^{-1}), (c) the lipid-dominated (2860–2880 cm^{-1}), (**d**, **g**) phase, with (**e**, **f**, **h**) constructed as overlay images. Scale bars are 5 μm. (Image from Pavillon et al. 2014)

difference in imaging speed of these two modalities. Raman imaging can be performed on a time scale on the order of minutes, while the DHM phase imaging can be as fast as video rate. This allows the detection of relatively fast moving objects in the cell. Typical speeds of intracellular transport or bacterial motion are on the order of micrometers per second, which are easily resolved by the DHM mode, but too fast for the Raman imaging. The Raman mode, however, has a unique ability to give insight into the nature of the dynamic intracellular objects. In our data of moving objects we have utilized the DHM imaging mode to observe intracellular objects and then used the Raman measurements to classify the types of moving objects, such as vesicles, nuclear components, or invasive objects such as bacteria, nanoparticles or adjuvants.

One example of this type of intracellular invasive object identification and tracking was done in our lab, where macrophages were exposed to hemozoin nanocrystals. Hemozoin is the byproduct of malaria infection, where the parasite biocrystallizes free heme to make a heme-based crystal. The uptake of the particles can produce an immune response, and can also act as an adjuvant in the response to other immune-triggering substances. Figure 14.3 shows Raman imaging of the macrophage hemozoin uptake, with the color channels determined automatically by PCA analysis. The images show the response can be visualized in terms of how endogenous compounds (see figure caption) move around in the cell in response to the presence of hemozoin. By comparison, the control cells look relatively homogenous. This in contrast to the cell imaging shown above, and is a result of the PCA analysis used here: the method determines the strongest contributions to the spectral contrast. When control data, 3 h, and 5 h post-incubation data is analyzed together, the differences within the cells at 3 and 5 h show the strongest contrast. If only control data is analyzed, then variance within the cell components, such as cytosolic components and nuclear material, is highlighted similar to the cell images shown above in Figs. 14.1 and 14.2.

We can also use the quantitative phase information to determine a number of different features in the cells that correlate with immune reactions or other processes in the cell. For macrophages exposed to LPS, toll-like receptors trigger a cascade of signals in the inflammatory response (Kawai and Akira 2010) the details of which are still an important topic of investigation. However, in a sample dish of relatively homogenous cultured cells, with tens of thousands of cells, each cell responds

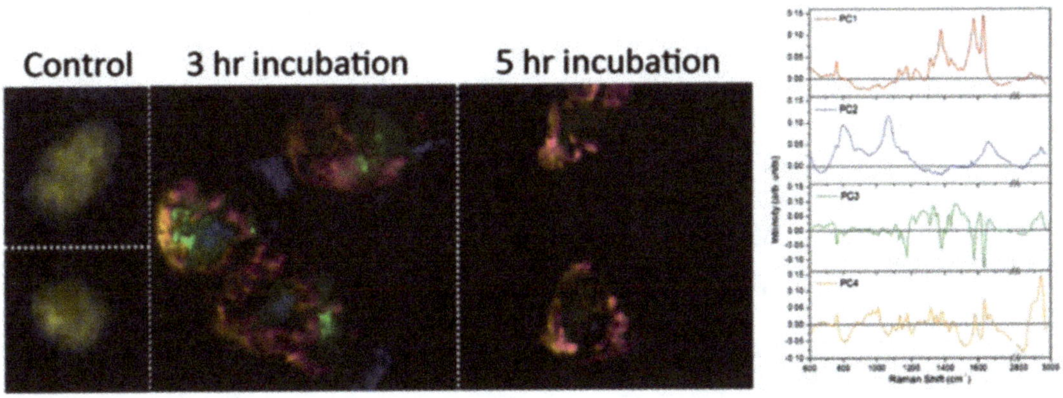

Fig. 14.3 Label-free Raman imaging of the uptake of malaria-related hemozoin by modified bone-marrow derived macrophages. The red channel shows hemozoin, appearing only at 3 and 5 h post-incubation, while the other channels show how the endogeneous cell components rearrange in response to the presence of the hemozoin. Color channels are assigned by principal components (PC1–PC4) determined from Raman spectral contrast. (See Hobro et al. 2015 for details)

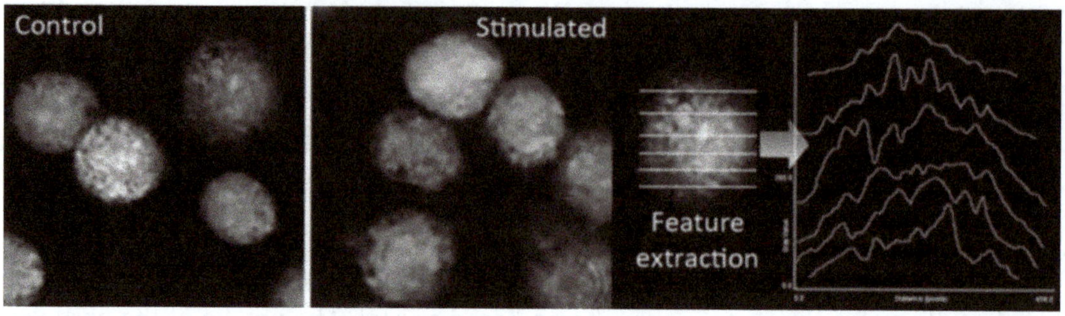

Fig. 14.4 Quantitative DHM phase images of J774 macrophages, in control conditions and when exposed to bacteria-related LPS. Morphological features as well as Raman spectral features can both be used to investigate, on a single-cell level, how individual cells respond to immune stimulation (Pavillon et al. 2018)

slightly differently. Using both Raman and quantitative phase data, it is possible to observe the effects of LPS stimulation on the composition and morphology of individual cells, with single-cell precision and relatively high throughput. The use of quantitative phase imaging for this application in particular has the potential to be high throughput since the imaging time for a field of view is in the order of milliseconds. Figure 14.4 shows the concept of imaging and processing macrophages using this approach.

Interestingly, more and more reports are now emerging of how individual cells respond differently, and the expression of different markers can be highly variable. The approaches shown here provide a means to evaluate these single cell level responses, without changing or modifying the sample. While not having the specificity of more traditional techniques such as labelling or invasive PCR type methods, these label-free techniques allow the evaluation of different cellular functions before, during, and after they occur, and can then be used over time to evaluate the progression as well as heterogeneity of cell responses. We also use complementary techniques such as ELISA or other wetlab techniques to validate these methods, and can use the resulting data to form a set of independent measurements, covering both population level responses (from ELISA) and single cell variations in response.

I sincerely appreciate the Uehara foundation funding for supporting this fundamental research and we look forward to future progress building on these results.

References

Hamada K et al (2008) Raman microscopy for dynamic molecular imaging of living cells. J Biomed Opt 13:44027

Hobro AJ, Kumagai Y, Akira S, Smith NI (2016) Raman spectroscopy as a tool for label-free lymphocyte cell line discrimination. Analyst 141:3756–3764

Hobro AJ et al (2015) Label-free Raman imaging of the macrophage response to the malaria pigment hemozoin. Analyst 140:2350–2359

Kawai T, Akira S (2010) The role of pattern-recognition receptors in innate immunity: update on Toll-like receptors. Nat Immunol 11:373–384

Okada M et al (2012) Label-free Raman observation of cytochrome c dynamics during apoptosis. Proc Natl Acad Sci 109:28–32

Pavillon N, Fujita K, Smith NI (2014) Multimodal label-free microscopy. J Innov Opt Health Sci 7:1330009

Pavillon N et al (2012) Early cell death detection with digital holographic microscopy. PLoS One 7:e30912

Pavillon N, Hobro AJ, Akira S, Smith NI (2018) Noninvasive detection of macrophage activation with single-cell resolution through machine learning. Proc Natl Acad Sci U S A 115(12):E2676–E2685

Spiller DG, Wood CD, Rand DA, White MRH (2010) Measurement of single-cell dynamics. Nature 465:736–745

Watanabe K et al (2015) Structured line illumination Raman microscopy. Nat Commun 6:10095

Chapter 15
Investigating In Vivo Myocardial and Coronary Molecular Pathophysiology in Mice with X-Ray Radiation Imaging Approaches

James T. Pearson, Hirotsugu Tsuchimochi, Takashi Sonobe, and Mikiyasu Shirai

15.1 Translating Imaging of Cardiac Function to Small Animals

Our current approaches to the study of cardiac function and the mechanisms that regulate it in both healthy and disease states rely heavily on biochemical assays of the expression of genes and proteins, extracted from some part of the myocardium. However, we know from studies of the anatomy and physiology of the heart over the past two centuries that in many regards the heart is far from uniform across different regions in its function from the cell to tissue levels. It is easy to forget, when considering molecular analyses, that heart disease too is more often than not, non-uniform in the way it affects the coronary vessels and cardiac muscle. The assessment of myocardial contractile-relaxation properties and coronary vascular function in specific regions of the heart in humans and large experimental animals are two areas in fundamental cardiovascular science and clinical diagnosis that have been greatly aided by the application of various invasive biophysical sensors and non-invasive or less invasive imaging techniques. However, rodents and in particular transgenic mice, are the most common subjects utilized for basic cardiovascular science to discover the mechanisms of disease development and progression and the efficacy of pharmacological and regenerative interventions. Nonetheless, the small physical size of the rodent heart and limitations in the spatial and or temporal resolution of many of the traditional techniques employed to study cardiac and coronary function

Electronic Supplementary Material The online version of this chapter (https://doi.org/10.1007/978-981-13-7908-6_15) contains supplementary material, which is available to authorized users.

J. T. Pearson (✉) · H. Tsuchimochi · T. Sonobe · M. Shirai
National Cerebral and Cardiovascular Center Research Institute, Suita, Japan
e-mail: jpearson@ncvc.go.jp

Y. Toyama et al. (eds.), *Make Life Visible*,
https://doi.org/10.1007/978-981-13-7908-6_15

has previously limited such assessments to global measures. Frequently, it has not been possible to make repeated measurements in the same animals in the past.

Herein, we describe our recent progress in the development of in vivo imaging approaches that permit repeated measurements of coronary vascular function utilizing microangiography and local cardiac actin-myosin cross-bridge dynamics utilizing synchrotron radiation (SR) based small angle X-ray scattering (SAXS). This combination of techniques is being used to investigate the important role of the coronary microcirculation in the origins of myocardial disease associated with diabetes, hypertension, obesity and heart failure. For detailed overviews of the cardiovascular application of these techniques, their merits and limitations, the reader is referred to our reviews on synchrotron imaging applications (Shirai et al. 2009, 2013). The high intensity X-ray radiation obtainable at third and fourth generation synchrotron facilities around the world is essential for in situ SAXS recordings from the beating heart in anaesthetised rodents. Lab X-ray sources, routinely used for protein crystallography and SAXS studies of ex vivo samples do not produce sufficient photon flux to enable in vivo recordings with the resolution of several milliseconds. While microangiography performed with SR tuned to energies selective for the elements of contrast imaging agents (such as iodine) facilitates the highest possible temporal and spatial resolution for vascular imaging (see Sect. 15.2.1), the current capabilities of optimized microfocus X-ray systems now permits in vivo imaging of microvessels and has some applications for coronary imaging. Our progress in this area is briefly presented in this chapter (see Sect. 15.3). Before describing how we can apply SAXS and microangiography in our ongoing studies in rats and now mice, we first discuss the motivation for utilizing these techniques.

> Synchrotron facilities with the capability of biomedical imaging, including the techniques described in this chapter, are available in many continents. The Lightsources.org webpages (http://www.lightsources.org/) is a useful community based entry point for explanations of synchrotron radiation principles, recent applications and descriptions of the synchrotron facilities available worldwide for non-commercial and commercial research. These webpages also describe access programs for each of these facilities.

15.2 The Importance of the Microvessels in Sustaining Cardiac Function

Conduit arteries, which includes the large main left and right coronary arteries and the medium to small artery side branches (>300 μm internal diameter, ID in humans) serve to distribute blood flow to all regions of the heart. However, the intramural resistance vessels, which primarily includes arterioles (<150 μm ID) and to a lesser extent, small arteries, distribute blood within the myocardial tissue. The majority of coronary resistance is produced by the arterioles, and is determined by the calibre (vessel ID) and the extent of deformation of these vessels during systolic

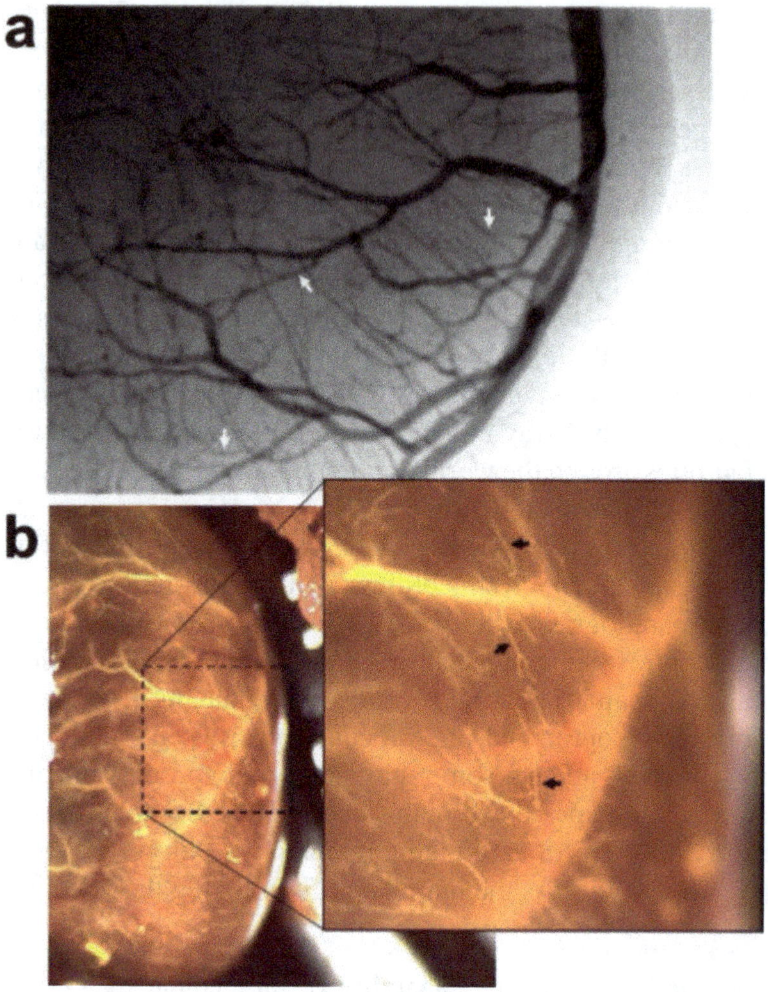

Fig. 15.1 Ex vivo mouse hearts filled with (**a**) barium gelatin mixture (angiogram) and (**b**) Microfil ® resin (microscope image) in the coronary arterial circulations reveals the extraordinary microvessel density within the obvious network of macrovessels. *Arrows* indicate 30 μm arterioles, which represent the limit of visualization utilising in vivo 2D X-ray angiography

contractions (Camici et al. 2012). As can be appreciated from Fig. 15.1, the capillary and arteriole microvessel network of the myocardium is very extensive. Interspersed between the muscle fibres the capillary density varies from a little over 2000/mm^2 in mice to more than 3000/mm^2 in dogs (Bassingthwaighte et al. 1974; Xu et al. 2016). Notably, utilizing clinical angiography in humans it is not possible to visualize the microvessels. The smallest vessels evident in clinical angiograms are small artery conduit vessels (Fig. 15.2).

Coronary regulation of the larger microvessels acts to adjust local blood flow to meet metabolic demands. An increase in cardiac work during stress and exercise is facilitated by an increase in coronary flow through the opening of side branches and more distal segments of the vascular tree (vasodilation). The ratio or the maximal increase in coronary flow above resting level is referred to as coronary flow reserve

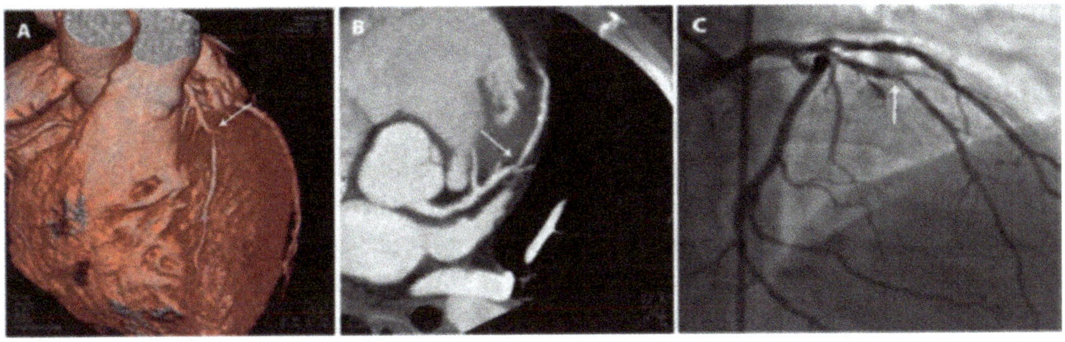

Fig. 15.2 Clinical CT (**a**, **b**) is not able to resolve microvessels, and the smallest visible vessels observed with clinical angiography (**c**) are small to medium arteries (>200 μm internal diameter). (Reproduced from Rao and Thompson 2011)

and is a useful index of the health of the coronary circulation. Coronary flow reserve can be determined by positron emission tomography, myocardial contrast echocardiography or invasively with electromagnetic flow probes, cine-angiography or the thermodilution technique. Regardless of the technique used, coronary flow reserve is an integrated measure of blood flow changes across the whole myocardium, including the large coronary arteries and the microvessels, and while very informative, it does not inform on how blood flow is distributed between vessel types or regions. However, direct visualization of coronary vascular responses during cine-angiography does permit analysis of regional changes in blood flow in terms of flow velocity, vessel calibre and visible vessel number. Hence, cine-angiography provides opportunities to investigate changes in coronary function in healthy and disease states.

Various studies now reveal that microvascular function impairment is an important contributor to the progression of many forms of heart failure, including hereditary and non-hereditary forms of hypertrophic cardiomyopathy (Olivotto et al. 2011; Camici et al. 2012), and the increasingly prevalent forms of heart failure with preserved ejection fraction (HFpEF) and angina (Franssen et al. 2016; Crea et al. 2017). There is growing evidence that endothelial dysfunction and ongoing vascular inflammation contribute not only to progressive rarefaction of coronary microvessels (Mohammed et al. 2015), but also increased stiffness and impaired relaxation of cardiac muscle (Franssen et al. 2016; Crea et al. 2017). Reduced nitric oxide bioavailability in the cardiomyocytes surrounding the microvessels is associated with diminished protein kinase G activity and reduced phosphorylation of the giant sarcomeric protein titin, and thus, increased passive tension (one component of muscle stiffening) of the sarcomeres and promotion of ventricular hypertrophy (Borbely et al. 2009; van Heerebeek et al. 2012; Paulus and Tschöpe 2013; Franssen et al. 2016). However, the roles of other vasodilators have not been considered in the current paradigm that links microvessel endothelial inflammation to the origins of HFpEF. It is well established that endothelium derived hyperpolarization factors (EDHF) are important for the regulation of microvessel flow and coronary flow reserve during exercise. Diabetes, obesity, hypertension and aging all impair microvessel EDHF production and or transmission of the hyperpolarization signal through the vessel wall (Park et al. 2008; Luksha et al. 2009; Jenkins et al. 2012; Behringer et al. 2013; Feher et al. 2014; Beyer et al. 2016; Chen et al. 2016; Garland and Dora 2016). Moreover, an imbalance of vasoconstrictor factors, including endothelin-1, rho-kinase and serotonin also contribute to vascular dysfunction in the same comorbidities, which in combination drive the development of HFpEF. Therefore, the roles of other vasodilators and vasoconstrictors in the deterioration of coronary flow reserve, myocardial contractile reserve and diastolic dysfunction remain to be investigated.

15.2.1 The Challenges Associated with Investigating Coronary Microvascular Function

How then do we assess the presence of endothelial dysfunction, particularly in the microvessels? Conventional cine-angiography using clinical radiography systems does not permit visualization of the coronary microvessels as low photon flux and collimation limit vessel resolution to vessels >200 μm ID (Shirai et al. 2013) (Fig. 15.2). Despite the advances in clinical computed tomography (CT) angiography with dual-energy multidetector systems, these systems still have a spatial resolution less than that of clinical cine-angiography, and therefore only medium to large arteries can be resolved. However, in rodents the coronary arterioles are 40–100 μm ID and can readily be visualized with SR microangiography (Jenkins et al. 2012; Pearson et al. 2017) (Fig. 15.3). This approach facilitates investigations of endothelial and smooth muscle function during pharmacological stimulation in anaesthetised rodents in vivo. The main advantage of this SR cine-angiography approach is that it enables in vivo analysis of vascular function at the same time in multiple arterial vessels across the micro- to macrovessel network under

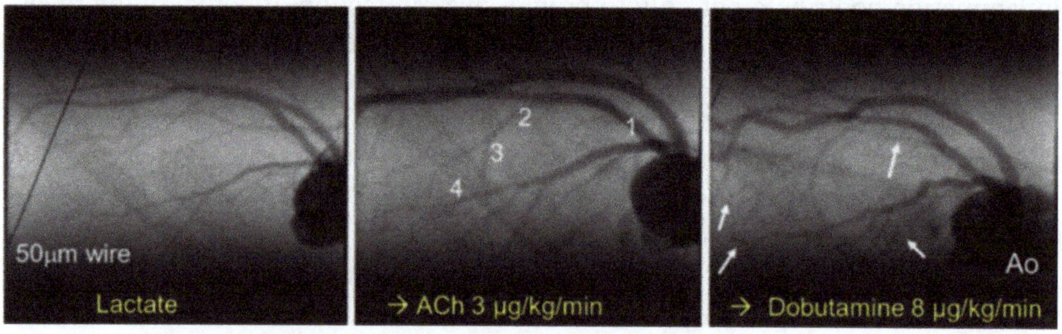

Fig. 15.3 Assessment of endothelial function in the coronary circulation in vivo in a male Sprague Dawley rat. (**a**) baseline vehicle infusion, (**b**) acetylcholine (ACh) administration, (**c**) dobutamine administration. Numerals show four branching orders of arterial vessels. ACh and dobutamine stimulation evoked dilation and an increase in visible vessel number (*white arrows*)

physiological conditions and with intact neurohormonal regulation, which is important for research translation. Further, it is possible to repeat imaging many times during pharmacological stimulation and the manipulation of cardiac loading conditions. An important limitation is the tradeoff for imaging at pixel resolutions of 10–15 μm is that generally available optic chips have arrays of 1024 × 1024 or 2048 × 2048 pixels, limiting the maximum observable field of view to 1–3 cm.

We utilize direct arterial injection of bolus amounts of commercial iodinated contrast agents. The increased viscosity of pure contrast agent requires that contrast be injected with a fast syringe pump via an arterial catheter that is as short as possible to reduce resistance to bolus delivery, and placed as close to target vessels as possible. Typically, paediatric radiography catheters can be used for adult and adolescent rats and hamsters, but for studies utilizing mice then tapered or step-down catheters are essential. Polyethylene or polyurethane catheters with an outer diameter of 1.2F (0.4 mm), such as a cut down version of the FunnelCath™, can successfully deliver contrast agent boluses in mice in ~1 s if the distal narrow tube is shortened (a simple manual test can confirm the ideal length for bolus injection) (Pearson et al. 2017). Furthermore, in the case of coronary angiography in rodents, ideal coronary cine-angiograms can only be obtained if the tip of the catheter is inserted retrograde via the right carotid artery (most direct route) up to a position immediately behind the aortic valve, otherwise left ventricle pumping greatly dilutes contrast concentration and entry into the coronary arteries. When inserting narrow gauge catheters in mice the use of a guidewire is sometimes needed to assist catheter insertion when vascular remodeling makes the artery wall increasingly fragile.

15.2.2 Protocols for Assessment of Coronary Endothelial Function

As demonstrated in Fig. 15.3 with current X-ray detectors it is possible to acquire coronary angiograms at physiological heart rates (300–700 bpm) free from motion artefacts, even at video frame rates, utilizing shutters placed in the X-ray beam to reduce single frame exposure times to 1–5 ms. High speed detectors operating at 50–100 Hz with high sensitivity phosphor plates eliminate the need for shutters for imaging acquisition, but such shutters serve to reduce surface entry radiation dose when image acquisitions are repeated many times in the same animals. Furthermore, motion-induced artefacts during coronary imaging are nearly eliminated by briefly sustaining lung volume at end inspiration (a breath hold 3–4 s), without significantly altering haemodynamics.

Single frames from cine-sequences acquired from two mice during a drug stimulation protocol (~1 h duration) are illustrated in Fig. 15.4. In this study (Pearson

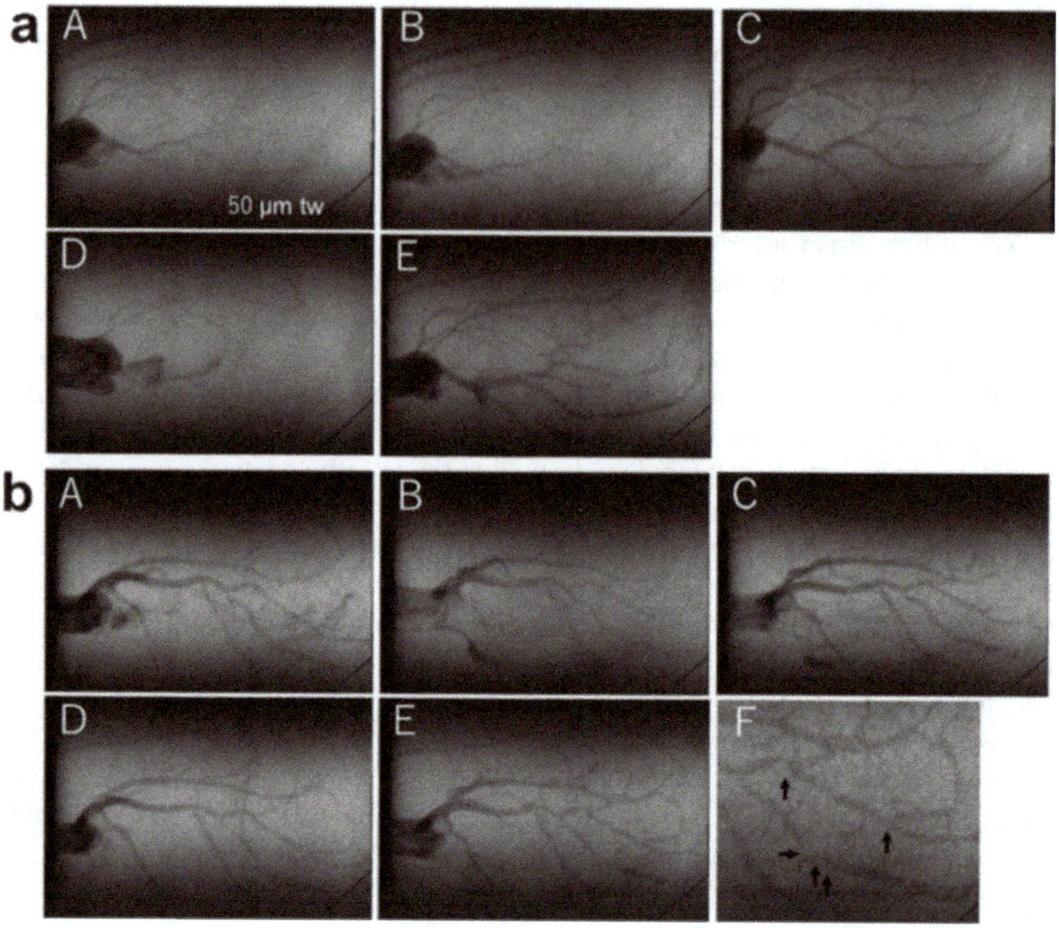

Fig. 15.4 Vascular responses to drug stimulation (**a**) in a mouse with SR-B1 protein present in blood vessels compared with (**b**) in a mouse deficient in SR-B1 protein. During baseline (A), ACh (B), sodium nitroprusside (C), blockade of nitric oxide and prostaglandins (D), blockade and ACh (E), enlargement of panel E illustrating stenoses (*black arrows*) in deficient mouse (F). (Reproduced from Pearson et al. 2017)

et al. 2017) we examined how the absence of a scavenger receptor class B (SR-B1) protein affected the global and regional regulation of coronary vasodilation in the microcirculation utilizing a transgenic mouse model exposed transiently to a high fat diet, which induces coronary plaque lesion formation. Not only were we able to show that SR cine-angiography could reveal partial occlusions (*black arrows* in b, stenoses confirmed by histology to be due to occlusive plaque formation, Fig. 15.4) in macrovessels, but also that smooth muscle dysfunction was present globally in non-occluded microvessels (Pearson et al. 2017).

We have successfully transferred coronary SR cine-angiography protocols to enable assessment of coronary vascular function in normal and transgenic mouse

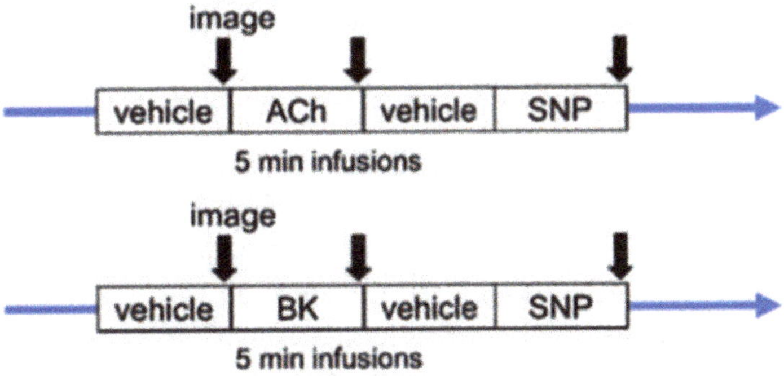

Fig. 15.5 Routine protocols for investigating endothelium-dependent and independent vasodilation in rodents with consecutive drug stimulations

models (Shirai et al. 2013). While assessment of coronary flow reserve can be performed with adenosine or dobutamine stress test in mice, as shown for a rat in Fig. 15.3, it is often desired to assess coronary endothelial function during disease progression and following pharmacological intervention. Two simple protocols are illustrated that allow the assessment of endothelial dysfunction in mice by evaluating the changes in coronary vessel calibre and visible vessel number mediated by endothelium-dependent and independent dilation induced by agonist stimulation (Fig. 15.5). Continuous infusion of acetylcholine (ACh) or bradykinin (BK) solutions (0.1 mg/ml) at flow rates of 3 μl/min in a 30 g mouse or 2 μl/min in a 20 g mouse (10 μg/kg/min) evoke endothelium-dependent dilation. It has been demonstrated many times that ACh and BK can evoke dilation through nitric oxide or endothelium-derived hyperpolarization factors (Batenburg et al. 2004, 2005; Bergaya et al. 2004; Jenkins et al. 2012; Chen et al. 2016). In order to establish whether the lack of a response to ACh stimulation is due to endothelial dysfunction in any given vascular bed it is common practice to subsequently stimulate the vessels with sodium nitroprusside (SNP, 10 μg/kg/min), a nitric oxide donor, after a suitable washout period. SNP evokes endothelium-independent dilation in the absence of smooth muscle dysfunction. Therefore, if a mouse shows dilation to SNP, but not ACh, then this is taken to be evidence of endothelial dysfunction. On the other hand, in models where vessels do not show dilation to SNP then this is taken to be evidence of smooth muscle dysfunction, at least in respect to nitrergic signaling within the smooth muscle. If vessels do not respond with dilation to either ACh or SNP it is not possible to establish that endothelial dysfunction is present since there is underlying smooth muscle dysfunction downstream of the endothelium, unless the same vessels also fail to dilate to BK, which can evoke hyperpolarization independent of nitric oxide. Hence, utilizing multiple endothelium-dependent agonists to investigate endothelial function is recommended where possible. If the presence of smooth muscle dysfunction is indicated by a lack of response to SNP, then further investigation of the mechanism involved can be achieved by also utilizing adenosine or large-conductance Ca^{2+}-activated K^+ channel agonists to determine which relaxation mechanisms are dysfunctional (Batenburg et al. 2005).

15.3 Progress in Vascular Imaging of Small Animals with Lab Systems

Preclinical microCT systems are commercially available that enable CT angiography in animals up to the size of rabbits. However, effective pixel size for single projection images on the CMOS flat-panel detectors with a field of view of several cm^3 is typically 100–200 μm. With such systems 2D angiography can at best reveal small arteries. Higher resolution acquisitions are only possible for ex vivo 3D acquisitions due to the prolonged scanning times (>5 min). Nonetheless, microfocus X-ray imaging systems are available that are suitable for real time imaging of the microvessels in vivo, but the challenge has been achieving fast imaging with sufficient absorption contrast to visualize vessels in organs that move, the heart and lungs. One such system that we have utilized for investigations of the hindlimb vasculature in peripheral arterial disease associated with diabetes is the Hitex system described in our recent study (Sonobe et al. 2015).

Utilising an optimised microfocus X-ray system (MFX-80HK, Hitex Ltd., Osaka, Japan) incorporating an off the shelf high speed camera with ultrasensitivity (FASTCAM Mini AX200, Photron, Japan) we have greatly improved the possibilities for real time cine-angiography in rats and mice (Fig. 15.6). The current capability of this system suggests that microvessel function studies approach the real resolution of SR microangiography in the hindlimb, brain and renal vessel beds (with frame averaging). However, limited photon counts at the detector result in blur and unsatisfactory vessel edge detection in single projection images of the coronary and pulmonary arteries below 100 μm. Further optimization of the image intensifier and X-ray source might lead to the development of a system that permits assessment of coronary endothelial function in vivo during closed-chest conditions in the laboratory.

15.4 Application of In Vivo SAXS to the Study of Myocardial Function in Mice

Various research groups currently employ SAXS for muscle diffraction studies of contraction-relaxation mechanisms in cardiac muscle ex vivo, which is complemented by cell approaches to investigate excitation-contraction coupling in isolated cardiomyocytes. This can be routinely achieved with dedicated lab X-ray SAXS systems, but real-time analysis of myofilament function is achieved with SR as an X-ray source. We and others have developed approaches for SAXS investigations in the beating heart in situ utilizing rats and more recently mice (Pearson et al. 2004, 2007; Yagi et al. 2004; Toh et al. 2006; Shirai et al. 2013).

Actin and myosin filaments form the bulk of sarcomeric proteins, along with titin, but only the lattice like arrangement of actin-myosin produces diffraction

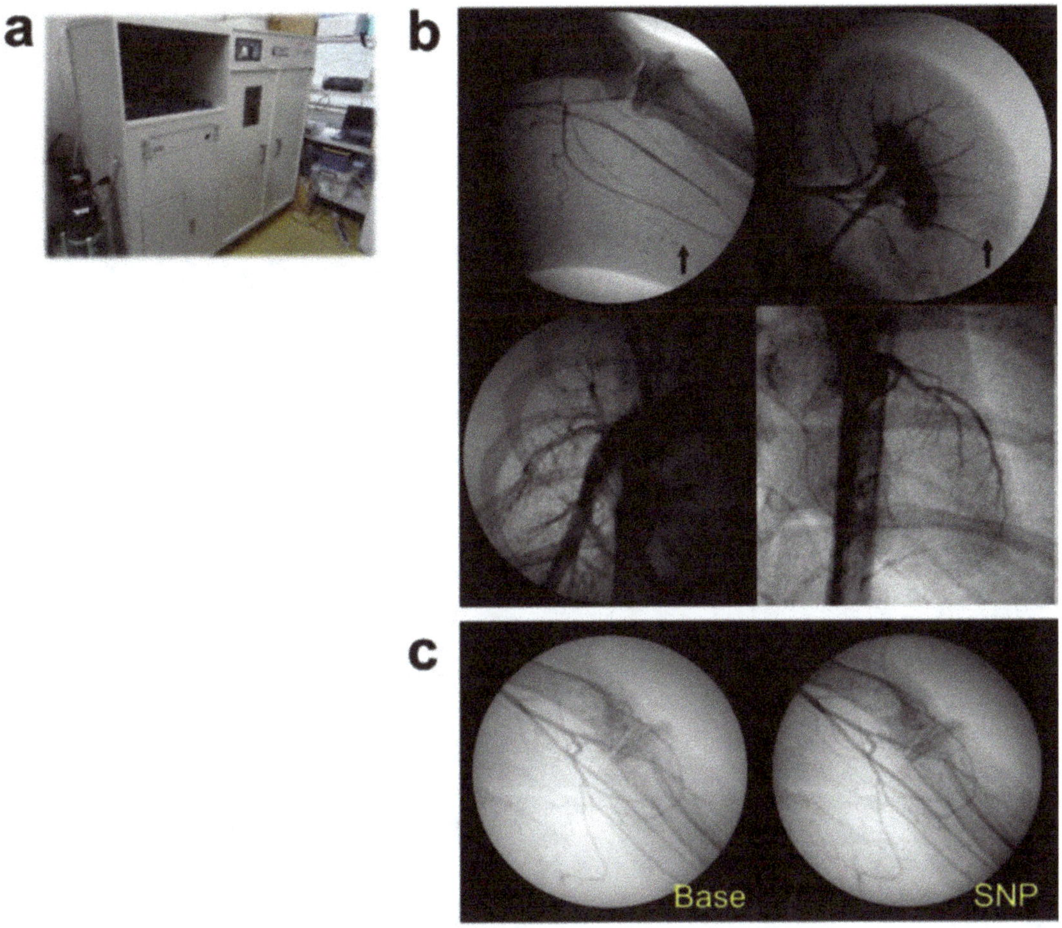

Fig. 15.6 (**a**) Microfocus X-ray video system (Hitex, Osaka, Japan) optimized for laboratory based imaging (iodine contrast agent) and examples of image quality achieved while imaging anaesthetised (**b**) rats (hindlimb, kidney, pulmonary and coronary arteries) and (**c**) mice (hindlimb), acquired at 250 frames/s, 60 kV and 80 μA. *Black arrows* indicate 50 μm arterioles in the hindlimb and renal cortex

reflections when a high energy X-ray beam (0.1 × 0.2 mm) is aligned perpendicular to the myocardial fibre direction (Shirai et al. 2013). The intensity of the two major reflections produced depends on the electron mass distribution around the filaments, which changes during the cross-bridge cycle as myosin heads shift between the myosin backbone and the surrounding actin filaments (Fig. 15.7). The diffraction pattern acquired at 10–15 ms intervals from a beam passing through the exposed heart of a supine anaesthetised rodent is sufficient to track the changes in myosin mass transfer over the cardiac cycle for several seconds (Pearson et al. 2004). The intensity of the 1,0 reflection decreases as myosin heads are extended towards actin and form force-developing cross-bridge attachments. This myosin mass transfer provides a simple index of the number of cross-bridge attachments formed, which is highly correlated with developed force and left ventricular pressure at systole.

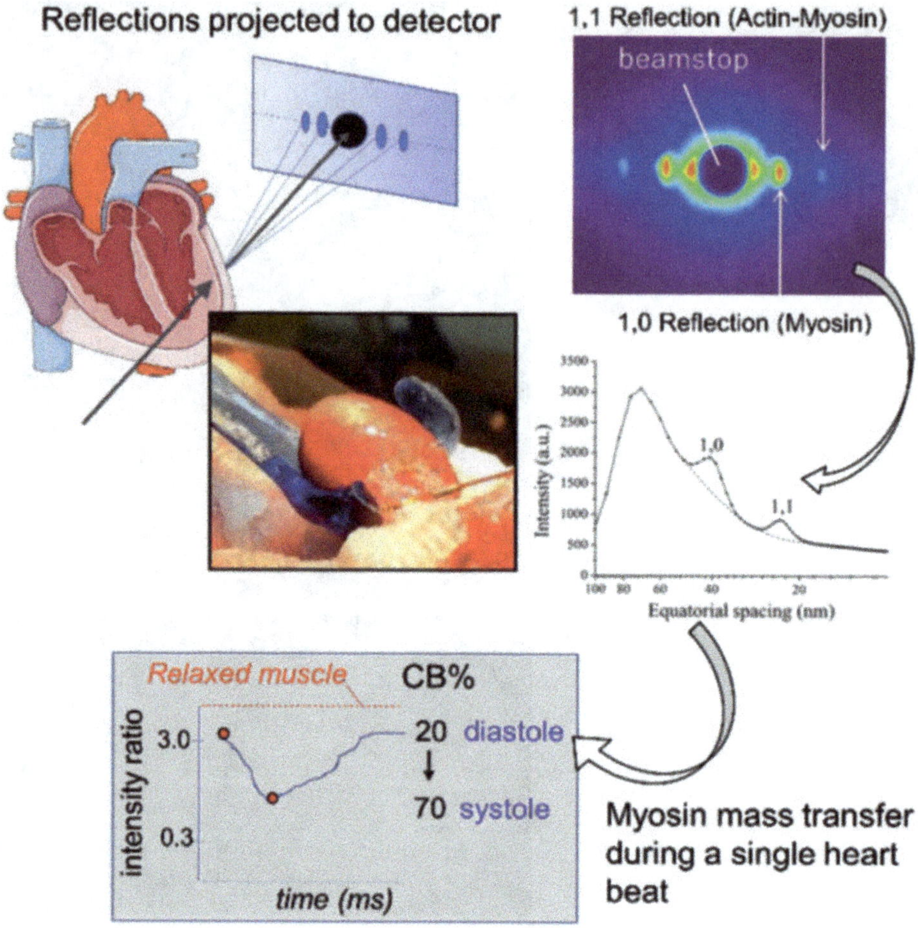

Fig. 15.7 In situ small angle X-ray scattering based investigations of regional cardiac contractile function. Diffraction pattern recorded in a 15 ms interval, and a typical intensity profile and the calculated intensity ratio change over the cardiac cycle

In recent years we and others have shown that this in vivo approach can be utilized to investigate regional differences in myocardial function and even differences across the myocardial wall from the epicardium to the subendocardium based on the trajectory of the X-ray beam (Jenkins et al. 2013; Shirai et al. 2013; Waddingham et al. 2015). Using this approach, we showed that altered kinase activity and changes in phosphorylation state of the various myofilaments in diabetes contributes to the early origins of diastolic dysfunction (Fig. 15.8). Further, others have shown with ex vivo SAXS that altered protein kinase activity in cardiac hypertrophy contributes to an increase in passive stiffness associated with more myosin heads remaining in the proximity of actin filaments (Sumita Yoshikawa et al. 2013).

Since the first SAXS studies on cross-circulated canine hearts, then spontaneously beating rat hearts, there has been only one study that investigated in situ cross-bridge interactions and myosin mass transfer simultaneous with electrocardiogram

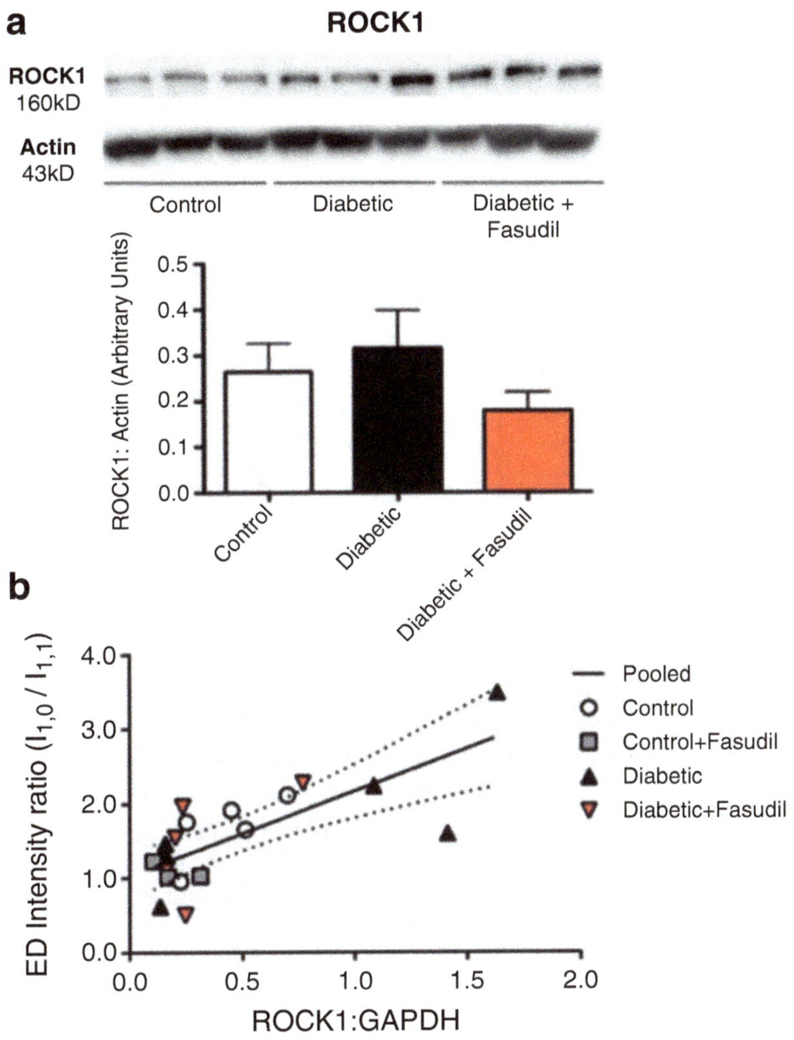

Fig. 15.8 (**a**) Direct relation between rho-kinase (ROCK1) protein expression in the myocardium of rats and (**b**) the measured diastolic (ED) intensity ratio determined from X-ray diffraction patterns. Results shown include non-diabetic (control) and diabetic rats treated with ROCK inhibitor fasudil. Reproduced from Waddingham et al. (2015)

in the mouse heart (Toh et al. 2006). Now we have been able to apply cardiac muscle diffraction recordings simultaneous with left ventricle pressure-volume recordings in transgenic mice, and again use this approach to measure myosin mass transfer across the cardiac cycle in different layers of the left ventricle (Fig. 15.9). Ongoing studies are now investigating myofilament dysfunction with aging in a knockin mouse model of human familial cardiac hypertrophy. This opens the possibilities of new investigations into cardiomyopathies and heart failure using cell-specific or receptor-ligand specific knock down or knockin and even conditional knockouts to

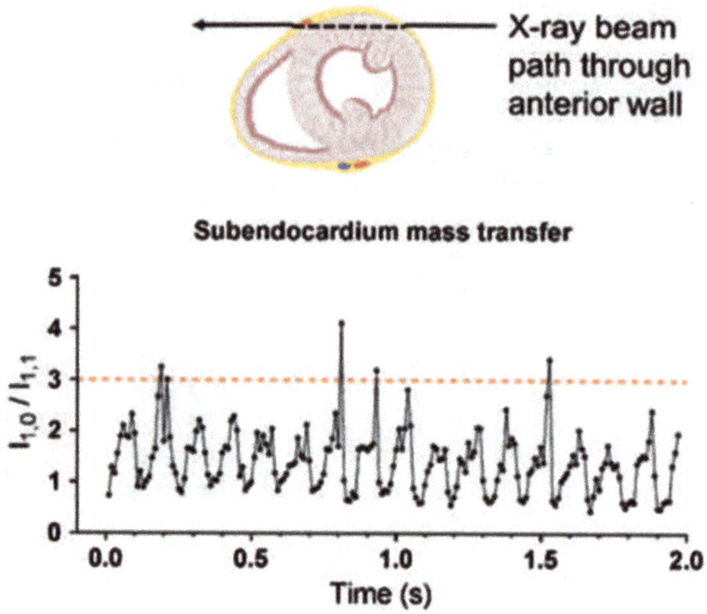

Fig. 15.9 Calculated equatorial reflection intensity ratio over the cardiac cycle in a normal wild type mouse over a 2-s recording (10 ms intervals). *red dashed line* indicates ratio obtained in the heart arrested in diastole (state with no cross-bridge attachments)

probe the underlying mechanisms associated with myofilament dysfunction due to altered myocardial energetics and calcium overload, changes in intracellular protein kinase signaling or increased myocardial oxidative stress and inflammation.

Acknowledgments The authors gratefully acknowledge support from the Uehara Memorial Foundation. All experiments performed at the Japan Synchrotron Radiation Research Institute with approval of the SPring-8 Animal Experiment Review Committee (proposals 2012A1674, 2013B1767, 2015A1354, 2015B1533, 2017A1324).

References

Bassingthwaighte JB, Yipintsoi T, Harvey RB (1974) Microvasculature of the dog left ventricular myocardium. Microvasc Res 7(2):229–249. https://doi.org/10.1016/0026-2862(74)90008-9

Batenburg WW, Garrelds IM, van Kats JP, Saxena PR, Danser AH (2004) Mediators of bradykinin-induced vasorelaxation in human coronary microarteries. Hypertension (Dallas, Tex : 1979) 43(2):488–492. https://doi.org/10.1161/01.hyp.0000110904.95771.26

Batenburg WW, Tom B, Schuijt MP, Danser AH (2005) Angiotensin II type 2 receptor-mediated vasodilation. Focus on bradykinin, NO and endothelium-derived hyperpolarizing factor(s). Vasc Pharmacol 42(3):109–118. https://doi.org/10.1016/j.vph.2005.01.005

Behringer EJ, Shaw RL, Westcott EB, Socha MJ, Segal SS (2013) Aging impairs electrical conduction along endothelium of resistance arteries through enhanced Ca2+-activated K+ channel activation. Arterioscler Thromb Vasc Biol 33(8):1892–1901. https://doi.org/10.1161/atvbaha.113.301514

Bergaya S, Hilgers RH, Meneton P, Dong Y, Bloch-Faure M, Inagami T, Alhenc-Gelas F, Levy BI, Boulanger CM (2004) Flow-dependent dilation mediated by endogenous kinins requires angiotensin AT2 receptors. Circ Res 94(12):1623–1629. https://doi.org/10.1161/01.RES.0000131497.73744.1a

Beyer AM, Zinkevich N, Miller B, Liu Y, Wittenburg AL, Mitchell M, Galdieri R, Sorokin A, Gutterman DD (2016) Transition in the mechanism of flow-mediated dilation with aging and development of coronary artery disease. Basic Res Cardiol 112(1):5. https://doi.org/10.1007/s00395-016-0594-x

Borbely A, van Heerebeek L, Paulus WJ (2009) Transcriptional and posttranslational modifications of titin: implications for diastole. Circ Res 104(1):12–14. https://doi.org/10.1161/circresaha.108.191130

Camici PG, Olivotto I, Rimoldi OE (2012) The coronary circulation and blood flow in left ventricular hypertrophy. J Mole Cell Cardiol 52(4):857–864. https://doi.org/10.1016/j.yjmcc.2011.08.028

Chen YC, Inagaki T, Fujii Y, Schwenke DO, Tsuchimochi H, Edgley AJ, Umetani K, Zhang Y, Kelly DJ, Yoshimoto M, Nagai H, Evans RG, Kuwahira I, Shirai M, Pearson JT (2016) Chronic intermittent hypoxia accelerates coronary microcirculatory dysfunction in insulin-resistant Goto-Kakizaki rats. Am J Physiology Reg Integ Comp Physiol 311(2):R426–R439. https://doi.org/10.1152/ajpregu.00112.2016

Crea F, Bairey Merz CN, Beltrame JF, Kaski JC, Ogawa H, Ong P, Sechtem U, Shimokawa H, Camici PG (2017) The parallel tales of microvascular angina and heart failure with preserved ejection fraction: a paradigm shift. Eur Heart J 38(7):473–477. https://doi.org/10.1093/eurheartj/ehw461

Feher A, Broskova Z, Bagi Z (2014) Age-related impairment of conducted dilation in human coronary arterioles. Am J Physiol Heart Circ Physiol 306(12):H1595–H1601. https://doi.org/10.1152/ajpheart.00179.2014

Franssen C, Chen S, Unger A, Korkmaz HI, De Keulenaer GW, Tschöpe C, Leite-Moreira AF, Musters R, Niessen HWM, Linke WA, Paulus WJ, Hamdani N (2016) Myocardial microvascular inflammatory endothelial activation in heart failure with preserved ejection fraction. JACC: Heart Failure 4(4):312–324. https://doi.org/10.1016/j.jchf.2015.10.007

Garland CJ, Dora KA (2016) EDH: endothelium-dependent hyperpolarization and microvascular signaling. Acta Physiol (Oxf) 219:152–161. https://doi.org/10.1111/apha.12649

Jenkins MJ, Edgley AJ, Sonobe T, Umetani K, Schwenke DO, Fujii Y, Brown RD, Kelly DJ, Shirai M, Pearson JT (2012) Dynamic synchrotron imaging of diabetic rat coronary microcirculation in vivo. Arterioscler Thromb Vasc Biol 32(2):370–U466. https://doi.org/10.1161/atvbaha.111.237172

Jenkins MJ, Pearson JT, Schwenke DO, Edgley AJ, Sonobe T, Fujii Y, Ishibashi-Ueda H, Kelly DJ, Yagi N, Shirai M (2013) Myosin heads are displaced from actin filaments in the in situ beating rat heart in early diabetes. Biophys J 104(5):1065–1072. https://doi.org/10.1016/j.bpj.2013.01.037

Luksha L, Agewall S, Kublickiene K (2009) Endothelium-derived hyperpolarizing factor in vascular physiology and cardiovascular disease. Atherosclerosis 202(2):330–344. https://doi.org/10.1016/j.atherosclerosis.2008.06.008

Mohammed SF, Hussain S, Mirzoyev SA, Edwards WD, Maleszewski JJ, Redfield MM (2015) Coronary microvascular rarefaction and myocardial fibrosis in heart failure with preserved ejection fraction. Circulation 131(6):550–559. https://doi.org/10.1161/circulationaha.114.009625

Olivotto I, Girolami F, Sciagra R, Ackerman MJ, Sotgia B, Bos JM, Nistri S, Sgalambro A, Grifoni C, Torricelli F, Camici PG, Cecchi F (2011) Microvascular function is selectively impaired in patients with hypertrophic cardiomyopathy and sarcomere myofilament gene mutations. J Am Coll Cardiol 58(8):839–848. https://doi.org/10.1016/j.jacc.2011.05.018

Park Y, Capobianco S, Gao X, Falck JR, Dellsperger KC, Zhang C (2008) Role of EDHF in type 2 diabetes-induced endothelial dysfunction. Am J Physiol Heart Circ Physiol 295(5):H1982–H1988. https://doi.org/10.1152/ajpheart.01261.2007

Paulus WJ, Tschöpe C (2013) A novel paradigm for heart failure with preserved ejection fraction. J Am Coll Cardiol 62(4):263–271. https://doi.org/10.1016/j.jacc.2013.02.092

Pearson JT, Shirai M, Ito H, Tokunaga N, Tsuchimochi H, Nishiura N, Schwenke DO, Ishibashi-Ueda H, Akiyama R, Mori H, Kangawa K, Suga H, Yagi N (2004) In situ measurements of crossbridge dynamics and lattice spacing in rat hearts by x-ray diffraction: sensitivity to regional ischemia. Circulation 109(24):2976–2979

Pearson JT, Shirai M, Tsuchimochi H, Schwenke DO, Ishida T, Kangawa K, Suga H, Yagi N (2007) Effects of sustained length-dependent activation on in situ cross-bridge dynamics in rat hearts. Biophys J 93(12):4319–4329. https://doi.org/10.1529/biophysj.107.111740

Pearson JT, Yoshimoto M, Chen YC, Sultani R, Edgley AJ, Nakaoka H, Nishida M, Umetani K, Waddingham MT, Jin H-L, Zhang Y, Kelly DJ, Schwenke DO, Inagaki T, Tsuchimochi H, Komuro I, Yamashita S, Shirai M (2017) Widespread coronary dysfunction in the absence of HDL receptor SR-B1 in an ischemic cardiomyopathy mouse model. Sci Rep 7(1):18108. https://doi.org/10.1038/s41598-017-18485-6

Rao SC, Thompson RC (2011) Coronary CT angiography as an alternative to invasive coronary angiography. In: Baskot B (ed) Coronary angiography – advances in noninvasive imaging approach for evaluation of coronary artery disease. InTech, Rijeka, p Ch. 06. https://doi.org/10.5772/21191

Shirai M, Schwenke DO, Eppel GA, Evans RG, Edgley AJ, Tsuchimochi H, Umetani K, Pearson JT (2009) Synchrotron-based angiography for investigation of the regulation of vasomotor function in the microcirculation in vivo. Clin Exper Pharmacol Physiol 36(1):107–116. https://doi.org/10.1111/j.1440-1681.2008.05073.x

Shirai M, Schwenke DO, Tsuchimochi H, Umetani K, Yagi N, Pearson JT (2013) Synchrotron radiation imaging for advancing our understanding of cardiovascular function. Circ Res 112(1):209–221. https://doi.org/10.1161/circresaha.111.300096

Sonobe T, Tsuchimochi H, Schwenke DO, Pearson JT, Shirai M (2015) Treadmill running improves hindlimb arteriolar endothelial function in type 1 diabetic mice as visualized by X-ray microangiography. Cardiovasc Diabetol 14:51. https://doi.org/10.1186/s12933-015-0217-0

Sumita Yoshikawa W, Nakamura K, Miura D, Shimizu J, Hashimoto K, Kataoka N, Toyota H, Okuyama H, Miyoshi T, Morita H, Fukushima Kusano K, Matsuo T, Takaki M, Kajiya F, Yagi N, Ohe T, Ito H (2013) Increased passive stiffness of cardiomyocytes in the transverse direction and residual actin and myosin cross-bridge formation in hypertrophied rat hearts induced by chronic β-adrenergic stimulation. Circ J 77(3):741–748. https://doi.org/10.1253/circj.CJ-12-0779

Toh R, Shinohara M, Takaya T, Yamashita T, Masuda S, Kawashima S, Yokoyama M, Yagi N (2006) An x-ray diffraction study on mouse cardiac cross-bridge function in vivo: effects of adrenergic β-stimulation. Biophys J 90(5):1723–1728. https://doi.org/10.1529/biophysj.105.074062

van Heerebeek L, Hamdani N, Falcao-Pires I, Leite-Moreira AF, Begieneman MP, Bronzwaer JG, van der Velden J, Stienen GJ, Laarman GJ, Somsen A, Verheugt FW, Niessen HW, Paulus WJ (2012) Low myocardial protein kinase G activity in heart failure with preserved ejection fraction. Circulation 126(7):830–839. https://doi.org/10.1161/circulationaha.111.076075

Waddingham MT, Edgley AJ, Astolfo A, Inagaki T, Fujii Y, Du C-K, Zhan D-Y, Tsuchimochi H, Yagi N, Kelly DJ, Shirai M, Pearson JT (2015) Chronic rho-kinase inhibition improves left ventricular contractile dysfunction in early type-1 diabetes by increasing myosin cross-bridge extension. Cardiovasc Diabetol 14:92. https://doi.org/10.1186/s12933-015-0256-6

Xu H, van Deel ED, Johnson MR, Opić P, Herbert BR, Moltzer E, Sooranna SR, van Beusekom H, Zang W-F, Duncker DJ, Roos-Hesselink JW (2016) Pregnancy mitigates cardiac pathology in a mouse model of left ventricular pressure overload. Am J Physiol Heart Circ Physiol 311(3):H807–H814. https://doi.org/10.1152/ajpheart.00056.2016

Yagi N, Shimizu J, Mohri S, Ji A, Nakamura K, Okuyama H, Toyota H, Morimoto T, Morizane Y, Kurusu M, Miura T, Hashimoto K, Tsujioka K, Suga H, Kajiya F (2004) X-ray diffraction from a left ventricular wall of rat heart. Biophys J 86(4):2286–2294

Chapter 16
Visualizing the Immune Response to Infections

Ulrich H. von Andrian

The immune system is tasked with detecting and responding to infections anywhere in the body. To accomplish this task requires the coordinated migration of immune cells and highly dynamic interactions of the migrating cells with their environment. Lymph nodes play a central role in this process by acting as local filter stations that prevent the spread of invading microbes and by providing a sophisticated environment to initiate and regulate innate and adaptive immune responses to antigens derived from pathogens, malignant cells and vaccines. To this end, lymph nodes harbor specialized antigen presenting cells and constantly recruit diverse lymphocyte subsets that engage in continuous immune surveillance and mount protective effector and memory responses.

Electronic Supplementary Material The online version of this chapter (https://doi.org/10.1007/978-981-13-7908-6_16) contains supplementary material, which is available to authorized users.

U. H. von Andrian (✉)
Department of Immunology, Harvard Medical School, Boston, MA, USA
e-mail: uva@hms.harvard.edu

Y. Toyama et al. (eds.), *Make Life Visible*,
https://doi.org/10.1007/978-981-13-7908-6_16

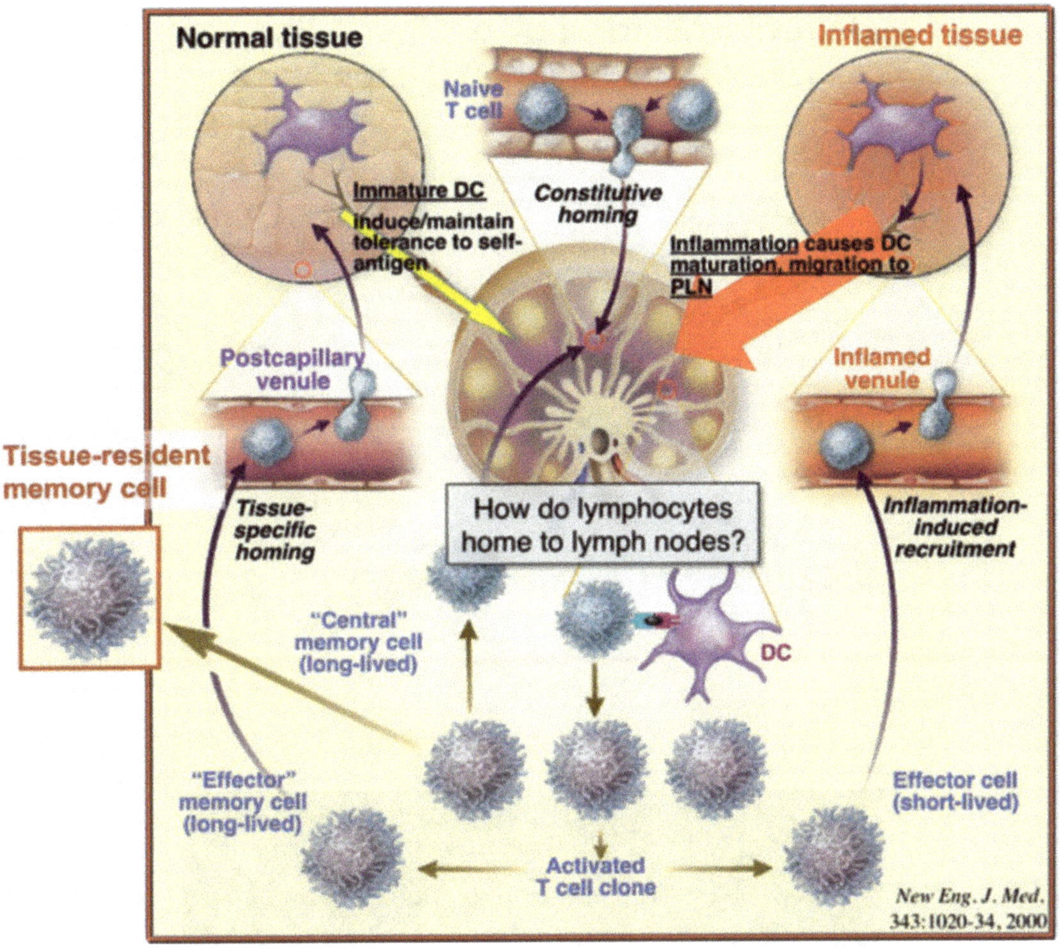

Our laboratory has developed intravital microscopy techniques that allow us to identify and track the intra- and extravascular trafficking and dynamic interactions of different immune cell subsets within lymph nodes of anesthetized mice. Using fluorescence imaging strategies, we have traced the dissemination of invading bacteria and viruses via the lymph and analyzed how lymph-borne pathogens are handled upon entering a lymph node. We have characterized how pathogen-derived antigens are presented to T and B lymphocytes and how the in vivo kinetics of antigen recognition impact anti-microbial immunity and the formation and quality of immunological memory.

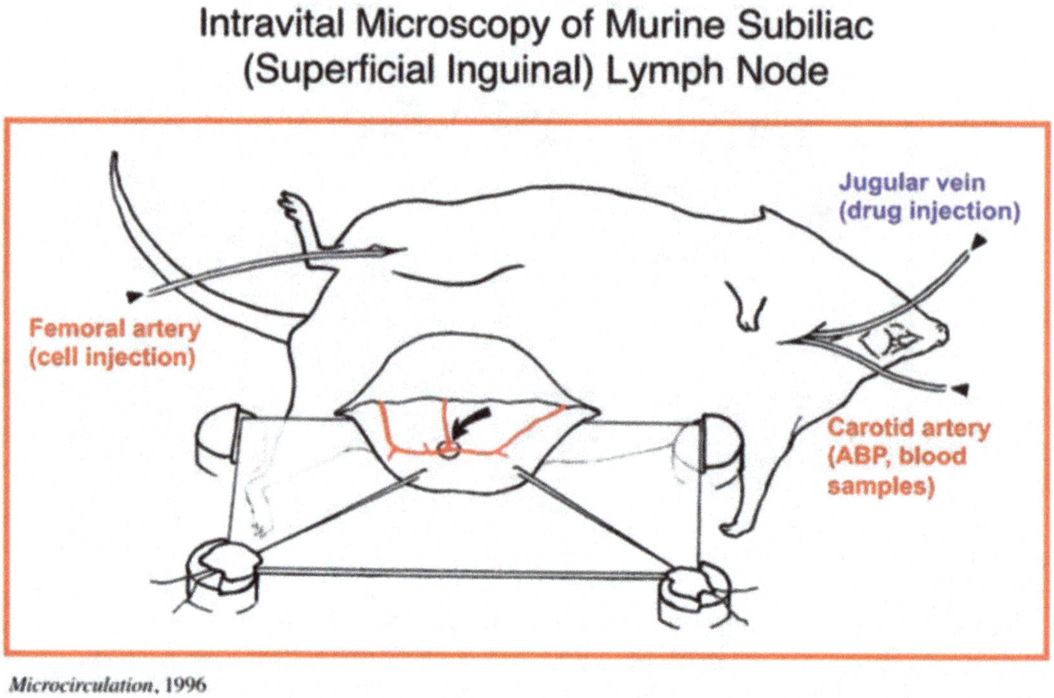
Intravital Microscopy of Murine Subiliac (Superficial Inguinal) Lymph Node
Jugular vein (drug injection)
Femoral artery (cell injection)
Carotid artery (ABP, blood samples)
Microcirculation, 1996

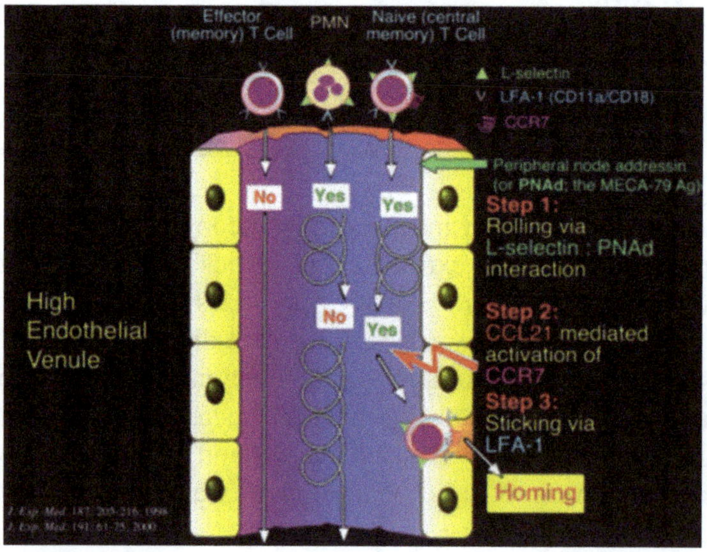
Effector (memory) T Cell
PMN
Naive (central memory) T Cell
L-selectin
LFA-1 (CD11a/CD18)
CCR7
Peripheral node addressin (or PNAd: the MECA-79 Ag)
No
Yes
Yes
No
Yes
High Endothelial Venule
Step 1: Rolling via L-selectin : PNAd interaction
Step 2: CCL21 mediated activation of CCR7
Step 3: Sticking via LFA-1
Homing

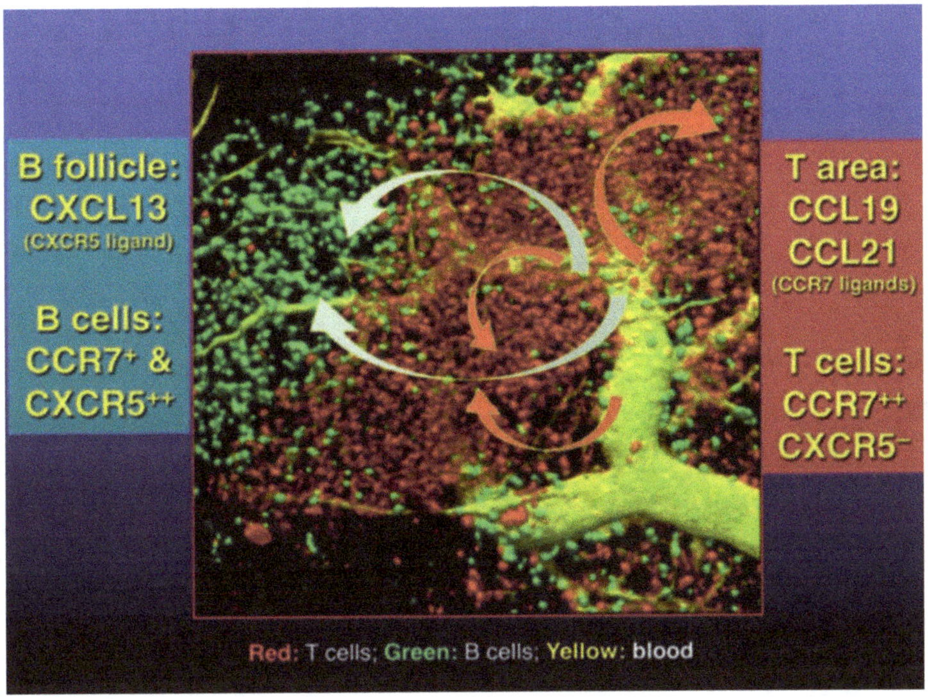

This lecture will provide an overview of our lymph node imaging strategies and summarize key insights that have been gained from their use to dissect the mechanisms and consequences of the multi-facetted immune responses to infections.

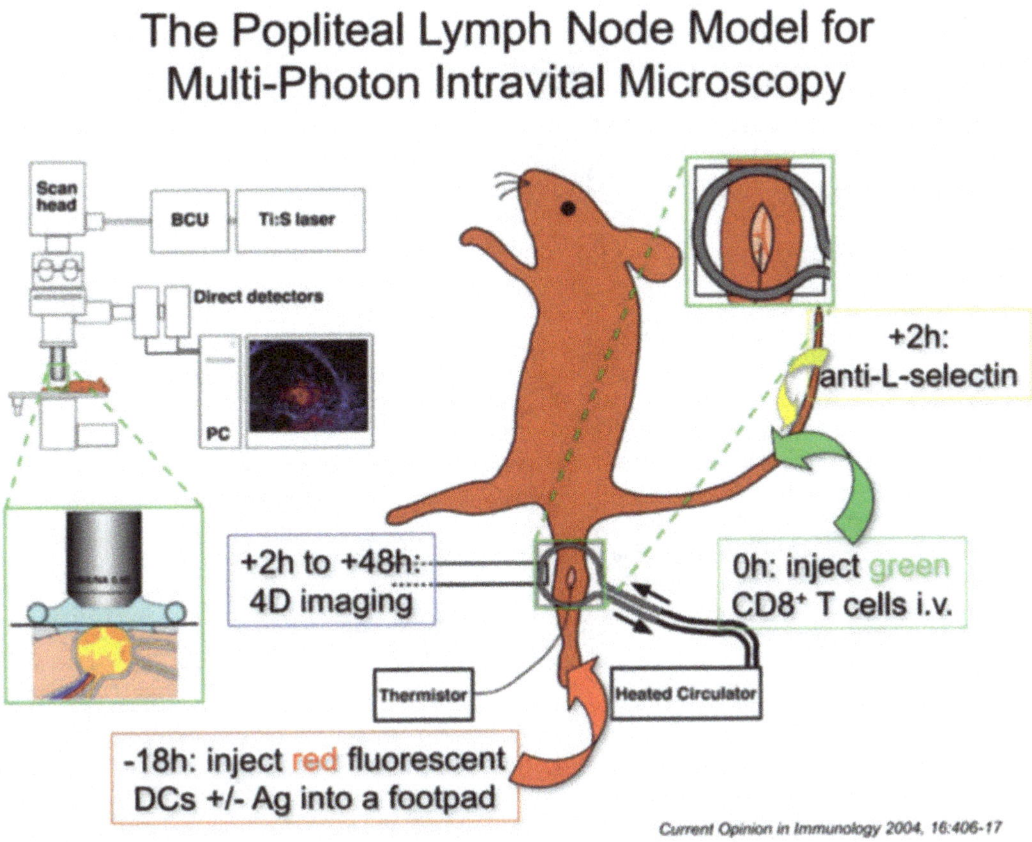

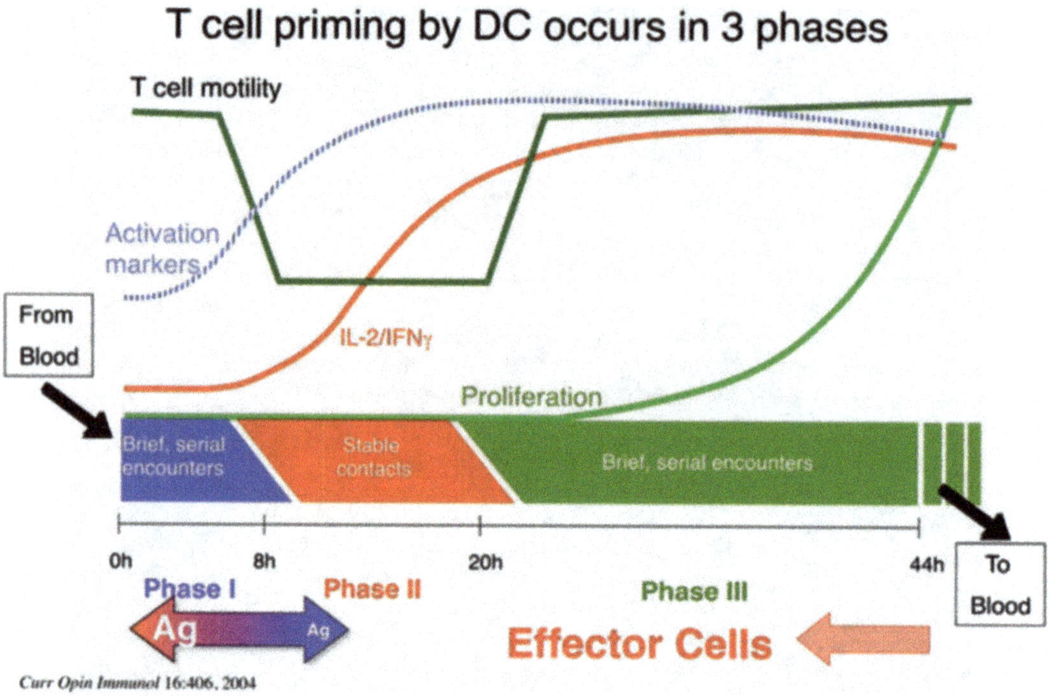
T cell priming by DC occurs in 3 phases
T cell motility
Activation markers
IL-2/IFNγ
Proliferation
From Blood
Brief, serial encounters
Stable contacts
Brief, serial encounters
0h
8h
20h
44h
To Blood
Phase I
Phase II
Phase III
Ag
Ag
Effector Cells
Curr Opin Immunol 16:406, 2004

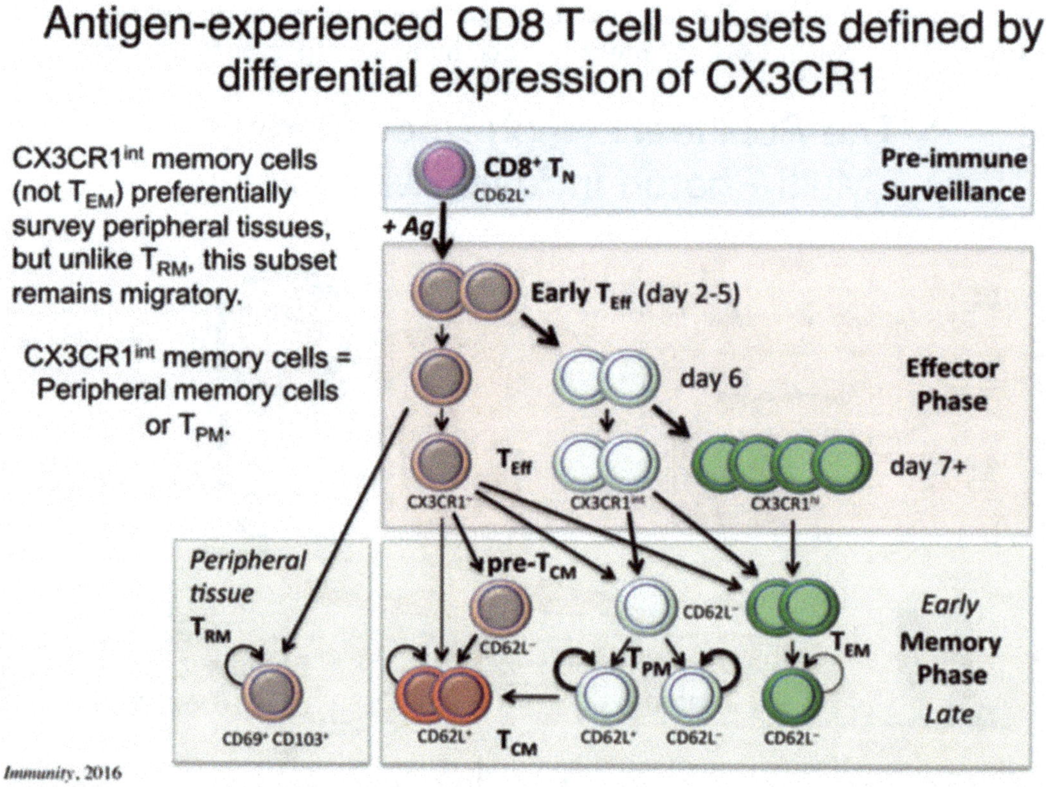
Antigen-experienced CD8 T cell subsets defined by differential expression of CX3CR1
CX3CR1^int memory cells (not T_EM) preferentially survey peripheral tissues, but unlike T_RM, this subset remains migratory.
CX3CR1^int memory cells = Peripheral memory cells or T_PM.
CD8+ T_N
CD62L+
Pre-immune Surveillance
+ Ag
Early T_Eff (day 2-5)
day 6
Effector Phase
T_Eff
day 7+
CX3CR1−
CX3CR1^int
CX3CR1^hi
Peripheral tissue
T_RM
pre-T_CM
CD62L−
CD62L−
T_PM
T_EM
Early
Memory
Phase
Late
CD69+ CD103+
CD62L+
T_CM
CD62L+
CD62L−
CD62L−
Immunity, 2016

Chapter 17
Imaging Sleep and Wakefulness

Takeshi Kanda, Takehiro Miyazaki, and Masashi Yanagisawa

17.1 Introduction: Behavioral Definition of Sleep

Sleep is considered to be a unique and essential phenomenon for life in all animals (Siegel 2008; Cirelli and Tononi 2008; Campbell and Tobler 1984). In fact, animals whose sleep is reduced for long periods eventually die under certain conditions (Rechtschaffen and Bergmann 2002; Driver et al. 2013; Shaw et al. 2002). The development of novel techniques for neuroscience research has rapidly increased our knowledge about the functions and mechanisms of sleep. First of all, what is the state of sleep? To answer this question, we must first define sleep. That is, a strict definition of sleep is the answer in and of itself. There are two major difficulties in defining sleep. First, while sleep seems to be a relatively simple behavior, it is not just a state of rest or immobility. For example, squirrels sleep immediately after arousal from hibernation, indicating that sleep is a distinct state with distinct functions from the energy-conserving rest state of hibernation. To distinguish between sleep and "non-sleeping" rest, sleep has been defined according to the following behavioral criteria: behavioral quiescence, characteristic stationary posture, rapid state reversibility, and elevated threshold to arousing stimuli (Piéron 1913). These criteria distinguish sleep not only from "non-sleeping" rest, but also from coma and anesthesia. Second, the sleep/wake cycle is linked with, but can be dissociated from,

T. Kanda (✉) · T. Miyazaki
International Institute for Integrative Sleep Medicine (WPI-IIIS), University of Tsukuba, Ibaraki, Japan
e-mail: kanda.takeshi.fu@u.tsukuba.ac.jp

M. Yanagisawa
International Institute for Integrative Sleep Medicine (WPI-IIIS), University of Tsukuba, Ibaraki, Japan

Department of Molecular Genetics, University of Texas Southwestern Medical Center, Dallas, TX, USA
e-mail: yanagisawa.masa.fu@u.tsukuba.ac.jp

Y. Toyama et al. (eds.), *Make Life Visible*,
https://doi.org/10.1007/978-981-13-7908-6_17

circadian rhythm. The sleep/wake cycle is controlled not only by the circadian rhythm, but also by homeostatic mechanisms (Borbély 1982). Homeostatic regulation is an additional criterion for defining sleep to distinguish between sleeping and circadian behaviors. In particular, animals exhibit recovery sleep after extended wakefulness. Based on these criteria, sleep can be defined behaviorally in diverse animal species, including genetic animal models such as the roundworm *Caenorhabditis elegans* (Raizen et al. 2008; Hill et al. 2014), fruit fly *Drosophila melanogaster* (Shaw et al. 2000; Hendricks et al. 2000), and zebrafish *Danio rerio* (Zhdanova et al. 2001; Yokogawa et al. 2007; Prober et al. 2006). Interestingly, according to these definitions, the jellyfish *Cassiopea spp*, which has a diffuse nervous system, also exhibits sleep-like behavior (Nath et al. 2017). On the other hand, some animals cannot be definitely judged to have sleep because they do not show behaviorally typical compensatory rebound sleep after sleep deprivation or reduced responsivity to stimuli during sleep-like behavior (Cirelli and Tononi 2008). Thus, the behavioral definition of sleep is highly variable, and could overlook sleep in certain animal species and several features of sleep, particularly the neurophysiological properties of sleep, as described below.

17.2 Oscillations in Sleep

Understanding the brain is critical for understanding sleep. In the early twentieth century, sleep in humans was reported to be controlled by several brain areas (von Economo 1931), which had also been experimentally investigated in non-human mammals (Jouvet 1962; Nauta 1946; Moruzzi and Magoun 1949). The brain not only controls sleep, but is also largely affected by sleep. Indeed, electroencephalogram (EEG), reflecting wide-range extracellular electrical activity in the brain, is currently used to provide a stricter definition of sleep (unless otherwise mentioned, EEG in this chapter refers to cortical EEG). The discovery of EEG brought two large changes to the concept of sleep: (1) the sleeping brain is not silent; (2) sleep comprises two main stages, non-rapid eye movement (NREM) and rapid eye movement (REM) sleep (Fig. 17.1). The first report of human EEG by Berger showed that

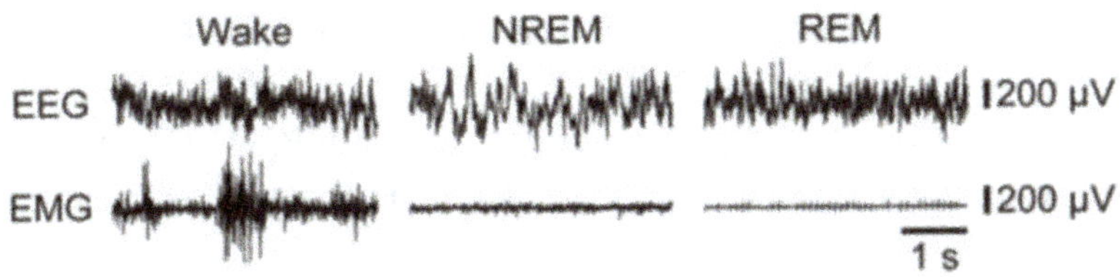

Fig. 17.1 EEG and EMG in a mouse during wakefulness (left), NREM (center), and REM sleep (right). EEG and EMG were recorded with screw electrodes inserted in the skull and stainless steel wires in the neck muscles, respectively. Note that EMG, especially of antigravity muscles, also reflects sleep/wake states: highest in wakefulness, lower in NREM, and lowest in REM sleep. (This figure is modified from Kanda et al. 2017)

EEG exhibits low-amplitude fast activity during wakefulness and large-amplitude alpha waves when the eyes are closed (Berger 1929). Adrian and Matthews later reported that slow waves are observed in EEG of deeply anesthetized animals (Adrian and Matthews 1934). Slow waves are also observed in EEG during sleep (Loomis et al. 1935a, b). Slow-wave activity (SWA, also known as delta wave activity, 1–4 Hz) is considered a hallmark of NREM sleep. Because of this feature, NREM sleep is also called slow-wave sleep. SWA is increased during recovery NREM sleep after sleep deprivation, suggesting that SWA reflects the homeostatic regulation of sleep (Borbély 1982; Tobler and Borbély 1986). The mechanism that underlies the generation of SWA, however, remains unknown. Aserinsky and Kleitman discovered another stage of sleep, REM sleep (Aserinsky and Kleitman 1953). Unlike in NREM sleep, EEG activity in REM sleep exhibits low-voltage desynchronized waves. As the name suggests, in REM sleep, electrooculogram shows high activity, whereas activity of electromyogram (EMG), reflecting the tone of antigravity muscles, shows lower activity during REM sleep than during NREM sleep (Fig. 17.1). Based on its unique characteristics, REM sleep is also called paradoxical sleep (PS) or active sleep. As described above, EEG activity closely reflects the state of sleep, including its homeostatic regulation. In addition, oscillatory activity in EEG during sleep occurs in mammals, as well as in amphibians, reptiles, and birds (Campbell and Tobler 1984). An EEG-based definition of sleep is more accurate but less applicable than the behavioral definition due to differences in nervous systems. EEG is usually recorded from the cerebral cortex, but most animal species have no nerve structure corresponding to the cerebral cortex of mammals. Importantly, however, although not recorded from mammalian cerebral cortex-like structures, electrophysiological oscillatory activity emerges in the sleeping central brain of the fly (Yap et al. 2017) and crayfish *Procambarus clarkii* (Mendoza-Angeles et al. 2007; Ramón et al. 2004), implying that neuronal oscillations during sleep is a common feature across animal species, including invertebrates.

17.3 Electrophysiological Insights into the Sleeping Brain

Oscillations associated with sleep are also observed in other electrophysiological events in the cortex, such as local electric potentials (LFP), extracellular multi- and single-unit activity, and membrane potentials. Cortical neurons exhibit changes in their firing patterns that correlate with the state of sleep/wakefulness: a tonic pattern during wakefulness, a burst-and-pause pattern during NREM sleep, and a rhythmic bursting pattern during REM sleep (Evarts 1964; Hubel 1959). In addition, short-term and synchronous cessation of firing occurs in cortical neurons during NREM sleep, which correlates with slow waves in EEG and LFP (Vyazovskiy et al. 2009, 2011; Destexhe et al. 1999; Nir et al. 2011). The active and silent periods of the cortical neuronal population in NREM sleep are referred to as ON and OFF periods, respectively (Vyazovskiy et al. 2009). Slow waves are detected not only in LFP, but also in the membrane potential and EEG during NREM sleep (Steriade et al. 1993a;

Achermann and Borbély 1997). Surprisingly, slow waves in LFP appear during both NREM sleep and REM sleep in the middle layer of the primary cortices (Funk et al. 2016). Intracellular recordings in the cortex reveal that oscillatory activity, which consists of periodic depolarizing (UP) and hyperpolarizing (DOWN) states, appears in both EEG and the membrane potential under anesthesia and during NREM sleep (Steriade et al. 1993a, b, 2001; Timofeev et al. 2001; Metherate et al. 1992). UP/DOWN oscillations in membrane potentials disappear during wakefulness and REM sleep (Steriade et al. 2001; Timofeev et al. 2001).

17.4 Imaging Techniques Show Novel Aspects of Sleep

Electrophysiology reveals various aspects of the state of sleep. The dynamics of extracellular ionic composition during sleep and wakefulness were recently revealed with ion-sensitive microelectrodes: extracellular Ca^{2+}, Mg^{2+}, and H^{+} increase, while K^{+} decreases, when falling asleep, and the opposite occurs upon awakening (Ding et al. 2016). These changes not only correlate with, but also cause, sleep/wake states. Infusion of high Ca^{2+}, Mg^{2+}, and H^{+}, and low K^{+} during wakefulness induces NREM sleep, while infusion of low Ca^{2+}, Mg^{2+}, and H^{+}, and high K^{+} during NREM sleep induces wakefulness (Ding et al. 2016). The development of innovative imaging techniques has greatly contributed to elucidating the physiological aspects of sleep. This chapter mainly deals with fluorescence imaging. The most notable progress in fluorescence imaging techniques is the development of genetically-encoded calcium indicators (Lin and Schnitzer 2016), which allow for visualization of neural activity in microstructures up to the whole brain with diverse microscopy techniques. Although anesthesia is often used during imaging experiments, anesthesia is similar to, but different, from sleep. Thus, experiments with unanesthetized animals are preferred for sleep research (Fig. 17.2). One advantage of fluorescence imaging, especially in vivo two-photon microscopy, is that it provides images with high spatial resolution of microstructures, such as, in sleep studies, the morphology and Ca^{2+} signals of the dendritic spines. Morphologic changes in the dendritic spines are thought to be a cellular basis of learning and memory (Lamprecht and LeDoux 2004; Kasai et al. 2010). Dendrite spines are tiny bumps on dendrites whose size correlates with the efficiency of synaptic transmission. In addition, stimulating dendrites induces long-term potentiation of synaptic transmission and increases the size of dendritic spines. Although sleep contributes to memory consolidation (Stickgold 2005; Walker and Stickgold 2004), it has been unclear whether spine turnover occurs during sleep after learning. Two-photon imaging of the rodent motor cortex revealed that, after motor learning, NREM and REM sleep induce Ca^{2+} signal–dependent formation and elimination of dendritic spines, respectively (Li et al. 2017; Cichon and Gan 2015). When no specific task, such as motor learning, is performed, however, a net loss of spines is observed during NREM sleep (Yang and Gan 2012; Maret et al. 2011), supporting the synaptic homeostasis hypothesis: synaptic weight is potentiated to enhance learning in the awake state, and synaptic

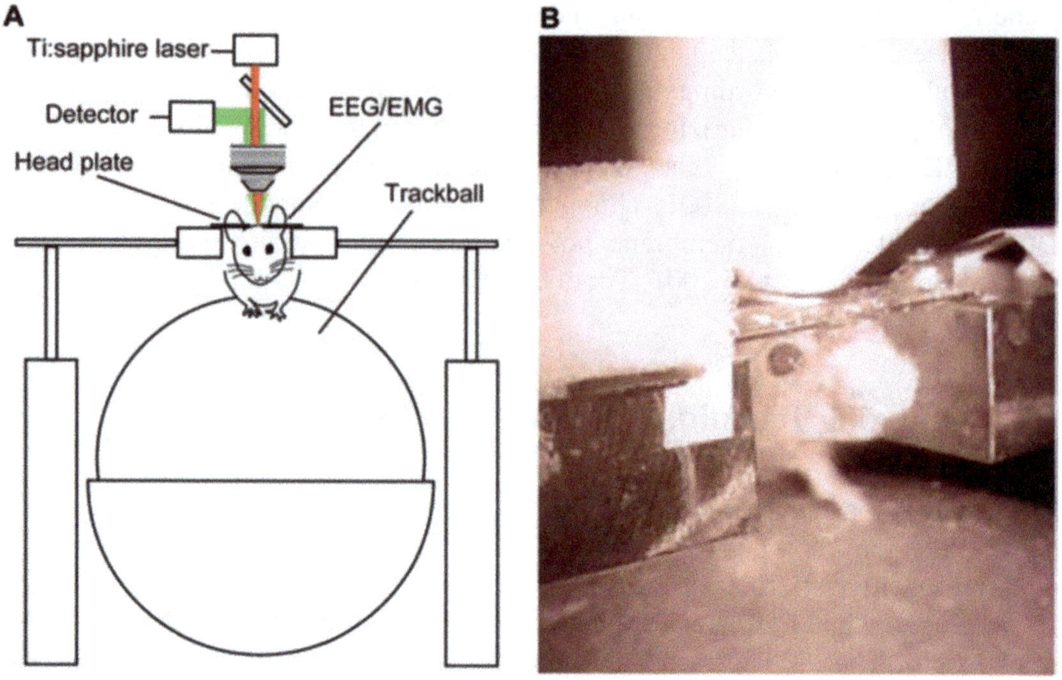

Fig. 17.2 Set-up for two-photon imaging from mouse brain during sleep and wakefulness. (**a**) Schematic showing arrangement of the head-restrained mouse, trackball, ball trackers, EEG/EMG electrodes, and custom-built two-photon laser-scanning microscope. (**b**) An infrared camera image depicting an awake mouse in the setup shown in (**a**). This setup allows for two-photon imaging in unanesthetized mice

downscaling occurs to save space and energy in sleep (Tononi and Cirelli 2006). Downscaling of synapses in sleep is driven by group I metabotropic glutamate receptors and Homer1a at postsynaptic densities (Diering et al. 2017). In the hippocampus, sharp-wave ripple oscillations trigger the downregulation of synaptic weights during NREM sleep (Norimoto et al. 2018). Another advantage of fluorescence imaging is the ability to visualize neural activity with cellular resolution in a wide-field, and in some cases the whole-brain. Whole-brain Ca^{2+} imaging during sleep and wakefulness in C. elegans revealed that sleep is a global quiescent brain state (Nichols et al. 2017). Ca^{2+} imaging in the mouse cortex revealed that neural activity is suppressed during NREM sleep as compared with wakefulness, and further suppressed during REM sleep (Niethard et al. 2016). Ca^{2+} imaging studies suggest that GABAergic neurons could contribute to suppress neural activity during sleep (Nichols et al. 2017; Niethard et al. 2016). Fluorescence imaging is also effective for studies of glial cells, especially astrocytes. The role of astrocytes in the regulation of sleep/wake states is still largely controversial, because there is no evidence that astrocytic Ca^{2+} dynamics correlate with sleep/wake cycles. Definitive conclusions await further in vivo imaging studies. Interestingly, astrocytes control interstitial fluid flow in the brain for clearance of the extracellular environment (Iliff et al. 2012), which increases during sleep and decreases during wakefulness (Xie et al. 2013). Thus, astrocytes might contribute to sleep function rather than sleep regulation.

17.5 Future Directions

Sleep has been energetically investigated using various techniques (Kanda et al. 2016). Electrophysiology can acquire accurate electric signals with high temporal resolution and signal-to-noise ratio, and has recently revealed new properties of sleep (Siclari et al. 2017; Watson et al. 2016). Imaging techniques combined with genetic engineering enables neuron-type–specific recordings (Fig. 17.3) that show activity patterns of specific neurons during sleep and wakefulness (Cox et al. 2016; Weber et al. 2018; Chen et al. 2018). Another advantage of imaging techniques is spatial analysis (Fig. 17.3). By combining mathematical analysis and imaging techniques, it is possible to capture the network structure of the brain spatially. In addition, imaging techniques can be used to measure the dynamics of neuromodulators in the brain, helping to elucidate brain states (Kanda et al. 2017; Wang et al. 2018). In mammals, sleep is well-defined by EEG. An electrophysiology-based definition of sleep is missing for animals other than mammals, however, whose sleep is defined by behaviors. If imaging techniques can be used to extract characteristic patterns of neuronal activity in sleeping animals, sleep can be defined by parameters that can be applied more universally than EEG. Further development of various imaging techniques will contribute to enhance our understanding of sleep.

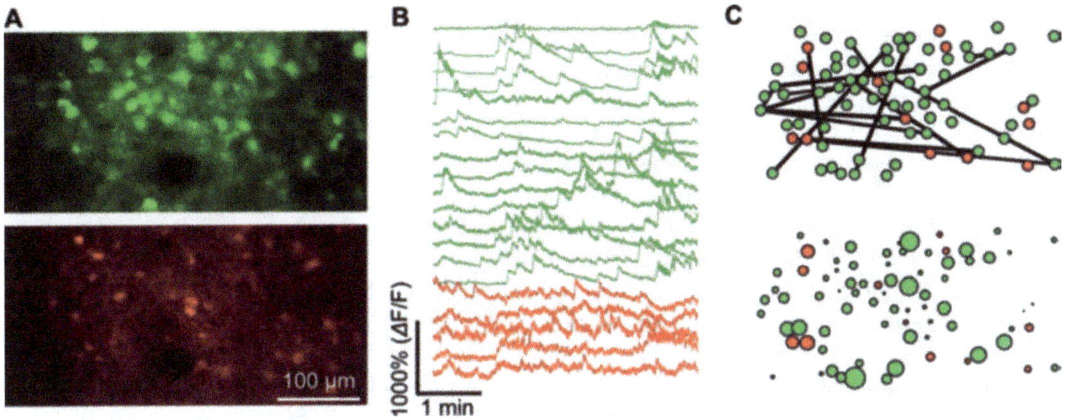

Fig. 17.3 In vivo two-photon Ca^{2+} imaging of cortical neurons. (**a**) A genetically encoded Ca^{2+} indicator, GCaMP6s (upper), and a fluorescent protein tandem dimer, Tomato (tdTomato) (lower), in the primary motor cortex layer 2/3. GCaMP6s was expressed in the primary motor cortex using an adeno-associated virus (AAV) vector. To identify GABAergic neurons, Vgat-tdTomato mice (Vgat-IRES-Cre; Rosa26-CAG-LSL-tdTomato-WPRE) were used. (**b**) Representative fluorescence signal (ΔF/F) traces from somata in (**a**). (**c**) Spatiotemporal analysis of Ca^{2+} signals in the field of (**a**). (Upper) Circle size represents the fluorescence intensity. (Lower) Green and red denote pyramidal neurons and interneurons, respectively. Black straight lines show the connectivity between neurons

References

Achermann P, Borbély AA (1997) Low-frequency (<1 hz) oscillations in the human sleep electroencephalogram. Neuroscience 81:213–222. https://doi.org/10.1016/S0306-4522(97)00186-3

Adrian ED, Matthews BH (1934) The interpretation of potential waves in the cortex. J Physiol 81:440–471

Aserinsky E, Kleitman N (1953) Regularly occurring periods of eye motility, and concomitant phenomena, during sleep. Science 118:273–274. https://doi.org/10.1126/science.118.3062.273

Berger H (1929) Über das Elektrenkephalogramm des Menschen. Arch Psychiatr Nervenkr 87:527–570

Borbély AA (1982) A two process model of sleep regulation. Hum Neurobiol 1:195–204

Campbell SS, Tobler I (1984) Animal sleep: a review of sleep duration across phylogeny. Neurosci Biobehav Rev 8:269–300. https://doi.org/10.1016/0149-7634(84)90054-X

Chen K-S, Xu M, Zhang Z, Chang W-C, Gaj T, Schaffer DV et al (2018) A hypothalamic switch for REM and non-REM sleep. Neuron 97:1–9. https://doi.org/10.1016/j.neuron.2018.02.005

Cichon J, Gan W-B (2015) Branch-specific dendritic Ca2+ spikes cause persistent synaptic plasticity. Nature 520:180–185. https://doi.org/10.1038/nature14251

Cirelli C, Tononi G (2008) Is sleep essential? PLoS Biol 6:e216. https://doi.org/10.1371/journal.pbio.0060216

Cox J, Pinto L, Dan Y (2016) Calcium imaging of sleep–wake related neuronal activity in the dorsal pons. Nat Commun 7:10763. https://doi.org/10.1038/ncomms10763

Destexhe A, Contreras D, Steriade M (1999) Spatiotemporal analysis of local field potentials and unit discharges in cat cerebral cortex during natural wake and sleep states. J Neurosci 19:4595–4608

Diering GH, Nirujogi RS, Roth RH, Worley PF, Pandey A, Huganir RL (2017) Homer1a drives homeostatic scaling-down of excitatory synapses during sleep. Science 355:511–515. https://doi.org/10.1126/science.aai8355

Ding F, ODonnell J, Xu Q, Kang N, Goldman N, Nedergaard M (2016) Changes in the composition of brain interstitial ions control the sleep-wake cycle. Science 352:550–555. https://doi.org/10.1126/science.aad4821

Driver RJ, Lamb AL, Wyner AJ, Raizen DM (2013) DAF-16/FOXO regulates homeostasis of essential sleep-like behavior during larval transitions in C. elegans. Curr Biol 23:501–506. https://doi.org/10.1016/j.cub.2013.02.009

Evarts EV (1964) Temporal patterns of discharge of pyramidal tract neurons during sleep and waking in the monkey. J Neurophysiol 27:152–171

Funk CM, Honjoh S, Rodriguez AV, Cirelli C, Tononi G (2016) Local slow waves in superficial layers of primary cortical areas during REM sleep. Curr Biol 26:396–403. https://doi.org/10.1016/j.cub.2015.11.062

Hendricks JC, Finn SM, Panckeri KA, Chavkin J, Williams JA, Sehgal A et al (2000) Rest in drosophila is a sleep-like state. Neuron 25:129–138. https://doi.org/10.1016/S0896-6273(00)80877-6

Hill AJ, Mansfield R, Lopez JMNG, Raizen DM, Van Buskirk C (2014) Cellular stress induces a protective sleep-like state in C. elegans. Curr Biol 24:2399–2405. https://doi.org/10.1016/j.cub.2014.08.040

Hubel DH (1959) Single unit activity in striate cortex of unrestrained cats. J Physiol 147:226–238.2. https://doi.org/10.1113/jphysiol.1959.sp006238

Iliff JJ, Wang M, Liao Y, Plogg BA, Peng W, Gundersen GA et al (2012) A paravascular pathway facilitates CSF flow through the brain parenchyma and the clearance of interstitial solutes, including amyloid β. Sci Transl Med 4:147ra111. https://doi.org/10.1126/scitranslmed.3003748

Jouvet M (1962) Recherches sur les structures nerveuses et les mécanismes responsables des différentes phases du sommeil physiologique. Arch Ital Biol 100:125–206

Kanda T, Tsujino N, Kuramoto E, Koyama Y, Susaki EA, Chikahisa S et al (2016) Sleep as a biological problem: an overview of frontiers in sleep research. J Physiol Sci 66:1–13. https://doi.org/10.1007/s12576-015-0414-3

Kanda T, Ohyama K, Muramoto H, Kitajima N, Sekiya H (2017) Promising techniques to illuminate neuromodulatory control of the cerebral cortex in sleeping and waking states. Neurosci Res 118:92–103. https://doi.org/10.1016/j.neures.2017.04.009

Kasai H, Fukuda M, Watanabe S, Hayashi-Takagi A, Noguchi J (2010) Structural dynamics of dendritic spines in memory and cognition. Trends Neurosci 33:121–129. https://doi.org/10.1016/j.tins.2010.01.001

Lamprecht R, LeDoux J (2004) Structural plasticity and memory. Nat Rev Neurosci 5:45–54. https://doi.org/10.1038/nrn1301

Li W, Ma L, Yang G, Gan W-B (2017) REM sleep selectively prunes and maintains new synapses in development and learning. Nat Neurosci 20:427–437. https://doi.org/10.1038/nn.4479

Lin MZ, Schnitzer MJ (2016) Genetically encoded indicators of neuronal activity. Nat Neurosci 19:1142–1153. https://doi.org/10.1038/nn.4359

Loomis AL, Harvey EN, Hobart G (1935a) Potential rhythms of the cerebral cortex during sleep. Science 81:597–598. https://doi.org/10.1126/science.81.2111.597

Loomis AL, Harvey EN, Hobart G (1935b) Further observations on the potential rhythms of the cerebral cortex during sleep. Science 82:198–200. https://doi.org/10.1126/science.82.2122.198

Maret S, Faraguna U, Nelson AB, Cirelli C, Tononi G (2011) Sleep and waking modulate spine turnover in the adolescent mouse cortex. Nat Neurosci 14:1418–1420. https://doi.org/10.1038/nn.2934

Mendoza-Angeles K, Cabrera A, Hernández-Falcón J, Ramón F (2007) Slow waves during sleep in crayfish: a time-frequency analysis. J Neurosci Methods 162:264–271. https://doi.org/10.1016/j.jneumeth.2007.01.025

Metherate R, Cox CL, Ashe JH (1992) Cellular bases of neocortical activation: modulation of neural oscillations by the nucleus basalis and endogenous acetylcholine. J Neurosci 12:4701–4711

Moruzzi G, Magoun HW (1949) Brain stem reticular formation and activation of the EEG. Electroencephalogr Clin Neurophysiol 1:455–473

Nath RD, Bedbrook CN, Abrams MJ, Sternberg PW, Gradinaru V, Correspondence LG et al (2017) The jellyfish cassiopea exhibits a sleep-like state. Curr Biol 27:1–7. https://doi.org/10.1016/j.cub.2017.08.014

Nauta WJH (1946) Hypothalamic regulation of sleep in rats; an experimental study. J Neurophysiol 9:285–316

Nichols ALA, Eichler T, Latham R, Zimmer M (2017) A global brain state underlies C. elegans sleep behavior. Science 356. https://doi.org/10.1126/science.aam6851

Niethard N, Hasegawa M, Itokazu T, Oyanedel C, Born J, Sato T (2016) Sleep-stage-specific regulation of cortical excitation and inhibition. Curr Biol 26:2739–2749. https://doi.org/10.1016/j.cub.2016.08.035

Nir Y, Staba RJ, Andrillon T, Vyazovskiy VV, Cirelli C, Fried I et al (2011) Regional slow waves and spindles in human sleep. Neuron 70:153–169. https://doi.org/10.1016/j.neuron.2011.02.043

Norimoto H, Makino K, Gao M, Shikano Y, Okamoto K, Ishikawa T et al (2018) Hippocampal ripples downregulate synapses. Science 0702:1–9. https://doi.org/10.1126/SCIENCE.AAO0702

Piéron H (1913) Le problème physiologique du sommeil. Masson, Paris

Prober DA, Rihel J, Onah AA, Sung R-J, Schier AF (2006) Hypocretin/orexin overexpression induces an insomnia-like phenotype in zebrafish. J Neurosci 26:13400–13410. https://doi.org/10.1523/JNEUROSCI.4332-06.2006

Raizen DM, Zimmerman JE, Maycock MH, Ta UD, You Y, Sundaram MV et al (2008) Lethargus is a Caenorhabditis elegans sleep-like state. Nature 451:569–572. https://doi.org/10.1038/nature06535

Ramón F, Hernández-Falcón J, Nguyen B, Bullock TH (2004) Slow wave sleep in crayfish. Proc Natl Acad Sci U S A 101:11857–11861. https://doi.org/10.1073/pnas.0402015101

Rechtschaffen A, Bergmann BM (2002) Sleep deprivation in the rat: an update of the 1989 paper. Sleep 25:18–24

Shaw PJ, Cirelli C, Greenspan RJ, Tononi G (2000) Correlates of sleep and waking in *Drosophila melanogaster*. Science 287:1834–1837. https://doi.org/10.1126/science.287.5459.1834

Shaw PJ, Tononi G, Greenspan RJ, Robinson DF (2002) Stress response genes protect against lethal effects of sleep deprivation in Drosophila. Nature 417:287–291. https://doi.org/10.1038/417287a

Siclari F, Baird B, Perogamvros L, Bernardi G, LaRocque JJ, Riedner B et al (2017) The neural correlates of dreaming. Nat Neurosci 20:1–52. https://doi.org/10.1038/nn.4545

Siegel JM (2008) Do all animals sleep? Trends Neurosci 31:208–213. https://doi.org/10.1016/j.tins.2008.02.001

Steriade M, Nuñez A, Amzica F (1993a) A novel slow (<1 Hz) oscillation of neocortical neurons in vivo: depolarizing and hyperpolarizing components. J Neurosci 13:3252–3265

Steriade M, Nuñez A, Amzica F (1993b) Intracellular analysis of relations between the slow (<1 Hz) neocortical oscillation and other sleep rhythms of the electroencephalogram. J Neurosci 13:3266–3283

Steriade M, Timofeev I, Grenier F (2001) Natural waking and sleep states: a view from inside neocortical neurons. J Neurophysiol 85:1969–1985

Stickgold R (2005) Sleep-dependent memory consolidation. Nature 437:1272–1278. https://doi.org/10.1038/nature04286

Timofeev I, Grenier F, Steriade M (2001) Disfacilitation and active inhibition in the neocortex during the natural sleep-wake cycle: an intracellular study. Proc Natl Acad Sci 98:1924–1929. https://doi.org/10.1073/pnas.98.4.1924

Tobler I, Borbély AA (1986) Sleep EEG in the rat as a function of prior waking. Electroencephalogr Clin Neurophysiol 64:74–76

Tononi G, Cirelli C (2006) Sleep function and synaptic homeostasis. Sleep Med Rev 10:49–62. https://doi.org/10.1016/j.smrv.2005.05.002

von Economo CF (1931) Encephalitis lethargica: its sequelae and treatment. Oxford University Press

Vyazovskiy VV, Olcese U, Lazimy YM, Faraguna U, Esser SK, Williams JC et al (2009) Cortical firing and sleep homeostasis. Neuron 63:865–878. https://doi.org/10.1016/j.neuron.2009.08.024

Vyazovskiy VV, Olcese U, Hanlon EC, Nir Y, Cirelli C, Tononi G (2011) Local sleep in awake rats. Nature 472:443–447. https://doi.org/10.1038/nature10009

Walker MP, Stickgold R (2004) Sleep-dependent learning and memory consolidation. Neuron 44:121–133. https://doi.org/10.1016/j.neuron.2004.08.031

Wang H, Jing M, Li Y (2018) Lighting up the brain: genetically encoded fluorescent sensors for imaging neurotransmitters and neuromodulators. Curr Opin Neurobiol 50:171–178. https://doi.org/10.1016/j.conb.2018.03.010

Watson BO, Levenstein D, Greene JP, Gelinas JN, Buzsáki G (2016) Network homeostasis and state dynamics of neocortical sleep. Neuron 90:839–852. https://doi.org/10.1016/j.neuron.2016.03.036

Weber F, Hoang Do JP, Chung S, Beier KT, Bikov M, Saffari Doost M et al (2018) Regulation of REM and non-REM sleep by periaqueductal GABAergic neurons. Nat Commun 9:354. https://doi.org/10.1038/s41467-017-02765-w

Xie L, Kang H, Xu Q, Chen MJ, Liao Y, Thiyagarajan M et al (2013) Sleep drives metabolite clearance from the adult brain. Science 342:373–377. https://doi.org/10.1126/science.1241224

Yang G, Gan W-B (2012) Sleep contributes to dendritic spine formation and elimination in the developing mouse somatosensory cortex. Dev Neurobiol 72:1391–1398. https://doi.org/10.1002/dneu.20996

Yap MHW, Grabowska MJ, Rohrscheib C, Jeans R, Troup M, Paulk AC et al (2017) Oscillatory brain activity in spontaneous and induced sleep stages in flies. Nat Commun 8:1815. https://doi.org/10.1038/s41467-017-02024-y

Yokogawa T, Marin W, Faraco J, Pézeron G, Appelbaum L, Zhang J et al (2007) Characterization of sleep in zebrafish and insomnia in hypocretin receptor mutants. PLoS Biol 5:2379–2397. https://doi.org/10.1371/journal.pbio.0050277

Zhdanova IV, Wang SY, Leclair OU, Danilova NP (2001) Melatonin promotes sleep-like state in zebrafish. Brain Res 903:263–268. https://doi.org/10.1016/S0006-8993(01)02444-1

Chapter 18
Abnormal Local Translation in Dendrites Impairs Cognitive Functions in Neuropsychiatric Disorders

Ryo Endo, Noriko Takashima, and Motomasa Tanaka

18.1 Introduction

Neurodegenerative disorders are associated with a wide spectrum of behavioral abnormalities including sensory, motor, memory and mental deficits (Orr and Zoghbi 2007). The neurodegenerative disease, frontotemporal lobar degeneration (FTLD), is characterized by neuronal atrophy in frontal and temporal brain lobes associated with marked deficits in cognitive behavior (Rascovsky et al. 2011; Irish et al. 2012). In FTLD brain, TAR DNA-binding protein 43 (TDP-43) is a major protein component of ubiquitin-positive hyper-phosphorylated inclusions (Neumann et al. 2006), suggesting that its aggregation is implicated in FTLD pathogenesis (Cohen et al. 2011; Ling et al. 2013). TDP-43 is a heterogeneous ribonucleoprotein containing two highly conserved RNA recognition motifs that are believed to selectively regulate RNA processing, such as exon splicing, mRNA transport and microRNA biogenesis (Lee et al. 2012) In neurons, TDP-43 is a constituent of neuronal RNA granules in dendrites (Lee et al. 2012; Wang et al. 2008) where it interacts with a complex of RNA binding proteins including fragile X mental-retardation protein (FMRP) and Staufen1, which collectively regulate mRNA transport and local translation (Wang et al. 2008), the processes that are critical for synaptic function and plasticity (Bramham and Wells 2007; Holt and Schuman 2013; Buffington et al. 2014). Considerable progress has been made to understand the molecular mechanism of neurodegeneration caused by TDP-43 aggregation (Baralle et al. 2013). However, it remains unclear how TDP-43 aggregation mediates complex behavioral phenotypes in FTLD including progressive impairment in mental function (Rascovsky et al. 2011; Irish et al. 2012). In this study, we investigate the causal mechanism for psychiatric symptoms in FTLD by testing the general hypothesis that, at least in some

R. Endo (✉) · N. Takashima · M. Tanaka
Laboratory for Protein Conformation Diseases, RIKEN Center for Brain Science, Wako, Saitama, Japan
e-mail: motomasa.tanaka@riken.jp

Y. Toyama et al. (eds.), *Make Life Visible*,
https://doi.org/10.1007/978-981-13-7908-6_18

neurodegenerative diseases, co-aggregation of casual disease factors like TDP-43, with genetic risk factors for psychiatric disease may alter cellular and behavioral phenotypes, resulting in overt manifestation of psychiatric symptoms.

18.2 Results

18.2.1 TDP-43 Forms Co-Aggregates with DISC1 in Neurons

We examined DISC1 as a possible binding partner for TDP-43 due to its aggregation-prone nature and well-established genetic role in mental illness (Leliveld et al. 2008; Brandon and Sawa 2011; Tanaka et al. 2017). First, we examined the co-immunoprecipitation of DISC1 and TDP-43 *in vivo*. DISC1 formed a complex with TDP-43 in both mouse and human brain and the binding interaction was higher in cerebral cortex than in cerebellum. DISC1 also bound to fused in sarcoma/translated in liposarcoma (FUS/TLS) and FMRP, both of which interact with TDP-43. Aggregation of a C-terminal fragment of TDP-43 in the cytosol is a hallmark of FTLD neurons (Neumann et al. 2006). Therefore, we examined whether DISC1 forms co-aggregates with the C-terminal fragment of TDP-43. Using a lentivirus system, we cultured cortical neurons that expressed an N-terminal Venus-tagged C-terminal fragment (residues 220–414) of TDP-43, termed TDP-220C that formed round-shaped aggregates in both cytosol and neurites typical of those observed in FTLD neurons (Fig. 18.1a) (Lee et al. 2012). These aggregates were ubiquitinated and highly phosphorylated (Ser409/Ser410) characteristic of aggregated TDP-43 in

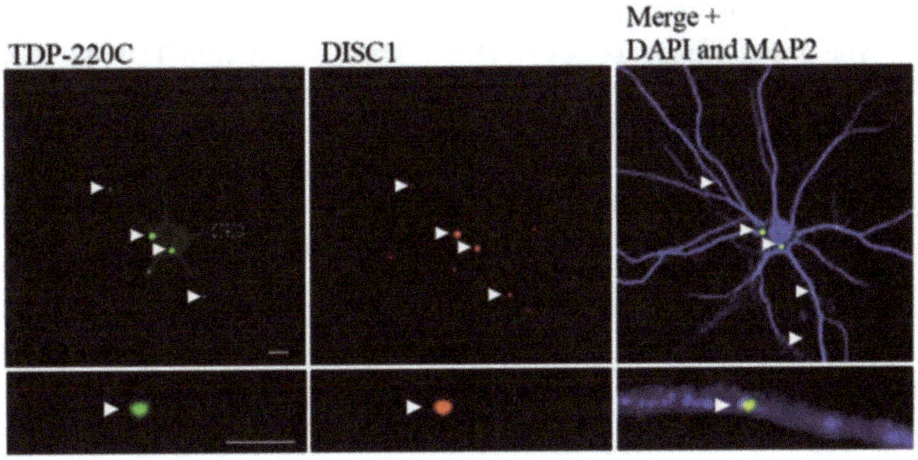

Fig. 18.1 DISC1 and TDP-43 form co-aggregates in neurons
Cultured cortical neurons were infected with a lentivirus expression vector encoding Venus-TDP-220C (green) and endogenous DISC1 was immunostained with an anti-DISC1 antibody (red). Nuclei were stained with DAPI (blue) and dendrites were stained with an anti-MAP 2 antibody (blue). A representative image is shown for the whole neuron (Top) and dendrite (Bottom), respectively. Scale bar represents 5 μm

neurons of FTLD brain (Neumann et al. 2006). Neurons with TDP-220C aggregates were immunostained with an antibody against DISC1, demonstrating that endogenous DISC1 co-localizes with TDP-220C aggregates (Fig. 18.1b). Furthermore, the filter trap assay showed that detergent-resistant insoluble DISC1 was increased in neurons expressing TDP-220C. Collectively, these results are consistent with the aggregation-prone nature of DISC1 (Leliveld et al. 2008; Tanaka et al. 2017), although physiological consequences of DISC1 aggregation in neuropsychiatric diseases remain poorly understood.

Several RNA-binding proteins such as TDP-43, FUS/TLS and FMRP were co-immunoprecipitated with DISC1. So, we asked whether RNA is critical for this interaction. To examine this possibility, we treated mouse brain homogenates with or without RNase, followed by co-immunoprecipitation with an anti-DISC1 antibody. RNase treatment abolished the binding of DISC1 to RNA-binding proteins, indicating RNA-dependence of the DISC1 association. This result suggests that DISC1 has a functional role in RNA metabolism to regulate neuronal functions. Furthermore, we investigated whether DISC1 regulates the abundance of synaptic proteins. When we examined amounts of postsynaptic proteins in synaptosomal fractions by western blotting, we found that the DISC1 depletion reduced levels of several key postsynaptic proteins in dendrites.

18.2.2 Role of DISC1 in Local Translation in Dendrites

To investigate whether the reduced levels of synaptic proteins in synaptosomal fractions might be caused by impaired local translation in dendrites, we examined the involvement of DISC1 in mRNA translation. Previous studies indicated that TDP-43 is associated with a translational machinery and polyribosomes (Higashi et al. 2013; Coyne and Siddegowda 2014). DISC1 can interact with TDP-43, therefore we examined whether DISC1 is also associated with a translational machinery by polysome gradient centrifugation analysis. DISC1 was detected in polyribosome fractions, as observed for TDP-43 (Coyne and Siddegowda 2014). After either EDTA or RNase treatment (Stefani et al. 2004), DISC1 in the polyribosome fractions co-migrated with TDP-43 and ribosomal S6 (RS6), indicating that, like TDP-43, DISC1 interacts with polyribosomes. Immunoprecipitation experiments demonstrated that DISC1 forms a complex with TDP-43 in the polyribosome fraction and that this binding was more significant in cerebral cortex than that cerebellum. Together, these data suggest that the DISC1-TDP-43 interaction is crucial for translation in cerebral cortex.

To further investigate the possible roles of DISC1 in local translation in dendrites, we examined whether DISC1 regulates translation of synaptic mRNAs in neurons by Surface Sensing of Translation (SUnSET), a method to monitor new protein synthesis by incorporation of puromycin into newly synthesized polypeptides (Schmidt et al. 2009). First, we assessed whether DISC1 might regulate local translation of synaptic mRNAs which are bound with DISC1. We labeled newly synthesized proteins in cultured cortical neurons with puromycin, and puromycin-incorporated proteins were immunoprecipitated from the synaptosomal fraction, followed by detection of newly synthesized postsynaptic NR2B and PSD95 proteins by western blotting. Remarkably, DISC1 knockdown significantly reduced synthesis of these synaptic proteins, which were restored by co-expression of an RNAi-resistant form of DISC1. These results suggest that DISC1 plays a critical role in dendrite local translation.

Neuronal stimulation induces local protein synthesis in dendrites (Ramocki and Zoghbi 2008; Ebert and Greenberg 2013). Therefore, we examined the effects of DISC1 depletion on new protein synthesis induced by neuronal stimulation. We evaluated new protein synthesis in a synaptosomal fraction with or without neuronal stimulation with KCl (Wang et al. 2008; Bading et al. 1993). In basal culture conditions without stimulation (5 mM KCl), newly synthesized protein levels were similar between control and DISC1-knockdown neurons. We confirmed that neuronal stimulation with 55 mM KCl enhanced protein synthesis in control neurons. In contrast, such an increase in new protein synthesis was not observed in DISC1-knockdown neurons, but the defect was restored by co-expression of the RNAi-resistant form of DISC1. To confirm the involvement of DISC1 in local translation in dendrites, we visualized puromycin-conjugated nascent polypeptides. We found the DISC1 depletion reduced new protein synthesis in dendrites under stimulation (Fig. 18.2), consistent with the observation by western blotting. Total mRNA levels in the synaptosomal fraction were not altered by the deletion of DISC1, suggesting that the decreased activity-dependent protein synthesis in DISC1-knockdown neurons is not caused by defects of mRNA transport but by impaired translation activity. Together, these results showed a novel function of DISC1 in regulating dendrite local translation that is dependent on neuronal activity.

18.2.3 TDP-43-DISC1 Co-Aggregation Inhibits Local Translation in Dendrites

Since endogenous DISC1 is readily sequestered into TDP-220C aggregates, we hypothesized that the co-aggregation between DISC1 and TDP-220C might impair local translation, similar to the DISC1 depletion. Overexpression of TDP-220C in neurons decreased synaptic protein levels in synaptosomal fractions, including surface-localized neuronal receptors. However, co-expression of DISC1 normalized the reduction of synaptic protein levels. Furthermore, the overexpression of TDP-220C in neurons impaired induction of new protein synthesis in synaptosomal fractions by neuronal stimulation, which was also restored by co-expression of DISC1. These rescue effects were not caused simply by reduction in TDP-220C protein levels due to the co-expression of DISC1. These results indicate that the loss of functional DISC1 mediates the impairment of local translation in the neurons containing TDP-220C aggregates. Together, our findings suggest that co-aggregation of DISC1 with TDP-220C selectively perturbs the role of DISC1 in local translation in dendrites.

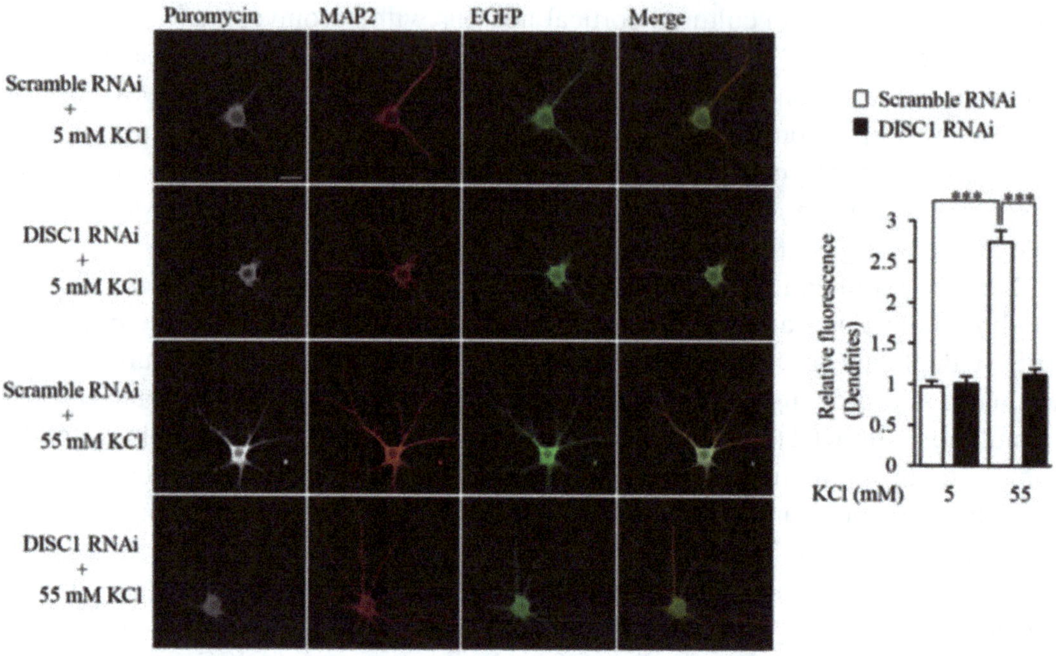

Fig. 18.2 Local translation in dendrites is regulated by DISC1
Neurons were immunostained with anti-puromycin (gray) and anti-MAP 2 (red) antibodies. The fluorescent intensities in MAP 2-labeled dendrites were measured and normalized by those in 5 mM KCl treated-control neurons (right). (n = 19,18,25,21 for Scramble RNAi +5 mM KCl, DISC1 RNAi +5 mM KCl, Scamble RNAi +55 mM KCl and DISC1 RNAi +55 mM KCl respectively. $F(3,79) = 74.17$, $P < 0.0001$, one-way ANOVA; $***P < 0.001$, Bonferroni's multiple comparison test *post hoc*). Scale bar represents 25 μm

18.2.4 DISC1-Dependent Behavioral Impairment and Rescue in TDP-220C Mice

We examined *in vivo* behavioral consequences of the co-aggregation of DISC1 with TDP-220C. To examine this issue, we stereotaxically injected adeno-associated virus (AAV) encoding N-terminally Venus tagged TDP-220C into the frontal cortex of mice (hereafter termed TDP-220C mice) at 6 weeks old. The AAV infection resulted in formation of highly phosphorylated TDP-220C aggregates in neurons of frontal cortex. We observed endogenous DISC1 and full-length TDP-43 sequestered into the TDP-220C aggregates. Protein levels of synaptic genes were significantly reduced in TDP-220C mice, consistent with the results from cultured neurons.

Next, we examined selected behavioral repertoire of TDP-220C mice after 2 weeks following AAV injection. TDP-220C mice showed significantly increased locomotor activity (hyperactivity) in the open field test while no change was observed in the time spent in a center region of the field between control and TDP-220C mice. In social interaction tests, control mice interacted with an unfamiliar stranger mouse than a familiar mouse for a longer time, but TDP-220C mice did not show significant differences (Fig. 18.3). Importantly, the time spent in each area was comparable for control and TDP-220C mice, indicating that the social interaction defect of TDP-

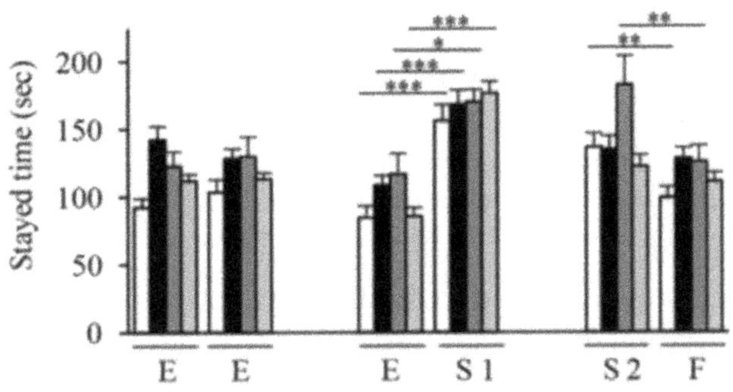

Fig. 18.3 Social deficits in FTLD model TDP-220C mice are mediated by DISC1 dysfunction
In the social interaction test, TDP-220C mice were less interested in novel stranger mice, which was rescued by the co-expression of DISC1. During the first encounter, all mice group spent more time in the area with first stranger mice (S1) compared to empty cage (E). During the second encounter, EGFP control mice spent more time with novel, unfamiliar mice (S2) than with familiar mice (F) whereas TDP-220C mice spend equal time with unfamiliar and familiar mice. This behavior was normalized by co-expression of DISC1. n = 23, 23, 21, 24 for EGFP (white), TDP-220C + EGFP (black), TDP 220C + DISC1 (dark gray), DISC1 + EGFP (light gray) mice, respectively (EGFP: $F(5,132) = 9.048$, $P < 0.0001$; TDP-220C + EGFP: $F(5,132) = 4.875$, $P = 0.0004$; TDP 220C + DISC1: $F(5,120) = 3.666$, $P = 0.004$; DISC1 + EGFP: $F(5,138) = 19.95$, $P < 0.0001$, one-way ANOVA, $*P < 0.05$, $**P < 0.01$, $***P < 0.001$, Bonferroni's multiple comparison test *post hoc*)

220C mice was not caused simply by their hyperactive phenotypes. We then examined whether the hyperactivity and the impaired sociability in TDP-220C mice could be normalized by DISC1 co-expression. We found that the rescue of the behavioral phenotypes could be achieved by DISC1 co-expression, indicating that restoration of DISC1 function was critical to normative behavior. Furthermore, we performed a Morris water maze test in order to evaluate the potential impact of TDP-220C-DISC1 co-aggregation on acquisition of spatial memory. TDP-220C mice, but not control mice, showed a significant learning impairment. We found that co-expression of DISC1 did not rescue the spatial learning impairment, indicating that the defect in the hippocampal-dependent learning task in TDP-220C mice is independent of DISC1 dysfunction. As an additional control, the grip strength test revealed that neuromuscular function was not affected in TDP-220C mice. Collectively, these results suggest that hyperactivity and disturbed sociability in TDP-220C mice are selectively mediated by the loss of DISC1 function due to the co-aggregation, providing support for the role of TDP-43/DISC1 interactions in mental conditions.

18.3 Discussion

In this study, we demonstrate that TDP-43, the causal protein in FTLD, co-aggregates with DISC1, a biological mediator for major mental illnesses, resulting in impaired local dendritic translation and disturbed social behaviors. The TDP-43-DISC1 co-aggregation compromised activity-dependent local dendritic translation and elicited mental deficits in FTLD model mice. Importantly, the psychiatric behaviors in the disease model mice were normalized by exogenous expression of DISC1 in frontal cortex, demonstrating that the loss of soluble, functional DISC1 due to co-aggregation is causally responsible for disturbed mental conditions in FTLD model mice. It has remained unclear why abnormal mental disorders are frequently observed in many neurodegenerative disorders. Given that local translation in dendrites is a critical process in higher brain functions (Buffington et al. 2014), our study has solved the long-standing puzzle of this neurological/psychiatric phenotypic overlap.

DISC1 was previously proposed to regulate synaptic plasticity and mental conditions, but the underlying molecular mechanisms have remained unclear (Tsuboi et al. 2015; Hayashi-Takagi et al. 2010). Our study reveals that DISC plays an unexpected role in determining activity-dependent local translation in dendrites, suggesting that DISC1 regulates the expression and hence function of postsynaptic genes in dendrites. Thus, our finding provides a candidate molecular basis for impaired synaptic plasticity and mental conditions observed in DISC1-knockdown neurons and DISC1 mutant mice (Hayashi-Takagi et al. 2010; Kvajo et al. 2011; Kuroda et al. 2011). Our results show that DISC1 regulates translation of mRNAs of critical synaptic genes, some of which are associated with psychiatric disorders. Our study validated, for TDP-43 and DISC1, the novel hypothesis that the co-aggregation of risk molecules for psychiatric diseases may account for latent psychiatric symptoms in neurodegenerative disorders.

Acknowledgments We thank Akira Sawa, Yoko Machida, Yusuke Komi, Shigeo Murayama, Masaki Takao, Hiroyasu Akatsu, Koko Ishizuka, Miles Houslay and the members of Tanaka Laboratory for helpful discussion. We are grateful to the Brain Bank for Aging Research at Tokyo Metropolitan Institute of Gerontology and Fukushimura Brain Bank, and the families of the patients for providing brain samples used in this study. DNA sequencing and preparation of polyclonal antibodies were performed at the Research Resource Center facility in RIKEN Brain Science Institute. Animals were maintained by RIKEN Brain Science Institute animal facility. This work was supported by The Uehara Memorial Foundation (M.T.), Grant-in-Aid for Scientific Research on Innovative Areas from Ministry of Education, Culture, Sports, Science and Technology, Japan (26116004 to M.T.) and RIKEN Aging Project (MT).

References

Bading H, Ginty DD, Greenberg ME (1993) Regulation of gene expression in hippocampal neurons by distinct calcium signaling pathways. Science 260:181–186

Baralle M, Buratti E, Baralle FE (2013) The role of TDP-43 in the pathogenesis of ALS and FTLD. Biochem Soc Trans 41:1536–1540

Bramham CR, Wells DG (2007) Dendritic mRNA: transport, translation and function. Nat Rev Neurosci 8:776–789

Brandon NJ, Sawa A (2011) Linking neurodevelopmental and synaptic theories of mental illness through DISC1. Nat Rev Neurosci 12:707–722

Buffington SA, Huang W, Costa-Mattioli M (2014) Translation control in synaptic plasticity and cognitive dysfunction. Annu Rev Neurosci 37:17–38

Cohen TJ, Lee VM, Trojanowski JQ (2011) TDP-43 functions and pathogenic mechanisms implicated in TDP-43 proteinopathies. Trends Mol Med 11:659–667

Coyne AN, Siddegowda BB (2014) Futch/MAP 1B mRNA is a translational target of TDP-43 and is neuroprotective in a Drosophila model of amyotrophic lateral sclerosis. J Neurosci 34:15962–15974

Ebert DH, Greenberg ME (2013) Activity-dependent neuronal signalling and autism spectrum disorder. Nature 493:327–337

Hayashi-Takagi A et al (2010) Disrupted-in-schizophrenia 1 (DISC1) regulates spines of the glutamate synapse via Rac1. Nat Neurosci 13:327–332

Higashi S, Kabuta T, Nagai Y, Tsuchiya Y, Akiyama H et al (2013) TDP-43 associates with stalled ribosomes and contribute to cell survival during cellular stress. J Neurochem 126:288–300

Holt CE, Schuman EM (2013) The central dogma decentralized: new perspectives on RNA function and local translation in neurons. Neuron 80:648–657

Irish M, Piguet O, Hodges JR (2012) Self-projection and the default network in frontotemporal dementia. Nat Rev Neurol 8:152–161

Kuroda K et al (2011) Behavioral alterations associated with targeted disruption of exon 2 and 3 of the Disc1 gene in the mouse. Hum Mol Genet 20:4666–4683

Kvajo M et al (2011) Altered axonal targeting and short-term plasticity in the hippocampus of Disc1 mutant mice. Proc Natl Acad Sci U S A 108:1349–1358

Lee EB, Lee VM, Trojanowski JQ (2012) Gains or losses: molecular mechanisms of TDP43-mediated neurodegeneration. Nat Rev Neurosci 13:38–50

Leliveld SR et al (2008) Insolubility of disrupted-in-schizophrenia 1 disrupts oligomer-dependent interactions with nuclear distribution element 1 and is associated with sporadic mental disease. J Neurosci 28:3839–3845

Ling SC, Polymenidou M, Cleveland DW (2013) Converging mechanisms in ALS and FTD: disrupted RNA and protein homeostasis. Neuron 3:416–438

Neumann M et al (2006) Ubiquitinated TDP-43 in frontotemporal lobar degeneration and amyotrophic lateral sclerosis. Science 314:130–133

Orr HT, Zoghbi HY (2007) Trinucleotide repeat disorders. Annu Rev Neurosci 30:575–621

Ramocki MB, Zoghbi HY (2008) Failure of neuronal homeostasis results in common neuropsychiatric phenotypes. Nature 455:912–918

Rascovsky K, Hodges JR, Knopman D, Mendez MF, Kramer JH et al (2011) Sensitivity of revised diagnostic criteria for the behavioural variant of frontotemporal dementia. Brain 134:2456–2477

Schmidt EK, Clavarino G, Ceppi M, Pierre P (2009) SUnSET, a nonradioactive method to monitor protein synthesis. Nat Methods 6:275–277

Stefani G, Fraser CE, Darnell JC, Darnell RB (2004) Fragile X mental retardation protein is associated with translating polyribosomes in neuronal cells. J Neurosci 24:7272–7276

Tanaka M et al (2017) Aggregation of scaffolding protein DISC1 dysregulates phophodiesterase 4 in Huntington's disease. J Clin Invest 127:1438–1450

Tsuboi D et al (2015) Disrupted-in-schizophrenia 1 regulates transport of ITPR1 mRNA for synaptic plasticity. Nat Neurosci 18:698–707

Wang IF, Wu LS, Shen CK (2008) TDP-43, the signature protein of FTLD-U, is a neuronal activity-responsive factor. J Neurochem 105:797–806

Chapter 19
Imaging Synapse Formation and Remodeling In Vitro and In Vivo

Shigeo Okabe

19.1 Synapse, Neuron, and Neural Network

The brain is a special organ dedicated for information processing that enables sensory perception, motor control and higher cognitive functions. Network of neurons is responsible for transmission, integration, and storage of information in the brain. Therefore, comprehensive description of complex neural network and extraction of the basic principles that govern the connectivity are essential in our understanding of brain function. This task is not simple and requires multiple-level analyses of the nervous system.

Neurons develop highly branched dendrites, which receive a large number of synaptic inputs, together with a long axon that enables connection with target neurons located in distant brain regions. Presynaptic axons contain synaptic vesicles and their exocytosis is coupled with arrival of action potentials (Munno and Syed 2003). Neurotransmitters released from presynaptic sites are immediately captured by postsynaptic receptors, which trigger either changes in postsynaptic membrane potential or activation of second messengers. Postsynaptic sites of neocortical pyramidal neurons form dendritic spines, which are tiny protrusions with a variety of morphology (Yuste and Bonhoeffer 2004). Neurotransmitter receptors on the cell surface are concentrated at postsynaptic densities (PSDs), a specialized region within dendritic spines (Okabe 2007). PSDs can be recognized as electron-dense structure by conventional transmission electron microscopy.

Electronic Supplementary Material The online version of this chapter (https://doi.org/10.1007/978-981-13-7908-6_19) contains supplementary material, which is available to authorized users.

S. Okabe (✉)
Department of Cellular Neurobiology, Graduate School of Medicine, University of Tokyo, Tokyo, Japan
e-mail: okabe@m.u-tokyo.ac.jp

Y. Toyama et al. (eds.), *Make Life Visible*,
https://doi.org/10.1007/978-981-13-7908-6_19

Connectivity of neurons is not homogeneous but distinct between different brain regions. In the neocortex, two types of neurons, excitatory neurons and inhibitory neurons, form local network. Excitatory pyramidal neurons release glutamate and inhibitory interneurons release γ-aminobutyric acid (GABA) from the axon terminal. The main information processing in the neocortex is mediated by connection between excitatory pyramidal neurons. Inhibitory interneurons regulate information processing by applying adequate suppression to the system. The most important question in the analyses of neocortical neuronal circuit is the relationship between neuronal connectivity and the mechanism of information processing. However, effective analytical methods that can achieve comprehensive and quantitative analyses of neural connectivity in the neocortex are not yet available at present.

On the level of the whole brain, reliable tracing technology of neuronal projections between distant brain regions is essential. This may be achieved by high resolution magnetic resonance imaging (MRI) in combination with injection of tracers and subsequent detection of labeled projections (Grandjean et al. 2017). Development of diffusion weighted imaging is rapid, but precise determination of axonal fibers is still difficult to achieve (Jbabdi et al. 2015). Physical tracers, such as fluorescent dyes and small molecules that can be taken up by living neurons, have been traditionally applied to neuron labeling, but these classical tracers cannot distinguish cell types, such as pyramidal neurons and interneurons, and also are not effective enough for complete detection of all axonal structures. Therefore, new genetic approaches for effective labeling of axons should be developed and applied for this purpose.

These arguments on the hierarchical architecture of the nervous system and the limitations of the available techniques indicate that it is important to develop new methodologies that integrate morphological and functional information on different scales. On the level of single synapses, high resolution imaging of synaptic structure and functional synaptic molecules are essential tools in modern neurobiology and in vitro imaging studies provided rich information about molecular mechanisms of synapse formation, maturation, elimination and remodeling. On the level of local neuronal circuits, morphological dynamics of axons, dendrites, and synapses in vivo can be recorded by two-photon excitation laser scanning microscopy in combination with appropriate surgical techniques for chronic imaging. In the following chapters, we will discuss these two major microscopic approaches to synapse dynamics.

19.2 In Vitro Imaging of Dynamic Synapses

In the initial attempt of understanding synapse development, researchers performed staining of neurons in culture or in fixed brain sections using antibodies specific for synaptic molecules and collected static images at different time points (Cohen-Cory 2002). In many cases, these studies utilized either the neocortex or the hippocampus as model systems and reported gradual increases in both presynaptic and postsynaptic immunoreactivity along the time course of development (Fletcher et al. 1991).

The electron microscopic observation also supported the data of immunohistochemistry (Harris et al. 1992). These morphological data were taken as evidence for the slow differentiation process of synapses after their formation and the concept of turnover of single synapses had not been introduced.

This situation was changed dramatically after introduction of the single synapse imaging technique applied to living neurons in dissociated culture system (Okabe 2017). Researchers initially predicted that nascent synapses are formed between neurons only in the early period of culture and these immature synapses gradually reach the mature stage in the following 2–3 weeks of the culture period. However, this prediction was not correct and live-cell imaging revealed continual formation of nascent synapses throughout the period of neuronal culture. For example, when a prominent PSD scaffold protein, PSD-95, tagged with GFP (PSD-95-GFP) is expressed in cultured hippocampal neurons, PSD-95-GFP is nicely localized to the PSDs within spines (Okabe et al. 1999). Distribution of PSD-95 puncta imaged at two time points with intervals of 24 h is markedly different, indicating that formation of individual synapses is a rapid process that takes place within a day. Quantitative analysis indicated that about 20% of synapses turnover within 24 h even when cultured neurons have been maintained for more than 3 weeks. More detailed analysis of both presynaptic molecular markers and postsynaptic spine structure further supported the idea of continual formation of nascent synapses in culture (Okabe et al. 2001). Namely, when new PSD-95 puncta appear, there is concomitant formation of presynaptic synaptophysin puncta and postsynaptic spine formation. These three processes are synchronized and complete within several hours, strongly suggesting that rapid establishment of the complete synaptic structure and molecular assembly is a highly frequent event throughout the development of neural circuits in culture system.

It should also be emphasized that synapse elimination is another important component of the synapse dynamics that takes place throughout the culture period (Fig. 19.1). Elimination rate of synapses is high in the mature neurons that have

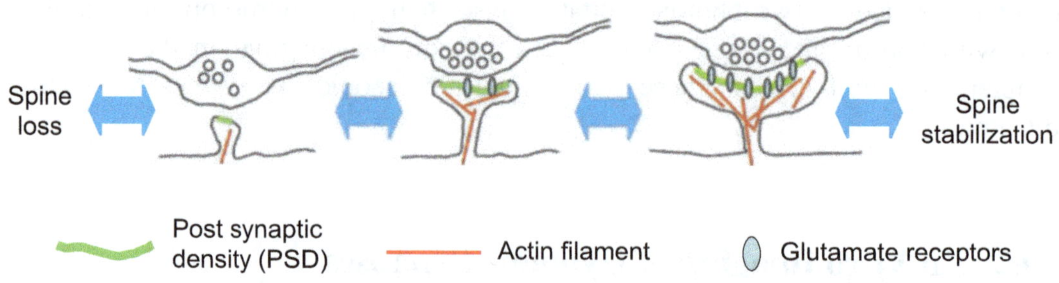

Fig. 19.1 Formation and subsequent stabilization of synapses. Synapse formation starts from appearance of nascent synaptic structure with a small PSD and a few synaptic vesicles. Subsequent increase in PSD size and accumulation of actin filaments in spines stabilizes postsynaptic structure. Recruitment of more synaptic vesicles in the presynaptic bouton and insertion of glutamate receptors are important in initiation of synaptic transmission. Not all of the newly generated synapses go through the entire process of synapse maturation in the developmental period. A large number of newly generated synapses reverse the direction and are lost after reduction of their structure

been maintained for more than 3 weeks in culture. Importantly, synapse formation and elimination are balanced and the subtraction of synapse elimination from formation is a good predictor for the overall trend of synapse density increase. Long-term observation of the synapse population on the same dendrites is possible by culturing neurons isolated from transgenic mouse lines expressing PSD-95-GFP or another abundant postsynaptic scaffolding protein, Homer1c, tagged with GFP (Ebihara et al. 2003). When the fate of single PSD structures is monitored over days, elimination of newly formed synapses and concomitant appearance of new synapses in the vicinity of lost synapses are frequently observed. This experiment confirmed the importance of the balance between synapse formation and elimination in setting the density of synapses within the optimal range.

How synapse density is regulated to be within the optimal range? To answer this question, candidate molecular pathways involved in the setting of spine density after maturation of the neural circuit should be identified. Our recent study of calcium-calmodulin-dependent protein kinase II-alpha (CaMKIIα) activity in regulation of spine density indicated that pyramidal neurons without CaMKIIα activity upregulate the rate of spine addition and show increase in spine density (Cornelia Koeberle et al. 2017). This CaMKIIα-dependent regulation of spine density is through the pathway of synaptic Ras GTPase-activating protein (synGAP) and the activity of the small GTPase Rap1. Because CaMKIIα protein content and its activity increase prominently in the postnatal period, this upregulation enhances Rap1 activity, which negatively regulates spine stability via increase in actin dynamics.

It is possible that the balance between formation and elimination of synapses is regulated not only by postsynaptic mechanisms, such as CaMKII activity, but also by the mechanisms involving presynaptic activity. Indeed, we identified presynaptic release of bone morphogenetic protein 4 (BMP4), a well-known signaling molecule for neuroepithelial differentiation in the early embryo, as a major regulator of synapse elimination in neural circuits of the hippocampus and the neocortex (Higashi et al. 2018). BMP4 is transported in dense-core vesicles along the axon, released locally in the vicinity of synapses in an activity-dependent manner, tethered to the plasma membrane of the perisynaptic region, and destabilizes nearby synapses. This effect is mediated through BMP receptors on the axonal surface and subsequent activation of canonical Smad pathway. This study clearly shows the existence of specific molecular pathway that controls synapse elimination with a spatial precision of single synapses.

19.3 In Vivo Imaging of Dynamic Synapses

Introduction of the technique of two-photon excitation laser scanning microscopy opened the way toward in vivo long-term monitoring of single synapses. In combination with appropriate surgical techniques to create optical windows over the brain parenchyma, single synapses can be followed for hours, days, and months in living animals (Grutzendler et al. 2002; Trachtenberg et al. 2002). Previous data collected in reduced preparations, such as dissociated neuron culture and slice preparations, can now be confirmed in the intact neuronal circuits in vivo. As in the case of synapse detection in culture, combination of structural markers, such as dendritic spines, and molecular markers, such as PSD-95-GFP, can increase the reliability of detecting spine synapses formed onto neocortical pyramidal neurons (Gray et al. 2006). One drawback in the approach of in vivo two-photon imaging is that only limited brain areas can be accessed by this technique, mainly because penetration of infrared light is limited to the cortical layer of less than 1000 μm in depth from the surface (Helmchen and Denk 2005). By using endoscope technology, synapse turnover in the hippocampus and other subcortical areas can be measured, but the technique is less reliable than the two-photon imaging, mainly due to the lower resolution (Attardo et al. 2015).

As stated previously, comparison of tissue sections with immunohistochemical staining of synaptic molecules revealed progressive increase in synaptic molecules in the early postnatal cortex. This increase in synaptic molecules is associated with increase in the density of synaptic structures detected by electron microscopy. These studies collectively indicate a stereotyped pattern of neural circuit development. On the other hand, synapse imaging studies in vitro revealed highly dynamic nature of individual synapses and persistent exchange of synapses even in the mature stage of neurons in culture. Therefore, one of the major questions is whether synapse turnover persists in the adult neocortex or hippocampus. The current agreement to this question is that, at least in the mouse neocortex, more than 90% of synapses are highly stabilized and can be maintained for several months (Zuo et al. 2005; Holtmaat et al. 2009). This observation indicates that synapse maturation in dissociated neurons does not reach the level of mature neocortex in vivo. This difference may be related to many factors that are not present in the culture environment, such as glial cells, neurovascular coupling, and synaptic connections with remote brain regions. Interestingly, recent in vivo imaging by the endoscopic technique reported continual remodeling of a large proportion of synapses in the mature hippocampus, suggesting regional heterogeneity in synapse stability (Attardo et al. 2015).

In vivo two-photon imaging can also be applied to developing neural circuits in the early postnatal period. However, it is not an easy task to create imaging windows without inducing activation of glial cells in young animals. The cranial bone is thin and soft and the animals are less resistant to inappropriate surgery and anesthesia. Our group successfully applied the technique of thinning the skull to the thickness appropriate for in vivo imaging at postnatal 2 and 3 weeks of mice and obtained the reliable data of spine turnover in the multiple neocortical areas (Isshiki et al. 2014). The data showed extensive turnover of spines positive with PSD-95-GFP and the turnover rate (up to 15–20% over 24 h) was comparable to that measured in dissociated neurons in culture. Importantly, the basic principle that the balance between formation and elimination of spines determines the net change in total spine density holds true in the case of in vivo synapse turnover. At postnatal 2 weeks, spine formation largely exceeds spine elimination, supporting rapid increase in the spine density.

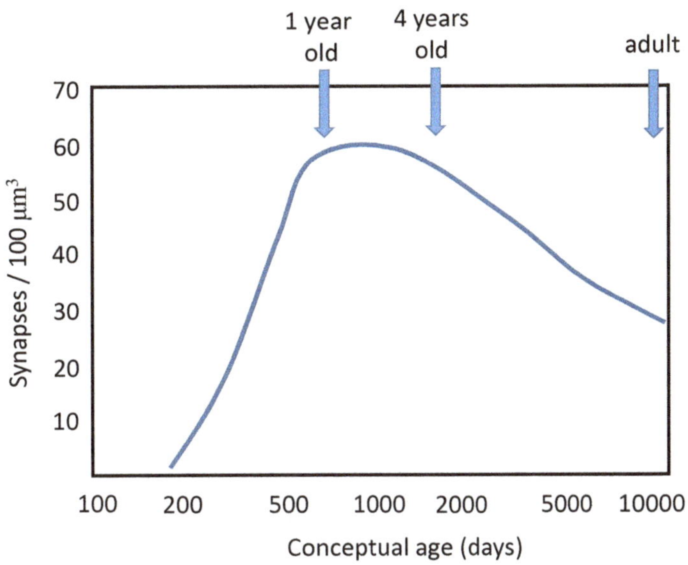

Fig. 19.2 The temporal profile of synapse density change in the human neocortex. The synapse density reaches the peak at 1–4 years after birth. After that, the density declines gradually in the rest of life. (modified from reference 21)

In turn, the two components are both suppressed and are balanced at postnatal 4 weeks, when the synapse density reaches the peak and starts to decline gradually afterwards.

Interestingly, this developmental profile of synapse density is common across different species including human, with different time scales. Previous studies show that the peak of spine density in the human neocortex is at the age of 1–4 years (Fig. 19.2) (Huttenlocher and Dabholkar 1997). The rate of spine increase is high before reaching the peak and the slow decline of spine density follows and persists thereafter. This specific temporal profile is preserved in both monkey (Elston et al. 2009) and mouse neocortex (Aceti et al. 2015). Synapse imaging data both in vitro and in vivo suggest that the initial phase of rapid construction of synaptic connectivity is regulated by the dynamic balance between synapse formation and elimination. Also this period corresponds to differentiation of specific functions in individual neocortical areas, such as sensory, motor, and association cortices, in response to the extrinsic signals from the environment. It is reasonable to assume that the intricate balance of synapse turnover in this early phase of circuit development profoundly affect the performance of the neocortical circuits thereafter.

19.4 In Vivo Imaging of Neocortical Circuits in Mouse Models of Developmental Disorders

Impairment in cortical information processing is thought to underlie behavioral deficits in autism spectrum disorders (ASDs). Advancement in the diagnostic techniques enabled screening of ASDs by 3 years of age. Because of relatively small changes in the cellular architecture and little signs of neurodegeneration in the patient brain, pathogenesis of ASDs is proposed to be associated with formation of inappropriate connectivity between cortical neurons (Bourgeron 2015). In support of this hypothesis, recent genetic studies of copy number variants (CNVs) and gene mutations reported that genes encoding synaptic cell adhesion molecules (postsynaptic cell adhesion molecules neurogilin-3 and -4, and their presynaptic binding partners neurexin-1), and PSD scaffolding molecules (Shank2 and Shank3) are involved in increasing the risk of ASDs. These genetic studies indicate that detection of proper synaptic binding partners and maintenance of postsynaptic structures are impaired by these genetic mutations and subsequent accumulation of mismatches in neuronal connectivity may lead to dysfunction of local neuronal circuits in the neocortex. Once the neocortical neuronal connectivity is stabilized in the mature brain, the impairment in the circuit becomes resistant to therapeutic intervention and the associated clinical symptoms, such as repetitive behavior and reduced social communication, may persist throughout life.

Recent progress in mouse molecular genetics enable us to create mouse models of ASDs. Several types of CNVs have been reported in ASD patients and the most frequently reported copy number variation in ASD, the duplication of 15q11-13, has been mimicked in mice by creating the genomic duplication in the corresponding genomic region of the mouse chromosome 7 (patDp/+ mice)(Nakatani et al. 2009). This mouse model shows impairment in social behaviors and imbalance of excitatory and inhibitory synaptic transmission, which are common phenotypes seen in mouse models of ASDs. Another reliable model of ASD was created by introducing a point mutation in the coding region of neuroligin 3 (NLG R451C mice) (Tabuchi et al. 2007). This point mutation is responsible for the alterations again in the balance of excitatory and inhibitory synapses in the neocortex, together with impairment in synaptic plasticity and social behaviors. These two models are heterogeneous in their genetic properties, but show similar impairments in the functions of neocortical circuits and behaviors. Therefore, it is reasonable to expect common alterations in neocortical synapse development in the early postnatal period. Initial quantitative analysis of spine and synapse, together with the analysis of their morphology, could not detect any significant change in these mutant mice, suggesting that the static analysis of spines and synapses is not sufficient to detect the phenotypes (Isshiki et al. 2014). In spite of little changes in spine synapse density and morphology, in vivo two-photon imaging of spine synapses in the neocortex of patDp/+ mice and NLG R451C mice revealed prominent upregulation of spine turnover at postnatal 3 weeks. This upregulation is more prominent in spines containing PSD-95 clusters, suggesting that spines with functional synaptic connectivity are more severely affected. In addition, the phenotype is specific to spines receiving intracortical projections while spines contacting with the thalamocortical projections are unaffected. This selective impairment in the intracortical connections may be responsible for behavioral phenotypes of the mutant mice, such as deficits in social behavior, which are thought to be related to functions in the association cortex. We observed similar upregulation of cortical spine synapses in the third ASD mouse model, BTBR mice. This strain also exhibits clear impairment in ASD-related behaviors, such as social interactions and repetitive behaviors (McFarlane et al. 2008). In Fmr1 knockout mice, a model of fragile X syndrome and syndromic autism, spine turnover in the neocortex is also reported to be upregulated (Pan et al. 2010). Taken together, these results indicate that higher synapse turnover in the early postnatal period is a shared synapse-level phenotype across ASD mouse models.

Based on our observation of synapse dynamics in multiple mouse models of ASDs, together with reports from other laboratories, we propose that multiple genetic and environmental risk factors operate in the early postnatal period and their effects converge towards upregulation of cortical synapse turnover, which subsequently induce increased misconnections of cortical neurons and its dysfunction (Fig. 19.3). Although it is widely accepted that the imbalance between excitatory and inhibitory synapses underlies the dysfunction of ASD brain, the relationship between enhanced synapse turnover and the excitatory-inhibitory imbalance has not yet been clarified (Han et al. 2012; Nakai et al. 2017). One possible explanation is that the late maturation of inhibitory neurons in the cortex requires an adequate level of excitatory inputs within the cortex, and this excitatory drive is reduced after initial increase in the misconnections caused by increased synapse turnover. This model is consistent with our observation of reduced activity in layer II/III neurons

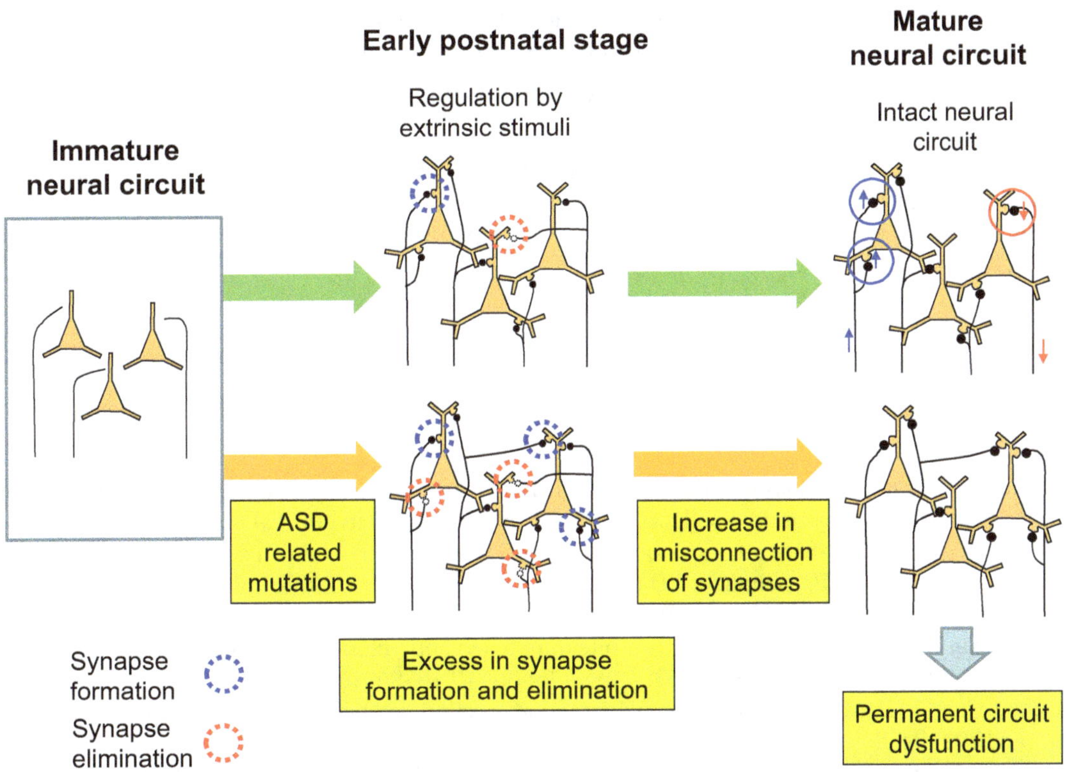

Fig. 19.3 A proposed model of neural circuit dysfunction in mouse models of ASD. Synaptic connections increase during the early postnatal period. Excess in synapse formation and elimination seen in the mouse models of ASD increases the probability of synaptic misconnection. This inhibits proper activation of neural circuits in the neocortex in the mature brain and leads to behavioral phenotypes

after enhancement of whisker-related sensory experience in both patDp/+ mice and NLG R451C mice. If the activity in the neocortex is reduced, inhibitory system may be less developed, and after maturation of the system, the local cortical circuits will become less resistant to the excess amount of sensory inputs. This scenario can explain higher probability of epileptic episodes in multiple mouse models of ASDs and also in ASD patients.

19.5 Perspectives

Progress in synapse neurobiology has been accelerated by development of novel imaging technologies. Fluorescent protein-based live cell imaging is a powerful approach toward detection of single synapses and their remodeling in culture. Application of two-photon excitation microscopy to visualization of synapse dynamics in the brain of living mice provided indispensable information about stability and lifetime of individual spine synapses. This technique was also proved to be useful in detection of synapse pathology in mice containing genetic mutations seen in human patients of neurodevelopmental disorders. In future, further advancements in both light microscopic and electron microscopic techniques of synapse visualization will promote our understanding of neural circuit construction and remodeling in development, maturation, and aging.

Acknowledgements This study was supported by the Uehara Memorial Foundation, Grants-in-Aid for Scientific Research (17H01387, 26250014 and 25117006), and Core Research for Evolutional Science and Technology from the Japanese Science and Technology Agency (JPMJCR14W2).

References

Aceti M, Creson TK, Vaissiere T et al (2015) Syngap1 haploinsufficiency damages a postnatal critical period of pyramidal cell structural maturation linked to cortical circuit assembly. Biol Psychiatry 77:805–815. https://doi.org/10.1016/j.biopsych.2014.08.001

Attardo A, Fitzgerald JE, Schnitzer MJ (2015) Impermanence of dendritic spines in live adult CA1 hippocampus. Nature 523:592–596. https://doi.org/10.1038/nature14467

Bourgeron T (2015) From the genetic architecture to synaptic plasticity in autism spectrum disorder. Nat Rev Neurosci 16:551–563. https://doi.org/10.1038/nrn3992

Cohen-Cory S (2002) The developing synapse: construction and modulation of synaptic structures and circuits. Science 298:770–776. https://doi.org/10.1126/science.1075510

Cornelia Koeberle S, Tanaka S, Kuriu T et al (2017) Developmental stage-dependent regulation of spine formation by calcium-calmodulin-dependent protein kinase IIα and Rap1. Sci Rep 7. https://doi.org/10.1038/s41598-017-13728-y

Ebihara T, Kawabata I, Usui S et al (2003) Synchronized formation and remodeling of postsynaptic densities: long-term visualization of hippocampal neurons expressing postsynaptic density proteins tagged with green fluorescent protein. J Neurosci 23:2170–2181. 23/6/2170 [pii]

Elston GN, Oga T, Fujita I (2009) Spinogenesis and pruning scales across functional hierarchies. J Neurosci 29:3271–3275. https://doi.org/10.1523/JNEUROSCI.5216-08.2009

Fletcher TL, Cameron P, De Camilli P, Banker G (1991) The distribution of synapsin I and synaptophysin in hippocampal neurons developing in culture. J Neurosci 11:1617–1626. https://doi.org/10.1103/PhysRevLett.114.173002

Grandjean J, Zerbi V, Balsters J et al (2017) The structural basis of large-scale functional connectivity in the mouse. J Neurosci:438–417. https://doi.org/10.1523/JNEUROSCI.0438-17.2017

Gray NW, Weimer RM, Bureau I, Svoboda K (2006) Rapid redistribution of synaptic PSD-95 in the neocortex in vivo. PLoS Biol 4:2065–2075. https://doi.org/10.1371/journal.pbio.0040370

Grutzendler J, Kasthuri N, Gan WBW-B (2002) Long-term dendritic spine stability in the adult cortex. Nature 420:812–816. https://doi.org/10.1038/nature01151.1

Han S, Tai C, Westenbroek RE et al (2012) Autistic-like behaviour in Scn1a +− mice and rescue by enhanced GABA-mediated neurotransmission. Nature 489:385–390. https://doi.org/10.1038/nature11356

Harris KM, Jensen FE, Tsao B (1992) Three-dimensional structure of dendritic spines and synapses in rat hippocampus (CA1) at postnatal day 15 and adult ages: implications for the maturation of synaptic physiology and long-term potentiation. J Neurosci 12:2685–2705. https://doi.org/10.1016/j.tcb.2009.06.001

Helmchen F, Denk W (2005) Deep tissue two-photon microscopy. Nat Methods 2:932–940. https://doi.org/10.1038/nmeth818

Higashi T, Tanaka S, IIda T, Okabe S (2018) Synapse elimination triggered by BMP4 exocytosis and presynaptic BMP receptor activation. Cell Rep 22(4):919–929

Holtmaat A, Bonhoeffer T, Chow DK et al (2009) Long-term, high-resolution imaging in the mouse neocortex through a chronic cranial window. Nat Protoc 4:1128–1144. https://doi.org/10.1038/nprot.2009.89.Long-term

Huttenlocher PR, Dabholkar AS (1997) Regional differences in synaptogenesis in human cerebral cortex. J Comp Neurol 387:167–178. https://doi.org/10.1002/(SICI)1096-9861(19971020)387:2<167::AID-CNE1>3.0.CO;2-Z

Isshiki M, Tanaka S, Kuriu T et al (2014) Enhanced synapse remodelling as a common phenotype in mouse models of autism. Nat Commun 5:4742. https://doi.org/10.1038/ncomms5742

Jbabdi S, Sotiropoulos SN, Haber SN et al (2015) Measuring macroscopic brain connections in vivo. Nat Neurosci 18:1546–1555. https://doi.org/10.1038/nn.4134

McFarlane HG, Kusek GK, Yang M et al (2008) Autism-like behavioral phenotypes in BTBR T+tf/J mice. Genes Brain Behav 7:152–163. https://doi.org/10.1111/j.1601-183X.2007.00330.x

Munno DW, Syed NI (2003) Synaptogenesis in the CNS: an odyssey from wiring together to firing together. J Physiol 552:1–11. https://doi.org/10.1113/jphysiol.2003.045062

Nakai N, Nagano M, Saitow F et al (2017) Serotonin rebalances cortical tuning and behavior linked to autism symptoms in 15q11-13 CNV mice. Sci Adv 3:e1603001. https://doi.org/10.1126/sciadv.1603001

Nakatani J, Tamada K, Hatanaka F et al (2009) Abnormal behavior in a chromosome- engineered mouse model for human 15q11-13 duplication seen in autism. Cell 137:1235–1246. https://doi.org/10.1016/j.cell.2009.04.024

Okabe S (2007) Molecular anatomy of the postsynaptic density. Mol Cell Neurosci 34:503–518. https://doi.org/10.1016/j.mcn.2007.01.006

Okabe S (2017) Fluorescence imaging of synapse dynamics in normal circuit maturation and in developmental disorders. Proc Jpn Acad Ser B Phys Biol Sci 93:483–497. https://doi.org/10.2183/pjab.93.029

Okabe S, Kim HD, Miwa A et al (1999) Continual remodeling of postsynaptic density and its regulation by synaptic activity. Nat Neurosci 2:804–811. https://doi.org/10.1038/12175

Okabe S, Miwa A, Okado H (2001) Spine formation and correlated assembly of presynaptic and postsynaptic molecules. J Neurosci 21:6105–6114. 21/16/6105 [pii]

Pan F, Aldridge GM, Greenough WT, Gan W-B (2010) Dendritic spine instability and insensitivity to modulation by sensory experience in a mouse model of fragile X syndrome. Proc Natl Acad Sci U S A 107:17768–17773. https://doi.org/10.1073/pnas.1012496107

Tabuchi K, Blundell J, Etherton MR et al (2007) A neuroligin-3 mutation implicated in autism increases inhibitory synaptic transmission in mice. Science 318:71–76. https://doi.org/10.1126/science.1146221

Trachtenberg JT, Chen BE, Knott GW et al (2002) Long-term in vivo imaging of experience-dependent synaptic plasticity in adult cortex. Nature 420:788–794. https://doi.org/10.1038/nature01273

Yuste R, Bonhoeffer T (2004) Genesis of dendritic spines: insights from ultrastructural and imaging studies. Nat Rev Neurosci 5:24–34. https://doi.org/10.1038/nrn1300

Zuo Y, Lin A, Chang P, Gan WB (2005) Development of long-term dendritic spine stability in diverse regions of cerebral cortex. Neuron 46:181–189. https://doi.org/10.1016/j.neuron.2005.04.001

Part III
Imaging-Based Diagnosis and Therapy

Chapter 20
How MRI Makes the Brain Visible

Denis Le Bihan

20.1 Progress of Imaging to Investigate the Anatomy of the Brain

It is fair to say that medical imaging started with Roentgen (1896), who got the first Nobel Prize in Physics in 1901 for the discovery of the X-ray. With X-rays, images of the inner body could be obtained for the first time, opening the way to the field of "radiology". However, with radiography mainly bones could be visualized due to their high calcium content, whose many electrons efficiently interact with X-rays. Over time some tissues or organs could be identified on radiographs, such as the lungs, mainly due to improvements in film sensitivity, but radiologists had to deal, rather successfully, with organ shadows more than real images of the organs, sometimes using tricks, such as the injection of iodine-based contrast agents filling vessels or organ cavities to make their shape readily visible.

The second big discovery came when it became possible to really see "wet" tissues, organs of the body, not only dry bones or organ shadows, by combining X-ray systems with sensors and computers, so-called "computed tomography" or CT. It was invented by Dr. Hounsfield (1973) who shared the Nobel Prize in 1979 with Dr. Cormack. The revolution was two-fold. First, the brain became visible within the skull for the first time in patients, completely noninvasively. Second, radiologists had in front of their eyes not projected shadows on a film, but virtual slices of the

---

Electronic Supplementary Material The online version of this chapter (https://doi.org/10.1007/978-981-13-7908-6_20) contains supplementary material, which is available to authorized users.

D. Le Bihan (✉)
NeuroSpin, CEA-Saclay Center, Gif-sur-Yvette, France

Y. Toyama et al. (eds.), *Make Life Visible*,
https://doi.org/10.1007/978-981-13-7908-6_20

organs which they could manipulate on a computer screen, revealing some contrast features in tissues, normal or diseased. But this also means that radiologists who until then had to mentally reconstruct organ three-dimensional anatomy, most often from antero-posterior body projections, had now to reconstruct space from transverse slices of the body, a real cognitive revolution for them.

That was, however, still not enough. Although it was possible to see some lesions, such as tumors in the brain, the structure of the brain itself could not be seen with great details, nor to say brain function. Along the way came Positron Emission Tomography (PET) which could provide some functional or metabolic images of the brain throughout the injection to the patients of short-live positron emitting tracers made using a nearby cyclotron (Ter-Pogossian et al. 1975). The images were generated using CT mathematical algorithm, but the spatial resolution of the images was too coarse to evaluate brain anatomy, and the making of dedicated radioisotopes was not trivial. Very recently though, PET has undergone a spectacular revival in medicine due to important technical improvements. Ultrasounds can also be used to make precise images of the inner body, but not so much in the brain which has always tried to keep its secrets under the protection of the skull, a serious obstacle to mechanical waves.

Then came Magnetic Resonance Imaging (MRI). With MRI, we can finally see the brain in great details because of a radical shift in the nature of the interaction between the physical mean used to produce images and the biological tissues. With MRI a very strong magnetic field is first used to magnetize water molecules, more precisely, the nuclei (protons) of the water hydrogen atoms. This is a perfect match for medical imaging, compared to X-rays, as our body organs are made of 70% water, even more in the brain. The hydrogen nuclei magnetization properties of water in the brain is not the same for white matter, grey matter or blood vessels. This magnetization can be revealed by using common radiowaves through the Nuclear Magnetic Resonance (NMR) principle, based on quantum mechanics, which was devised by Bloch and Purcell (1952 Nobel Prize) and is commonly used in physics and chemistry. However, the wavelength of the photons associated to those radiowaves is way too large (in contrast to X-ray photons) to allow any fine localization suitable for imaging. The trick to localize the nuclear magnetization is to make the magnetic field to vary in a controlled manner in space (and time) through so-called magnetic field gradients which modulate the frequency of the radiowaves in space (and time) (Lauterbur 1973). Nuclear magnetization, thus, becomes spatially encoded and computer algorithms can produce images showing the spatial distribution of water hydrogen magnetization properties, that is Magnetic Resonance images. Dr. Paul Lauterbur, a chemist, and Sir Peter Mansfield, a physicist, were awarded the Nobel Prize in Medicine in 2003 for their invention of MRI.

By manipulating the magnetization of water molecules, tailoring radiowaves, radiologists are like magicians which can create at will contrasts between tissues within the body and notably the brain. Engineers have greatly improved technical features of MRI scanners, so it is common nowadays to see the blood vessels with amazing details within the brain, or visualize the beating heart or respiration. The brain is finally revealing its detailed anatomical structure with submillimetric resolution in 3 dimensions completely noninvasively. The images can be very impressive, mimicking photos from real brain specimen. We should not forget, however, that those images are only virtual, magnetic avatars of brain water, not real anatomy. Parts of the brain may get heavily distorted or even vanish in some patients when the magnetic field is perturbed, for instance by iron-containing mascara present on eye lids.

The advent of CT and more importantly of MRI was a revolution because it became possible, for the first time, to investigate the brain of patients where they were still alive, and not through dissection post-mortem, a tremendous revolution for health care, of course. Those images have confirmed the existence of a strong link between a lost function and the localization of a lesion, as first envisioned at the end of the nineteenth century by French surgeon Paul Broca with his famous patient suffering from aphasia (Broca 1861). Brain MRI has completely changed the way we can study the brain, normal or diseased.

Because MRI does not use any ionizing radiation, we can obtain images without any danger of fetuses during pregnancy and get images of the developing brain. Neurons are produced at a very high rate during pregnancy, up to 250,000 neurons per minute, to reach a capital of about 100 billion neurons at birth. MRI reveals how the brain shape evolves when neurons produced at the center of the fetal brain migrate to the future brain surface which becomes more and more complex, with sulci and gyri, as it must accommodate such a large number of neurons. MRI studies can thus be used to collect large amount of data which can infer or confirm theories about brain development, and the interactions between genes and environment. Indeed, although humans share many features in the brain anatomy there are large differences between people if we look at their brain in details.

For example, the location, length and shape of the central sulcus can vary a lot, sometimes by as much as 1.5 cm. We do not understand yet the exact mechanisms (and reasons) of this variability. Our genes are probably partly responsible, but there could also be mechanical reasons occurring during brain development. Another famous example is the brain of taxi drivers, at least London taxi drivers, where a study was carried out. London taxi drivers are trained hard for 2 years, navigating in the streets of London. Amazingly, the size of the hippocampus, our inner GPS, is bigger in those taxi drivers than in the common population (Maguire et al. 2000). It means that by practicing navigation, taxi drivers shape and increase the size of their hippocampus. Pianists for whom coordination between the two hands is very important have a little more gray matter (which is interpreted as containing more neurons) in the related parts of the brain (Gaser and Schlaug 2003, Parsons et al. 2005). Of course, those changes are tiny, not directly visible on the images at naked eye, but revealed by artificial intelligence computer algorithms which compare the MRI images of those brains with databases of MRI images collected in large cohort of normal subjects or patients. Time may come in the near future when such "phrenology" algorithms may reveal to us or others some intimate features of our personal life or genetic imprints on our brain from MRI images, which rises important ethical issues. From those studies, it is easy to see that that we deeply and specifically modify our brains depending on our life and history. Indeed, plasticity can change the anatomy of our brain very rapidly. A study has shown that in young subjects who got trained to juggle balls for a few weeks some parts of the brain had already developed, mainly in the regions of the brain involved when visualizing movement in space (Draganski et al. 2004).

20.2 Imaging Brain Function with Functional MRI (fMRI)

Plain MRI reveals exquisite details about brain's anatomy, but what about brain function? For many years, one way to see the brain working was through awake patients in the neurosurgery suit, simulating parts of the brain through electrodes. This approach is still currently used today by neurosurgeons after awakening their patients to very precisely determine the location where they have to perform their surgery to avoid functional damages. Looking at the activity of brain regions without opening the skull has been a dream. This dream has come true with functional MRI. Brain activity and blood flow are closely linked (neurovascular coupling hypothesis) as was suggested at the end of the nineteenth century by Roy and Sherrington (1890): Regions of the brain where there is activity have an increased energy demand and increased blood flow: If we have a way to see local changes in blood flow in the brain, we will have a chance to see its activity. Indeed, MRI can be made very sensitive to blood flow variations. Blood are made of red blood cells which contain hemoglobin, a complex molecule which hold an atom of iron. The magnetization status of the iron atom within the strong magnetic field of the MRI scanner depends on the oxygen load of hemoglobin. In short, one may consider that hemoglobin-filled red blood cells travelling in small blood vessels become tiny flowing magnets in the magnetic field of the MRI magnet, which will change locally the magnetic field around those vessels. The nearby water molecules are sensitive to those changes in the magnetic field, and their magnetization will change. The effect is tiny, but again, with dedicated computer software, one can produce images reflecting those changes in the water magnetization near the vessels occurring in the regions where the brain has been activated (Ogawa et al. 1992; Kwong et al. 1992; Bandettini et al. 1992). This is really a wonderful discovery which was made by Seiji Ogawa who called his method "BOLD" for Blood Oxygen Level Dependent (Ogawa et al. 1990).

BOLD fMRI is easy to perform and very powerful. For instance, when asking someone placed in complete darkness in a MRI scanner to just think about a cat or another animal we can see on the fMRI images that their primary visual cortex gets activated from the changes in the magnetization of the water molecules there, revealing the implication of the primary visual cortex not only to see the real world but also our mental images (Klein et al. 1990). Consequently, it was observed by Sadato et al. (1998) that congenitally blind people reading Braille with their fingers also activate their primary visual cortex. This means that literally they "see" and read with their fingers. From this result, one may consider that there are local circuits in the brain that are genetically programmed to perform generic, low-level basic tasks used to process information coming from various inputs. Yet, the way we use them varies from person to person, depending on how those basic circuits are connected. Blind people have the visual circuits, but they are connected differently because they do not receive visual inputs. For normal people, the connections are mainly with the eyes (but not specifically, as activation from fingers appears after a few days of Braille reading practice), while for blind people the connections are with other senses, touch from the fingers or audition from the ears.

We can see even further into our brain. The visual cortex is retinotopic: If we look at a vertical flashing bar, we activate the visual cortex in a particular way, different from the way activated by looking at a horizontal object, and this is visible on fMRI images. As it has been shown that real and mental vision shares some circuits it is not so surprising to see that similar pattern differences are observed in fMRI images when subjects in total darkness just think about a vertical or horizontal bar. Indeed, we can predict with high success which orientation subjects were thinking about, horizontal or vertical, when the MRI images were acquired. With high resolution fMRI it has now become possible to "read" on the visual cortex of volunteers the activation patterns produced by their imagination of alphabetic letters. With little training computer algorithms can decode such patterns and reveal those letters with incredible accuracy.

The potential of this "mind reading" ability is enormous. Owen et al. have shown amazing fMRI images obtained in a young lady who was in a vegetative state because of a car accident (Owen et al. 2006). Once installed in the scanner the team asked the patient "What is your name?" While, of course, no response could be observed physically, the fMRI images revealing that her language Broca's area became clearly activated, implying that this lady had understood the question and responded in her mind. To the question "Could you think that you are playing tennis?" or "Could you imagine you are navigating into your house" fMRI showed activation of regions which are activated in normal people performing the same thinking tasks. Similar results have been found in 15–20% of the patients in a similar state, opening the way to cognitive interactions with those patients.

20.3 Imaging Brain Tissue Microstructure with Diffusion MRI (dMRI)

Diffusion MRI is a specific imaging modality on its own, which has its early roots in the 1905 physics PhD thesis of Einstein on molecular diffusion (Einstein 1956). Einstein showed that the diffusion process, known macroscopically from the Fick laws, was, indeed, the results of microscopic Brownian motion of atoms and molecules, proving indirectly the existence of those atoms and molecules, the existence of which was only a hypothesis at the time. In 1985 it was shown that MRI could be used to produce images of Brownian motion and water molecular diffusion (Le Bihan and Breton 1985). The spatial resolution of MRI images is around millimeters, far from the scale which would be necessary to get information on the nature of tissues and lesions from individual cells which are 100 to 1000 times smaller. According to Einstein's diffusion equation, at the brain temperature (37 °C), water molecules diffuse on distances in the order of 15 μm during 50 milliseconds (typical time interval used with MRI). By measuring water diffusion, even at the MRI image scale, one could get precious information on what water molecules have encountered in the tissue, such as cell membranes, fibers, etc., acting as probes for us of the microscopic scale. In order to encode diffusion-driven molecular motion in MRI images one has to rely on the magnetic field gradients used for MRI, but pushed to a much greater level. The magnetic field is changed in space for very short time intervals, based on a method which was introduced for NMR, before the advent of MRI, by Stejskal and Tanner (1965). The problem was to combine the spatial encoding at microscopic (diffusion) and macroscopic (MRI) level which was solved in 1985, leading to the first "diffusion MRI" images of the brain of normal subjects and patients (Le Bihan et al. 1986). Those images revealed a completely new kind of contrast, not available with standard MRI, giving insight into the microstructure of tissues.

Diffusion MRI is now installed on almost all MRI scanners and widely used in the clinical field. The first major application of diffusion MRI has been acute stroke, but applications are now extending to oncology, psychiatry, etc. Ischemic brain stroke, caused by the obliteration of a cerebral blood vessel by a clot, is the third common cause of death and the first cause of long-term disability by far. After stroke, 30% patients who survive need daily assistance, and 70% have impaired occupational capacity. The cognitive and societal cost is huge for healthcare, but also for productivity loses. In 1990, Moseley et al. (1990a), working on a model of acute stroke in the cat and using the new diffusion MRI method discovered that the diffusion coefficient of water was going quickly (minutes) and sharply down during stroke at the acute phase following the obliteration of a brain blood vessel. In short, in the regions of the brain where neurons were dying due to a lack of blood irrigation, the diffusion of water molecules was slowing down in relation to the swelling of dying brain cells (cytotoxic edema). For the first time, an objective marker of acute stroke was available, showing at the acute phase (within minutes and hours after the stroke onset) that a stroke had occurred and where exactly in the brain. Stroke can now get instantaneously cured if diagnosed in emergency by dissolving the clots that caused the ischemic event using thrombolytic agents, saving the fate or even the life of many patients worldwide. The health problem now is to get enough stroke centers disposing of MRI scanners available to emergencies and to educate the public to the early symptoms, as millions of neurons are dying every minute after the stroke onset.

Diffusion MRI is also now making a big impact in oncology, as it can accurately detect malignant lesions completely noninvasively. In regions of the body where cells proliferate, as in cancer, water Brownian motion decreases. Sensitivity to malignant lesions has been shown to be very high. Because the diffusion MRI images are very crisp and accurate, this method is increasingly being used, especially in the breast and prostate, as a method to detect cancer, sometimes automatically using artificial intelligence algorithms. Diffusion MRI can also be used for monitoring treatment efficacy, giving information on whether therapy is effective or not at an early stage, before actual changes to the tumor size can be detected, saving several weeks or months if a switch to another treatment has to be made, as has been shown for brain glioblastoma.

Another major and unexpected breakthrough of diffusion MRI has been to give access, for the first time as there is no other approach available, to the brain connections. Brownian motion of water molecules seen with diffusion MRI is faster along the white matter fibers than perpendicular to them (Moseley et al. 1990b). In the early 1990s it was shown that by measuring water diffusion in two perpendicular directions the orientation of the white matter fibers in the brain could be determined. The images were very crude at that time, but it was the first demonstration that images of the orientation of the connection fibers in the brain could be obtained (Douek et al. 1991). Soon after, with P. Basser and J. Mattiello we developed the concept of diffusion tensor imaging (DTI) which fully exploits the sensitivity of diffusion MRI to orientation in space (Basser et al. 1994), allowing the orientation of the brain white matter fibers to be determined accurately for each point of the image. By connecting all those points together using dedicated mathematical algorithms one gets stunning 3D images of the connections themselves (Poupon, 1998; Mori et al. 1999; Conturo et al. 1999). Those images are now found in anatomy textbooks and atlas of the human brain connections in adults and children have been made available from DTI. It takes just a few minutes of brain scanning to get those connectivity maps, and applications are growing in neuroscience and medicine, revealing some unchartered territories. For instance, one can see that 2–4 months old babies have already connection fibers more developed in the arcuate fasciculus of the left hemisphere, before they acquire language skills (Dubois et al. 2009). Pianists also develop connections in specific areas of the brain depending on the number of hours spent practicing in their life (Bengtsson et al. 2005). During childhood a few thousand hours are enough to deeply modify those connections. Between 11 and 17 years of age, it takes more hours of practice to another set of regions. By adult age, other regions are affected, but at the price of a great many hours of practice, even in professional pianists. In dyslexia, it has been shown that some connections could be faulty in regions of the temporal lobe implied in reading (Klingberg et al. 2000). When dyslexic patients improve their reading abilities through some rehabilitation, one can observe improvements in those connections with dMRI. Indeed, brain connectivity seems to play a major role is some psychiatric illnesses, such as schizophrenia, as faulty connections have been found in some patients between frontal regions where thoughts originate and temporal auditory regions (Skelly et al. 2008), resulting in time asynchrony and explaining perhaps why “inner voices” (like mental images in the visual cortex) are perceived by those patients, as if watching a movie with the sound and the images out of synchrony, which is very uncomfortable.

Diffusion functional MRI (DfMRI) (Le Bihan et al. 2006) can also be used as an alternative for BOLD-fMRI. BOLD-fMRI, as we have seen, relies on the neurovascular coupling hypothesis and does not reflect neuronal activity directly, which may fail in certain conditions which impair neurovascular coupling. On the other hand, DfMRI is thought to be more directly linked to neuronal activation, as the diffusion MRI signal is exquisitely sensitive to minute changes occurring in the tissue microstructure upon various physiological or pathological changes (Le Bihan 2014). Studies on rodents have evidenced that while the BOLD fMRI response is abolished by blocking the neurovascular response the DfMRI response is maintained, strongly suggesting that the DfMRI signal is not of vascular origin and that its mechanism differs from that of BOLD (Tsurugizawa et al. 2013). In addition, the DfMRI response is faster (time to reach the activation peak and time to return to baseline) than the hemodynamically driven BOLD signal response, as revealed by visual stimulation experiments in human subjects (Le Bihan et al. 2006). Based on earlier reports that the water apparent diffusion coefficient (ADC) decreases in relation to cell swelling and that neural swelling is one of the responses associated with neural activation, it has been hypothesized that the decrease in the water ADC observed during neural evoked responses would originate from the dynamic swelling of neurons or neuron parts, in line with a neuromechanical coupling hypothesis. This hypothesis is supported by the observation with microscopic MRI in *Aplysia* neuronal preparations that water diffusion decreases at the tissue level, while increasing inside neuron bodies, when cells of are exposed to swelling inducers, such as hypotonic solution or ouabain (an inhibiter of Na^+/K^+ pumps) and after neuronal activation induced by perfusion with a solution containing dopamine (Abe et al. 2017a). During activation neural cell swelling can be evidenced from optical microscopy imaging. Furthermore, water diffusion increases in specific brain regions in anesthetized rats, reflecting the decrease neuronal activity observed with local field potentials (LFPs), especially in regions involved in wakefulness (Abe et al. 2017b). In contrast, BOLD signals showed non-specific changes reflecting systemic effects of the anesthesia on overall brain hemodynamics status. Electrical stimulation of the central median (CM) thalamus nucleus where this anesthesia-induced water diffusion increase has been observed leads the animals to transiently wake up. Infusion in CM of furosemide, a specific neuronal swelling blocker, leads water diffusion to increase further locally and increases the current threshold necessary for the awaking of the animals under CM electrical stimulation. Oppositely, induction of cell swelling in CM through infusion of a hypotonic solution (−80 mOsm aCSF) leads to a local water diffusion decrease and a lower current threshold to wake up the animals. Strikingly, the local water diffusion changes produced by blocking or enhancing cell swelling in CM are also mirrored remotely in areas functionally connected to the CM, such as the cingulate and somatosensory cortex. Together, those results strongly suggest that neuronal swelling, possibly at the dendritic spine level is a significant mechanism underlying DfMRI and likely brain function at an elementary level.

20.4 Future of MRI

By gaining an order of magnitude in the spatial and temporal resolution of the images obtained by MRI we should be able not only to "better" see inside our brain, confirming or invalidating our current assumptions on how it works, but also to generate new assumptions, today impossible to anticipate, and perhaps to reach a holy grail: decoding the functioning of our brain. As suggested by MRI studies in animals at ultra-high magnetic fields (> 10 Tesla), the sensitivity and, thus, the spatial and temporal resolution of the images increase together with the magnetic field. New contrast mechanisms could also be explored. There is no physical limit to this increase in magnetic field, only technical challenges which can be solved. With such an ultra-high field (UHF) MRI system in hands one would be within reach to acquire with timescales compatible within human tolerances images at a scale of one hundred micrometers at which everything remains to discover.

The brain is a spatially very inhomogeneous organ. A key question is to understand how the specific three-dimensional organization of our brain cells, neurons and glial cells, in clusters or networks within the layers of the brain cortex, and their short- and long-term dynamic interactions via their short and long range connections, are responsible for the emergence of a genetically determined set of elementary operations which, combined together and under the effect of exposure to environment result in higher order function, language, calculus, or even consciousness. Infants can today learn to manipulate cell phones with some success in a few hours, though, there are certainly no "cell phone" brain areas, nor to say "cell phone" genes. The segregation of cells in a set of functional areas along the cortical surface separated with abrupt boundaries has been known since Brodmann gave an account of his observation under a microscope of the single half-brain of an old lady at the onset of the twentieth century, and found out the existence of about 60 distinct areas which he labeled by numbers (for instance, area 17 is the primary visual cortex). A recent MRI study has extended this set of brain regions to almost 200 (Glasser et al. 2016). In some way, this is conceptually equivalent to the discovery of our 46 chromosomes and their link to heredity in the mid-1880s. At a more microscopic level it was later discovered that the vector of heredity was the DNA molecule, an assembly of nucleotides, present in the chromosomes. Similarly, we know neurons (as well as glial cells) compose Brodmann's areas and support brain function. But it was not until Crick and Watson had the vision that information was hidden at an intermediate spatial scale, between DNA's nucleotides and chromosomes scales, in the three-dimensional organization (double helix) of the DNA molecule that the existence of the genetic code emerged. Could there be a "neural code" carried by the three-dimensional organization of brain cells?

To find out we must explore this "mesoscale" which is today out of reach. We can explore the human brain in vivo roughly at millimeter resolution (hundreds of thousands of cells at best) and, at the other extremity of the spectrum, we can record the activity of a limited set of neurons in animals, which can be used in feed theoretical models of small neural networks. But what really happens between those two scales, around clusters of a few thousands of cells, remain Terra Incognita, and it would be naive to assume the landscape at this scale is a mere sum of what is visible at an inferior scale. Synergies across scales is in order and this quest for a "neural code" is one of the major challenges of contemporary science, together with the exploration of matter, of the universe, or the control of thermonuclear fusion. Key questions are: "How do neuron clusters work and exchange information? How is information stored? What are the respective role of genes and environment in the cortical localization, genesis and functioning of those clusters? How are they formed and maintained or altered during the brain development stage and after?" Obviously, this intimate knowledge of normal brain functioning mechanisms will lead to a better understanding of its dysfunctions, neurological or psychiatric pathologies in a broad sense, which will probably open new therapeutic possibilities (such as brain reprogramming).

Those challenging views led in the early 2000s the French Atomic Energy Commission (CEA) to launch a program to conceive and build a "human brain explorer", the first human MRI scanner operating at 11.7 T (Le Bihan and Schild 2017). This scanner was envisioned to be part of an ambitious project aimed at pushing the limits of neuroimaging, from mouse to man, using UHF MRI. With such a unique instrument brain connections and brain activity could be seen at a resolution of hundreds of micrometers, ions, metabolites, neurotransmitters could be detected and measured, giving access in vivo and noninvasively to brain chemistry or genes at work in the developing brain. This 11.7 T magnet was designed by the physicists and engineers of CEA based on specifications defined by teams at NeuroSpin. The magnet was part of a larger endeavor to develop Molecular Imaging at Ultra-High Field financed through a French-German initiative (hence the name "Iseult" for the project) involving academic (CEA and Julich University), industrial (Siemens, Bruker, Guerbet and Alstom MSA) and governmental organizations across both countries (AII, then Oséo and BPI for France, BMBF for Germany). The 11.7 T magnet has been finalized at the Alstom-GE facility in Belfort and delivered to NeuroSpin in Saclay in May 2017 for a commissioning in 2019. The first images of the human brain at 11.7 T might not be obtained until a few years later, however, due necessary developments in MRI technology to accommodate issues associated with the increase in frequency (the system will operate at 500 MHz) and approval for safety by regulatory agencies. Nonetheless, this prototype 11.7 T MRI scanner dedicated to advanced brain research, with the unprecedented resolution and new contrasts it will allow, will certainly open a new window of opportunities to make the brain even more visible and better understand some brain disorders, develop new disease biomarkers or novel therapeutic means.

References

Abe Y, Nguyen KV, Tsurugizawa T, Ciobanu L, Le Bihan D (2017a) Modification of water diffusion by activation-induced neural swelling in Aplysia Californica. Sci Rep 7:6178

Abe Y, Tsurugizawa T, Le Bihan D (2017b) Water diffusion closely reveals neural activity status in rat brain loci affected by anesthesia. PLoS Biol, 10.1371/journal.pbio.2001494 15(4):e2001494

Bandettini PA et al (1992) Time course EPI of human brain function during task activation. Magn Reson Med 25:390–397

Basser p J et al (1994) MR diffusion tensor spectroscopy and imaging. Biophys J 66:259–267

Bengtsson SL et al (2005) Extensive piano practicing has regionally specific effects on white matter development. Nat Neurosci 8:1148–1150

Broca MP (1861) Remarques sur le siège de la faculté du langage articulé, suivies d'une observation d'aphémie. Bull Mem Soc Anat Paris 36:330–357

Conturo TE et al (1999) Tracking neuronal fiber pathways in the living human brain. PNAS 96:10422

Douek P et al (1991) MR color mapping of myelin fiber orientation. J Comput Assit Tomogr 15:923–929

Draganski B et al (2004) Neuroplasticity: changes in grey matter induced by training. Nature 22:311–312

Dubois J et al (2009) Structural asymetries in the infant language and sensori-motor networks. Cereb Cortex 19(2):414–423

Einstein A, in Furthe R, Cowper AD (eds) (1956) Collection of papers translated from the German, Investigations on the Theory of Brownian Motion, Dover

Gaser C, Schlaug G (2003) Brain structures differ between musicians and non-musicians. J Neurosci 23:9240–9245

Glasser MF et al (2016) A multi-modal parcellation of human cerebral cortex. Nature 536:171–178

Hounsfield GN (1973) Computerized transverse axial scanning (tomography): Part1. Description of the system. BJR 46(552):1016–1022

Klein I et al (1990) Transient activity in the human calcarine cortex during visual-mental imagery: an event-related fMRI study. J Cogn Neurosci 12:15–23

Klingberg T et al (2000) Microstructure of temporo-parietal white matter as a basis for reading ability: evidence from diffusion tensor magnetic resonance imaging. Neuron 25:493–500

Kwong KK et al (1992) Dynamic magnetic resonance imaging of human brain activity during primary sensory stimulation. PNAS 89:5675–5679

Lauterbur PC (1973) Image formation by induced local interactions: examples employing nuclear magnetic resonance. Nature 242(5394):190–191

Le Bihan D, Schild T (2017) Human brain MRI at 500MHz, scientific perspectives and technological challenges. Supercond Sci Technol 30:033003

Le Bihan D (2014) Diffusion MRI: what water tells us about the brain. EMBO Mol Med 6:569–573

Le Bihan D, Breton E (1985) Imagerie de diffusion in vivo par résonance magnétique nucléaire. C R Acad Sci Paris 301(II):1109–1112

Le Bihan D et al (1986) MR imaging of intravoxel incoherent motions: application to diffusion and perfusion in neurologic disorders. Radiology 161:401–407

Le Bihan D, Urayama S, Aso T, Hanakawa T, Fukuyama H (2006) Direct and fast detection of neuronal activation in the human brain with diffusion MRI. PNAS 103:8263–8268

Maguire EA et al (2000) Navigation-related structural change in the hippocampi of taxi drivers. PNAS 97:4398–4403

Mori S et al (1999) Three-dimensional tracking of axonal projections in the brain by magnetic resonance imaging. Ann Neurol 45:265

Moseley ME et al (1990a) Diffusion-weighted MR imaging of anisotropic water diffusion in cat central nervous system. Radiology 176:439–446

Moseley ME et al (1990b) Early detection of regional cerebral ischemic injury in cats: evaluation of diffusion and T2-weighted MRI and spectroscopy. Magn Reson Med 14:330–346

Ogawa S, Lee TM, Kay AR, Tank DW (1990) Brain magnetic resonance imaging with contrast dependent on blood oxygenation. PNAS 87:9868–9872

Ogawa S et al (1992) Intrinsic signal changes accompanying sensory stimulation: function brain mapping with magnetic resonance imaging. PNAS 89:5951–5955

Owen AM et al (2006) Detecting awareness in the vegetative stat. Science 313:1402–1403

Parsons LM et al (2005) The brain basis of piano performance. Neuropsychologia 43:199–215

Poupon C et al (1998) Regularization of MR diffusion tensor maps for tracking brain white matter bundles. LNCS-1496. Springer, MICCAI, MIT, pp 489–498

Rontgen WC (1896) On a new kind of rays. Science 3(59):227–231

Roy CS, Sherrington CS (1890) On the regulation of blood-supply of the brain. J Physiol 11:85–158

Sadato N et al (1998) Neural networks for Braille reading by the blind. Brain 121:1193–1194

Skelly LR, Calhoun V, Meda SA, Kim J, Mathalon DH, Pearlson GD (2008) Diffusion tensor imaging in schizophrenia: relationship to symptoms. Schizophr Res 98:157–162

Stejskal EO, Tanner JE (1965) Spin diffusion measurements: spin echoes in the presence of a time-dependant field gradient. J Chem Phys 42:288–292

Ter-Pogossian MM, Phelps ME, Hoffman EJ, Mullani NA (1975) A positron-emission transaxial tomograph for nuclear imaging (PET). Radiology 114(1):89–98

Tsurugizawa T, Ciobanu L, Le Bihan D (2013) Water diffusion in brain cortex closely tracks underlying neuronal activity. PNAS 110:11636–11641

Chapter 21
Application of Imaging Technology to Humans

Takahiro Matsui and Masaru Ishii

21.1 Introduction

Through the history of clinical medicine, detailed observation of patient symptoms has been most important for both diagnosis and treatment, and several attempts to observe the human body more precisely have been conducted for a long time. Of the numerous brilliant inventions, histopathology established by Rudolf Ludwig Karl Virchow continues to occupy the central position of definite diagnosis. However, there still exist some problems with typical histopathological diagnostic procedures. First, histological analysis with biopsy procedure inevitably needs some tissue damage. Second, it takes much time to make a diagnosis after biopsy because of the various steps necessary to make pathological specimens, such as fixation, dehydration, embedding, and staining. Therefore, it is desirable to develop a new histological diagnostic system for use in real time, with a less invasive way. On the other hands, the development of imaging technology has greatly influenced life science research in recent years. Especially, intravital imaging technique has a strong impact because it enables to observe life phenomena visually while keeping animals alive. Multiphoton excitation microscopy (MPM) is one of the major tools used to observe deep regions of the living body using fluorescence and multiphoton absorption process. In the field of life science research, MPM is now widely used for intravital imaging of deep tissues such as brain (Meyer-Luehmann et al. 2008) and bone marrow (Ishii et al. 2009). Now life science and clinical medicine are inseparably connected, and the development of new imaging techniques such as MPM recalls the application to humans in the field of clinical medicine. Especially, malignant neoplasms are extremely important diseases that continue to be a major cause of death all over the world, and have a large number of patients. So detailed diagnosis of

T. Matsui · M. Ishii (✉)
Department of Immunology and Cell Biology, Osaka University Graduate School of Medicine, Suita, Osaka, Japan
e-mail: mishii@icb.med.osaka-u.ac.jp

Y. Toyama et al. (eds.), *Make Life Visible*,
https://doi.org/10.1007/978-981-13-7908-6_21

cancer at the cellular level through the application of imaging technology is thought to be of great interest all over the world and have much potential demand. However, there are many obstacles before application of MPM to the clinic. One of the most serious hurdles is that it is difficult to label fluorescently cells in human body, because fluorescent dyes are often toxic. It is obviously impossible as well to perform genetic fluorescent labeling unlike laboratory animals such as mice. In recent years, several articles have been reported the methods of imaging living tissues that do not require any labeling. For example, Raman spectroscopy obtains images by detecting Raman scattered light generated when a sample is irradiated with laser light. Depending on the vibrational properties and component distribution such as proteins, lipids, DNA and so on, image contrast generates without any labeling (Freudiger et al. 2008). Photoacoustic microscopy is also known as an efficient tool for non-labeling imaging. It images tissue by photoacoustic effect, a phenomenon in which molecules absorbing light energy emit heat and acoustic waves are generated by volume expansion due to the heat (Yao et al. 2015). There are some reports indicating the usefulness of imaging for human using these techniques described above (Ji et al. 2013; Hsu et al. 2016), and these facts recall the possible utility of non-labeling MPM (NL-MPM) imaging for human. Moreover, fluorescent imaging including MPM is considered superior to these techniques in spatiotemporal resolution. Here, we introduce our attempt of colorectal carcinoma diagnosis by non-labeling imaging for human colorectal tissues using MPM (Matsui et al. 2017).

21.2 MPM Technique Enables to Visualize the Histological Features of Fresh, Unstained Human Colorectal Mucosa and Can Be Used for Histopathological Diagnoses

First, imaging analysis of fresh, unstained normal human colorectal mucosal tissues was performed with an MPM imaging system under 780 nm excitation. Without any labeling, it was possible to visualize the histological features of the colorectal tissues in detail, such as ductal structures of epithelial cells and hematopoietic cells in the lamina propria (Fig. 21.1a). In the NL-MPM images, we were able to recognize three different components by the different color patterns: epithelial cells, hematopoietic cells, and basement membrane. Spectral analyses revealed that autofluorescent substances and second harmonic generation (SHG), which is a nonlinear optical phenomenon, made color variation among those three components and made MPM images. The images of our NL-MPM imaging for fresh tissue and conventional hematoxylin and eosin (HE) staining procedures for fixed sections were morphologically very similar (Fig. 21.1b). Such similarity was also observed in NL-MPM imaging of colorectal carcinoma tissue, which showed irregular and atypical ductal structure and nuclear enlargement in epithelial cells like HE staining

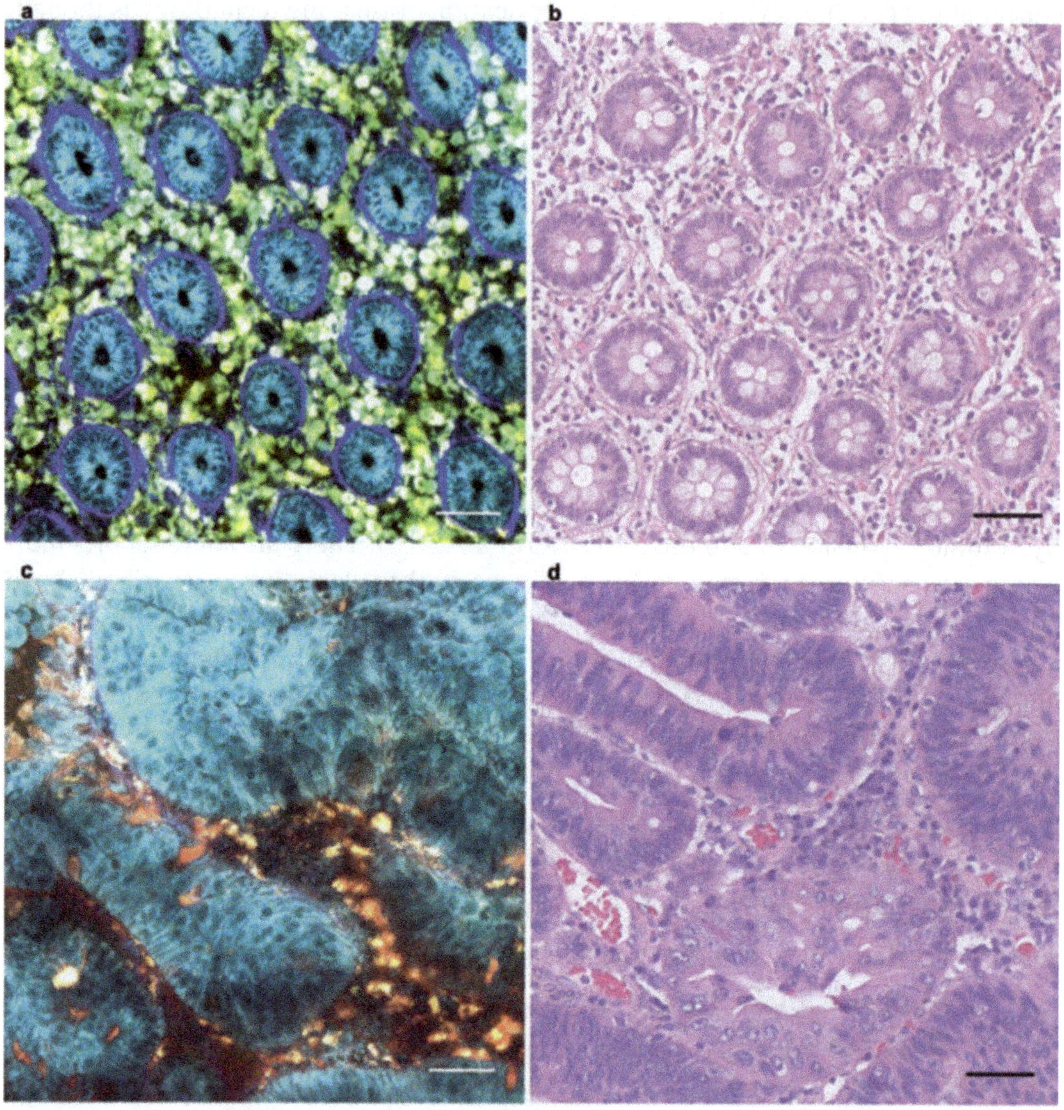

Fig. 21.1 Non-labeling MPM imaging of human normal colorectal mucosa and colorectal carcinoma. (**a**) MPM imaging of human normal colorectal mucosa. (**b**) HE staining of normal colorectal mucosa, using the same sample as in (**a**). (**c**) MPM images of colorectal cancer tissue. (**d**) HE-stained images of colorectal cancer tissue, using the same samples as in (**c**). Bar: 50 μm. (These figures were quoted from Matsui et al. 2017)

images (Fig. 21.1c, d). These facts made us to think that it might be possible to perform histopathological diagnosis by NL-MPM imaging, instead of HE staining. In fact, it was possible for experienced pathologists to make correct diagnoses based only on the NL-MPM images in the blind manner. These facts indicated that NL-MPM images of fresh unstained colorectal tissues were as useful as conventional HE staining of resected/fixed specimens for differential diagnosis of cancerous versus non-cancerous regions.

21.3 Classification by Numerical Parameters Enables to Distinguish NL-MPM Images to Normal and Cancerous Tissues Quantitatively

One of the most important advantages of fluorescent images is the ability to perform quantitative analyses. It is relatively easy to measure and analyze fluorescent signals compared to bright-field images of HE staining (Kikuta et al. 2013; Egawa et al. 2013). This means that we are able to perform histopathological diagnosis immediately and quantitatively by using MPM images. In order to handle image data quantitatively, it is necessary to extract numerical parameters from the images. In this colorectal NL-MPM imaging, two independent numerical parameters were established: nuclear diameters of epithelial cells and intensity of SHG signal from basement membrane. Nuclear diameters in cancer tissues were statistically larger than those in non-cancerous tissues, while SHG signals from basement membrane were diminished in cancer region compared to normal mucosa. Using both NL-MPM imaging and spectral analysis, these features could easily be quantified and defined as index N (represent nuclear dimeters) and index S (represent the intensity of SHG signals), respectively. In examination with multiple samples, most of NL-MPM images of the non-cancerous areas showed low index N and high index S values. In contrast, most areas from cancer lesions showed high index N and low index S values. After threshold values are set from these results, the utility of these two indices as diagnostic tools for distinguishing normal and malignant lesions in colorectal mucosa was evaluated, which showed 96% sensitivity and 84% specificity, respectively (Fig. 21.2). The kappa coefficient between the HE-based conventional diagnosis and the two indices described above was 0.82. From these results, it was shown that we could distinguish cancerous and non-cancerous tissues in fresh, human unstained colorectal mucosa quantitatively, using MPM images and the two indices.

21.4 Conclusion

We have described the diagnostic approach of cancer tissue using NL-MPM imaging as an example of imaging technology application to humans. Although we described the analysis of colon tissue, similar analysis is possible in other organs, depending on the distribution of auto-fluorescent substances as well as the degree of nonlinear optical phenomena (Ulrich et al. 2013; Miyamoto and Kudoh 2013). The usefulness of observing and diagnosing human tissues with imaging system lies in its rapidity and quantitativeness. Deep observation capability is also another useful advantage for MPM imaging, although the observation range is limited now (up to typical depth of 120 μm in colorectal mucosa). In life science research, imaging technologies have made it possible to perform quantitative assessment of life phenomena in real time, and have contributed greatly to elucidation of life phenomena.

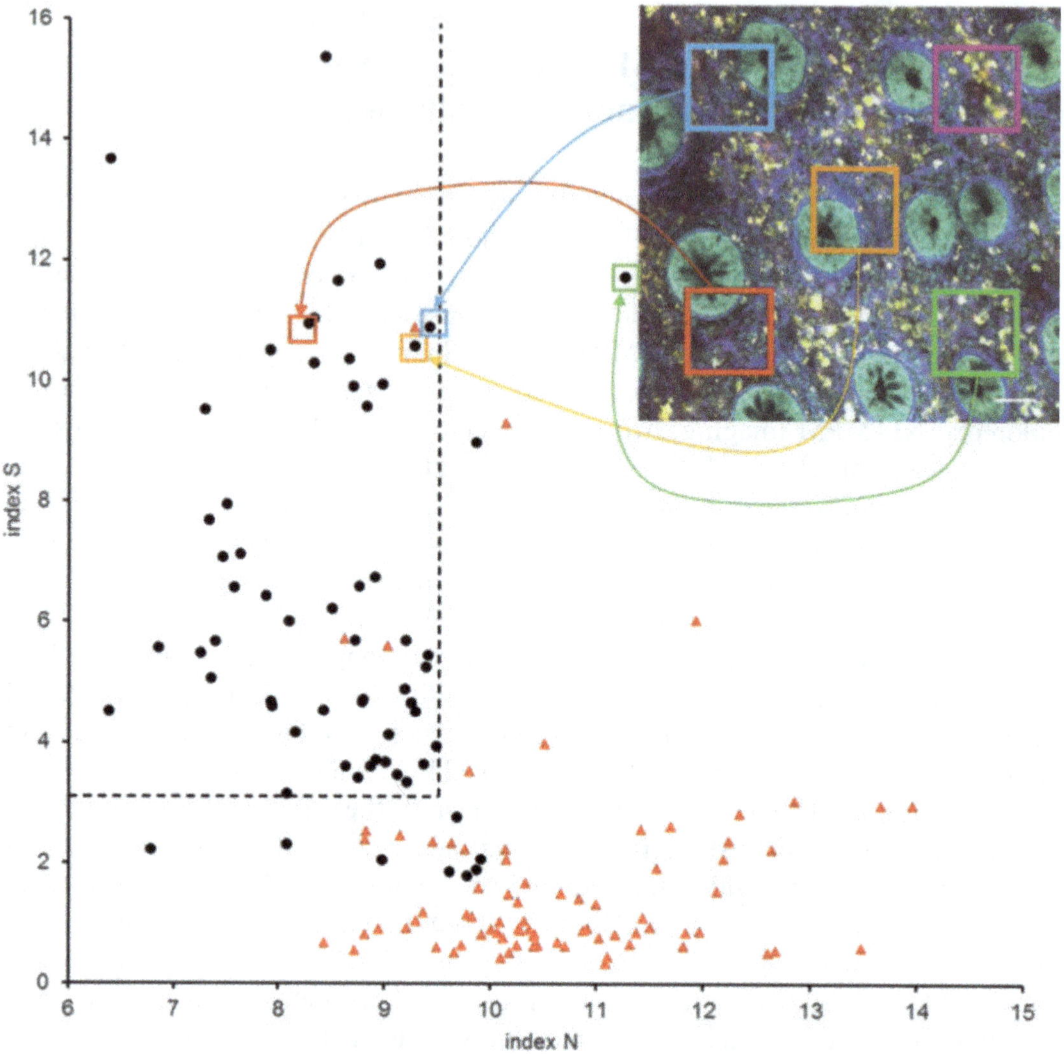

Fig. 21.2 Classification analysis of MPM images from normal and cancer tissues using the two indices N and S. Five areas (square ROI with a side length of 100 μm) were determined in advance in the x-y coordinate plane for the original image files, the two indices N and S were calculated with each ROI, and scatter plot was drawn. Final diagnoses of normal (black dot, n = 64) or cancer tissue (red triangle, n = 80) were made using HE-stained sections from the same specimens imaged by MPM. Areas that showed an index N ≤ 9.5 and index S > 3.1 (upper left area of the dashed line) were deemed normal in the classification analysis. Areas that contained no epithelial cell nuclei in the ROI (e.g., the pink ROI) were omitted from the analysis. Bar: 50 μm. (This figure was quoted from Matsui et al. 2017)

The usefulness of imaging procedures is also considered high in experiments targeting humans and clinical medicine. We hope that further development of imaging technology will introduce the breakthrough into clinical medicine as well and contribute to the happiness of humans.

References

Egawa G, Nakamizo S, Natsuaki Y, Doi H, Miyachi Y, Kabashima K (2013) Intravital analysis of vascular permeability in mice using two-photon microscopy. Sci Rep 3:1932. https://doi.org/10.1038/srep01932

Freudiger CW, Min W, Saar BG, Lu S, Holtom GR, He C et al (2008) Label-free biomedical imaging with high sensitivity by stimulated Raman scattering microscopy. Science 322(5909):1857–1861. https://doi.org/10.1126/science.1165758

Hsu HC, Wang L, Wang LV (2016) In vivo photoacoustic microscopy of human cuticle microvasculature with single-cell resolution. J Biomed Opt 21(5):56004. https://doi.org/10.1117/1.JBO.21.5.056004

Ishii M, Egen JG, Klauschen F, Meier-Schellersheim M, Saeki Y, Vacher J et al (2009) Sphingosine-1-phosphate mobilizes osteoclast precursors and regulates bone homeostasis. Nature 458(7237):524–528. https://doi.org/10.1038/nature07713

Ji M, Orringer DA, Freudiger CW, Ramkissoon S, Liu X, Lau D et al (2013) Rapid, label-free detection of brain tumors with stimulated Raman scattering microscopy. Sci Transl Med 5(201):201ra119. https://doi.org/10.1126/scitranslmed.3005954

Kikuta J, Wada Y, Kowada T, Wang Z, Sun-Wada GH, Nishiyama I et al (2013) Dynamic visualization of RANKL and Th17-mediated osteoclast function. J Clin Invest 123(2):866–873. https://doi.org/10.1172/JCI65054

Matsui T, Mizuno H, Sudo T, Kikuta J, Haraguchi N, Ikeda JI et al (2017) Non-labeling multiphoton excitation microscopy as a novel diagnostic tool for discriminating normal tissue and colorectal cancer lesions. Sci Rep 7(1):6959. https://doi.org/10.1038/s41598-017-07244-2

Meyer-Luehmann M, Spires-Jones TL, Prada C, Garcia-Alloza M, de Calignon A, Rozkalne A et al (2008) Rapid appearance and local toxicity of amyloid-beta plaques in a mouse model of Alzheimer's disease. Nature 451(7179):720–724. https://doi.org/10.1038/nature06616

Miyamoto K, Kudoh H (2013) Quantification and visualization of cellular NAD(P)H in young and aged female facial skin with in vivo two-photon tomography. Br J Dermatol 169(Suppl 2):25–31. https://doi.org/10.1111/bjd.12370

Ulrich M, Klemp M, Darvin ME, Konig K, Lademann J, Meinke MC (2013) In vivo detection of basal cell carcinoma: comparison of a reflectance confocal microscope and a multiphoton tomograph. J Biomed Opt 18(6):61229. https://doi.org/10.1117/1.JBO.18.6.061229

Yao J, Wang L, Yang JM, Maslov KI, Wong TT, Li L et al (2015) High-speed label-free functional photoacoustic microscopy of mouse brain in action. Nat Methods 12(5):407–410. https://doi.org/10.1038/nmeth.3336

Chapter 22
Theranostic Near-Infrared Photoimmunotherapy

Hisataka Kobayashi

22.1 Introduction

Targeted cancer therapies offer the promise of highly effective tumor control with fewer side-effects than conventional cancer treatments. In this approach, drugs or radioisotopes are directed to a tumor by coupling to monoclonal antibodies (mAbs) against specific targets on the cancer cell surface. These antibody–drug conjugates (ADCs) have had modest commercial success, but side-effects remain problematic. We have greatly advanced targeted cancer detection that assists surgical or endoscopic therapy by developing a series of optical imaging probes ('activatable probes') that only fluoresce when they are bound to or inside tumors (Kobayashi et al. 2010; Kobayashi and Choyke 2011), enabling precise tracking of cancer cells and drugs in the tissue (Urano et al. 2009). With these probes, cancer-specific fluorescence has been achieved in animal models and in fresh surgical specimens from cancer patients.

From a physics perspective, excitation energy can be dissipated in the form of fluorescent light for diagnosis. Alternatively, it can be exchanged for heat, oxidation or photochemical reactions to induce cytotoxic treatment. Our work is to be differentiated from conventional photodynamic therapy (PDT). PDT has been in limited clinical use for several decades. Photofrin (porfimer) is the most commonly employed PDT agent and has been used to treat endobronchial, esophageal and bladder cancers. Photofrin and related compounds passively permeate into cells based on their

Electronic Supplementary Material The online version of this chapter (https://doi.org/10.1007/978-981-13-7908-6_22) contains supplementary material, which is available to authorized users.

H. Kobayashi (✉)
Molecular Imaging Program, National Cancer Institute/National Institutes of Health, Bethesda, MD, USA
e-mail: Kobayash@mail.nih.gov

Y. Toyama et al. (eds.), *Make Life Visible*,
https://doi.org/10.1007/978-981-13-7908-6_22

hydrophobicity which is non-specific but slightly favors uptake in cancer cells and when exposed to light in the presence of oxygen, generate reactive oxygen species. Reactive oxygen species are typically toxic to the cell, resulting in cell death, however, this typically occurs within the cytoplasm and results in apoptosis rather than necrosis. Although PDT is used in specific cases, widespread adoption has been limited because the current compounds distribute rather non-specifically and permeate into normal cells leading to off-target toxicities. For instance, patients are often unable to go outside into direct sunlight for several months and even room light for several days. Incidental exposure to strong light, for instance, from a copy machine, can be catastrophic. Moreover, PDT is notorious for inducing serious inflammatory changes at the treatment site, limiting its utility. This relates to the non-specific biodistribution and slow clearance rates (half-life of 23 days) of PDT agents. More general use of PDT is thus limited by its potential side effects. Targeted PDT has been attempted but delivery issues related to the large number of photosensitizer molecules in each conjugate, limits the achievable concentrations of the photosensitizer.

By extending the target-cell specific fluorescence imaging methodology from ‘see’ for cancer detection to ‘kill’ for cancer therapy, we then developed a new form of ADC comprised of an mAb attached to a photoabsorbing phthalocyanine-based chemical, termed IRDye700DX (IR700). When this conjugate is injected and the target cancer tissue is illuminated with harmless near-infrared light of wavelength 690 nm, the IR700 part of the molecule becomes activated and splits, turning hydrophobic, which compromises the cell membrane, thereby killing the cancer cell. This approach is safer than other conventional ADCs because it only kills illuminated cells that bind mAb–IR700 conjugates. Since 690 nm light penetrates skin and tissue to several centimeters in depth without damaging any normal cells, the therapy can access most organs from the surface or via endoscopy or fine optical fiber insertion through a transparent catheter needle without surgery. Moreover, the loss of fluorescence upon activation allows therapeutic effects to be monitored in real time. We termed this new form of phototherapy ‘near-infrared photoimmunotherapy’ (NIR-PIT) (Mitsunaga et al. 2011) (Fig. 22.1).

22.2 NIR-PIT Can Selectively Kill Various Cancer Cells

We have shown that this approach works for numerous molecular targets and cancer types. By simply changing the antibody, NIR-PIT can target a broad array of cancer-specific target molecules including the proteins EGFR, HER2, PSMA, CD25, CEA, Mesothelin, GPC3, CD20 and PD-L1, among others. When NIR-PIT was employed for targeting cancer cells to be killed in animal models, we observed significant tumor shrinkage after a single administration of the conjugate and NIR light, and repeated exposure to NIR light produced a more than 80% reduction of the exposed tumors with prolonged disease-free survival and without evident adverse side-effects. Since NIR-PIT can achieve spatially selective killing of target cells, it can be used to eliminate cells containing cancer stem cell markers such as CD44 (Jin et al. 2016) and CD133 (Jing et al. 2016) as we have demonstrated for

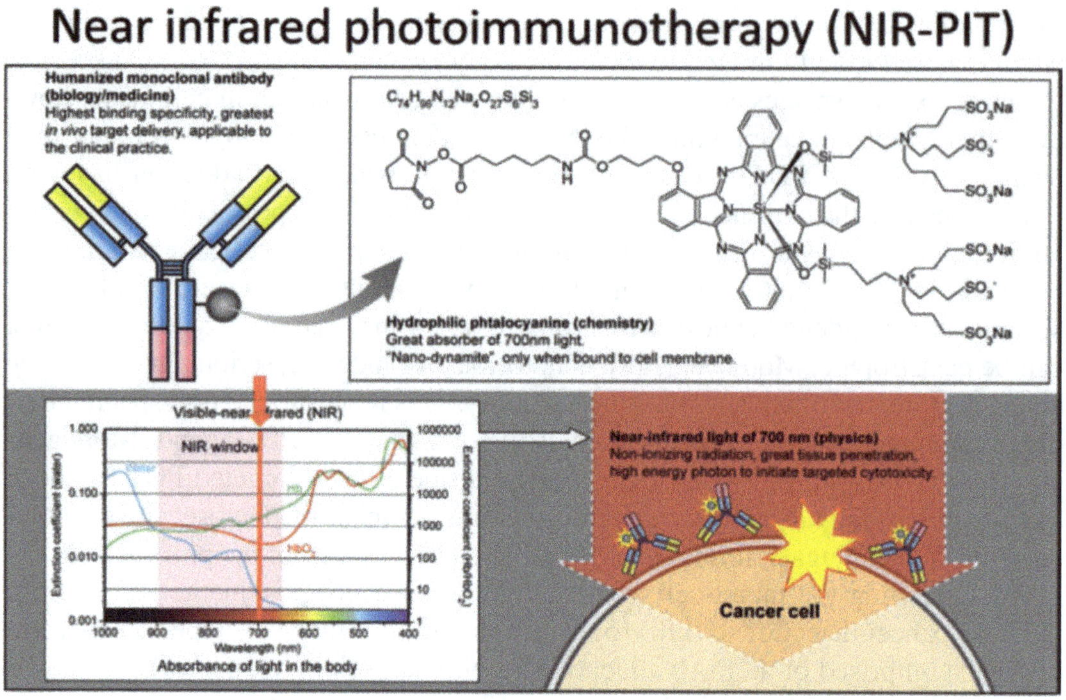

Fig. 22.1 Scheme explaining the basis of near-infrared photoimmunotherapy (NIR-PIT)

breast cancer and glioblastoma stem cells, respectively, without harming normal stem cells expressing these markers in other parts of the body. Targeting cancer stem cells in this way suppresses tumor regrowth for long periods (Fig. 22.2).

22.3 NIR-PIT Rapidly Enhances Nano-Drug Delivery

In addition, NIR-PIT has a desirable side-effect: it initially causes enlargement of the tumor vasculature, increasing blood flow and permeability that induces enhanced delivery of various size of nano-drugs ranging from 5 to 300 nm in diameter.

To date, the delivery of nano-sized therapeutic agents to cancers has been disappointing based as it is on enhanced permeability and retention (EPR) caused by the relatively leaky nature of cancer vasculature. As a result of EPR, there is a modest delivery of nano-sized agents which, although promising as a class of drugs, have demonstrated limited success in oncology. For instance, the EPR effect is estimated to increase nano-drug delivery 20–30% in most cases and 200% in the best case scenario compared with normal tissues. However, after NIR-PIT we observed dramatically increased permeability and retention in the treated tumor bed. We termed this phenomenon, super-enhanced permeability and retention effects (SUPR). Post NIR-PIT SUPR dramatically enhances the delivery of nano-sized agents into treated tissue by up to 24-fold compared with conventional EPR effects (Sano et al. 2013). SUPR occurs because the initial NIR-PIT only kills antigen expressing tumor cells in the perivascular space while leaving the tumor vessels intact, enabling a striking increase in blood volume and, therefore, nano-drug perfusion into the tumor bed

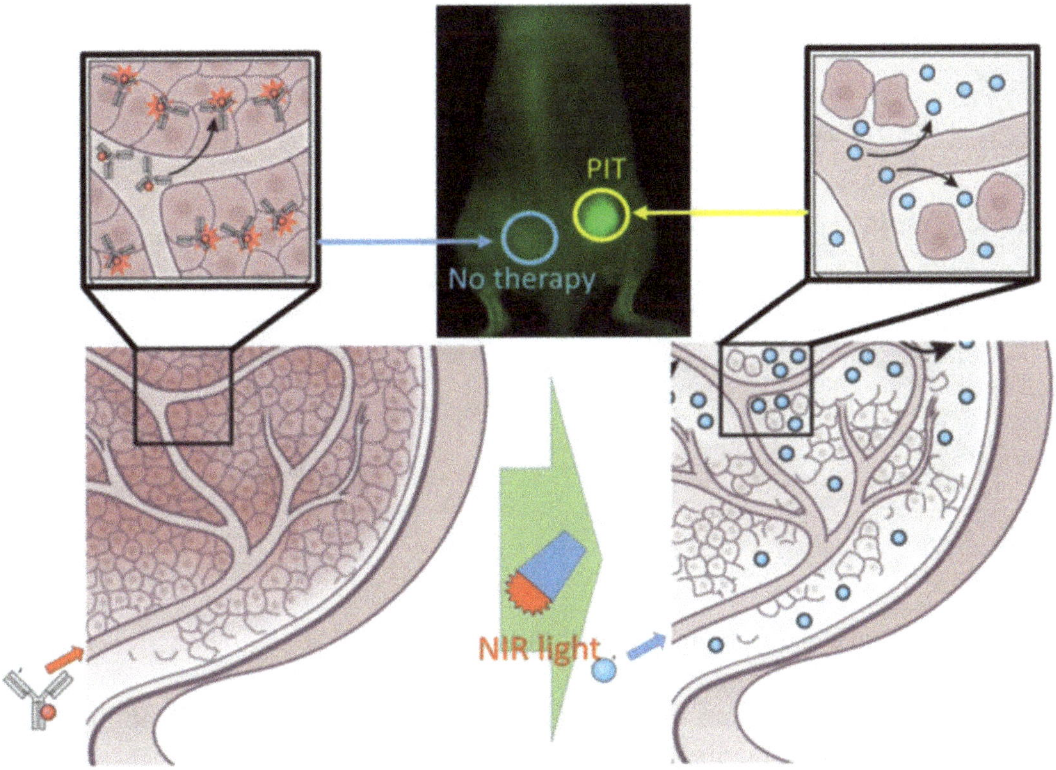

Fig. 22.2 Scheme explaining the mechanism of near-infrared photoimmunotherapy (NIR-PIT) induced super-enhanced permeability and retention (SUPR) effects

within tumor vessels. This permits the delivery of dramatically higher concentrations of nano-sized drugs into treated tumors with minimal uptake in untreated regions. Thus, after NIR-PIT the delivery of nano-drugs into tumors results in highly efficient tumor killing of cells surviving NIR-PIT with minimal side effects to other organs as therapeutic effects can be achieved at much lower doses (Fig. 22.3).

22.4 NIR-PIT Initiates Anti-Tumor Host Immunity and Promotes Rapid Healing

Three-dimensional dynamic quantitative phase-contrast microscopy (QPM) and dual selective plane illumination microscopy (dSPIM) of tumor cells undergoing PIT showed rapid swelling in treated cells immediately after light exposure suggesting rapid water influx into cells, followed by irreversible morphologic changes such as bleb formation, and rupture of cellular membrane and vesicles. Furthermore, biological markers of ICD including relocation of HSP70/90 and calreticulin from cytosol to cellular membrane, and release of calreticulin, ATP and High Mobility Group Box 1 (HMGB1), were clearly detected immediately after NIR-PIT. When NIR-PIT was performed in a mixed culture of cancer cells and immature dendritic

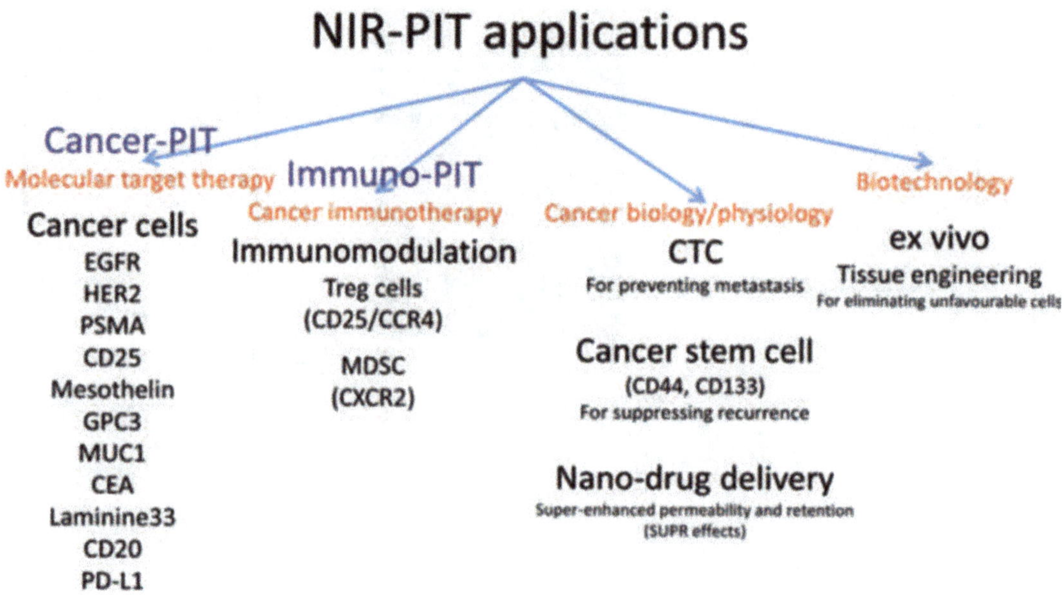

Fig. 22.3 Diagram of the applications of NIR-PIT

cells, maturation of immature dendritic cells was strongly induced rapidly after NIR-PIT against cancer cells.

Because cell membranes across mammalian species exhibit virtually identical physico-chemical properties, they are equally susceptible to the photochemical damage induced by NIR-PIT. Thus, new NIR-PIT conjugates can be developed *in vitro*, *ex vivo* or in animal models with a very high likelihood of successful translation to human patients. This translatability is an important advantage of our chemistry- and photophysics-based approach to cancer treatment. NIR-PIT technology opens the doors for many clinical applications and we hope it will lead to new treatments for numerous different cancer types. In addition, we have found that intact tissue stem cells in the tumor bed greatly contribute to clean wound healing, vital for improving the prognosis and quality of life of cancer patients treated with NIR-PIT.

22.5 Targeting Systemic Metastases

Furthermore, NIR-PIT also shows great promise as an indirect cancer immunotherapy. NIR-PIT achieved spatially selective depletion of tumor-associated immunosuppressing regulatory T cells (Tregs), which inhibit anti-tumor attack (and autoimmunity) by cytotoxic CD8+T cells that proliferate within a tumor. Eliminating Tregs locally in a tumor bed allows the adjacent cytotoxic CD8+T and natural killer (NK) cells to instantly attack the tumor within 1 h. Remarkably, Treg-targeting NIR-PIT also caused the selective systemic regression of untreated distant metastatic tumors with the same cell origin as the treated tumor within 2 days, presumably because once awakened, cytotoxic CD8+T cells were no longer susceptible to

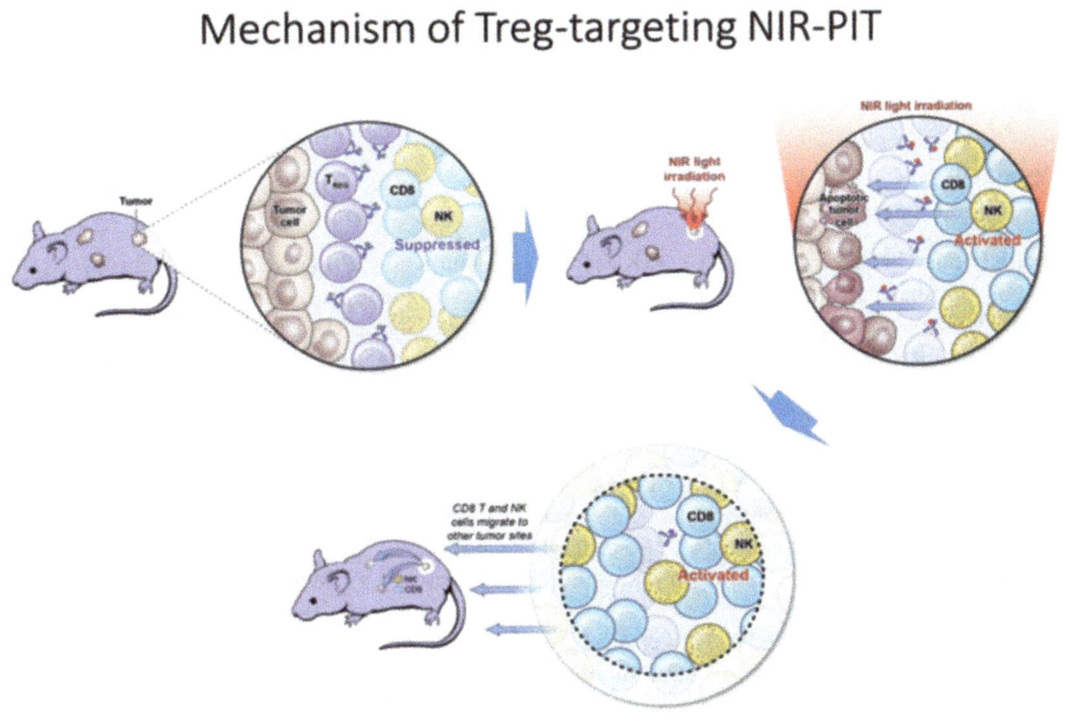

Fig. 22.4 Scheme explaining the functional mechanism of Treg-targeting near-infrared photoimmunotherapy (NIR-PIT)

Treg-induced inactivity (Sato et al. 2016). In contrast, awakened cytotoxic CD8+T cells did not attack normal cells or other cancer cells, ensuring that Treg-targeting NIR-PIT was a highly cell-selective cancer therapy with minimal autoimmune adverse side-effects of the type seen with systemic cancer immunotherapies that activate host-immunity throughout the body (Fig. 22.4).

22.6 Perspective

NIR-PIT shows immense promise for practical and clinical applications. Several NIR-PIT-related patents were licensed to the start-up biotech company Aspyrian Therapeutic Inc., which started a phase I clinical trial in June 2015 and currently advanced to phase II, using the cetuximab–IR700 conjugate (RM-1929) to treat head and neck cancer patients who had failed to respond to all conventional cancer therapies including surgery, chemotherapy and radiation therapy (https://clinicaltrials.gov/ct2/show/NCT02422979). Similar trials are planned for lung, esophageal, bladder and pancreatic cancer, some precancerous conditions including leukoplakia and papillomatosis, and others by targeting cancer cells or immune-suppressor cells in the near future. We have engaged researchers internationally to further explore the possibilities of NIR-PIT and to expedite its introduction into the clinic.

Acknowledgements This research was supported by the Intramural Research Program of the National Institutes of Health, National Cancer Institute, Center for Cancer Research.

References

Jin J, Krishnamachary B, Mironchik Y, Kobayashi H, Bhujwalla ZM (2016) Phototheranostics of CD44-positive cell populations in triple negative breast cancer. Sci Rep 6:27871

Jing H, Weidensteiner C, Reichardt W, Gaedicke S, Zhu X, Grosu AL, Kobayashi H, Niedermann G (2016) Imaging and selective elimination of glioblastoma stem cells with theranostic near-infrared-labeled CD133-specific antibodies. Theranostics 6:862–874

Kobayashi H, Choyke PL (2011) Target-cancer-cell-specific activatable fluorescence imaging probes: rational design and in vivo applications. Acc Chem Res 44:83–90

Kobayashi H, Ogawa M, Alford R, Choyke PL, Urano Y (2010) New strategies for fluorescent probe design in medical diagnostic imaging. Chem Rev 110:2620–2640

Mitsunaga M, Ogawa M, Kosaka N, Rosenblum LT, Choyke PL, Kobayashi H (2011) Cancer cell-selective in vivo near infrared photoimmunotherapy targeting specific membrane molecules. Nat Med 17:1685–1691

Sano K, Nakajima T, Choyke PL, Kobayashi H (2013) Markedly enhanced permeability and retention effects induced by photo-immunotherapy of tumors. ACS Nano 7:717–724

Sato K, Sato N, Xu B, Nakamura Y, Nagaya T, Choyke PL, Hasegawa Y, Kobayashi H (2016) Spatially selective depletion of tumor-associated regulatory T cells with near-infrared photoimmunotherapy. Sci Transl Med 8:352ra110

Urano Y, Asanuma D, Hama Y, Koyama Y, Barrett T, Kamiya M, Nagano T, Watanabe T, Hasegawa A, Choyke PL et al (2009) Selective molecular imaging of viable cancer cells with pH-activatable fluorescence probes. Nat Med 15:104–109

Dr. Hisataka Kobayashi is the Chief Scientist of the Molecular Imaging Program, National Cancer Institute/NIH in Bethesda, Maryland, with over 30 years' experience in R&D of bio-medical imaging and drug delivery, especially targeting cancer for diagnosis and therapy. Dr. Kobayashi holds an MD in Radiology, and a PhD in Immunology/Internal Medicine from Kyoto University, Kyoto, Japan, and has written or contributed to more than 270 articles and 50 invited reviews and book chapters, and has given more than 290 invited lectures and talks on basic and clinical bio-imaging.

Chapter 23
Integrated Imaging on Fatigue and Chronic Fatigue

Yasuyoshi Watanabe, Masaaki Tanaka, Akira Ishii, Kei Mizuno, Akihiro Sasaki, Emi Yamano, Yilong Cui, Sanae Fukuda, Yosky Kataoka, Kozi Yamaguti, Yasuhito Nakatomi, Yasuhiro Wada, and Hirohiko Kuratsune

23.1 Introduction

Fatigue is defined as a condition or phenomenon of decreased ability and efficiency of mental and/or physical activities, caused by excessive mental or physical activities, diseases, or syndromes. It is often accompanied by a peculiar sense of

---

Electronic Supplementary Material The online version of this chapter (https://doi.org/10.1007/978-981-13-7908-6_23) contains supplementary material, which is available to authorized users.

Y. Watanabe (✉) · K. Mizuno · A. Sasaki · E. Yamano · Y. Wada
RIKEN Center for Life Science Technologies, Kobe, Hyogo, Japan

RIKEN Center for Biosystems Dynamics Research, Kobe, Hyogo, Japan

Osaka City University Graduate School of Medicine, Osaka, Japan

RIKEN Compass to Healthy Life Research Complex Program, Kobe, Hyogo, Japan
e-mail: yywata@riken.jp

M. Tanaka · A. Ishii · K. Yamaguti
Osaka City University Graduate School of Medicine, Osaka, Japan

Y. Cui · Y. Kataoka
RIKEN Center for Life Science Technologies, Kobe, Hyogo, Japan

RIKEN Center for Biosystems Dynamics Research, Kobe, Hyogo, Japan

RIKEN Compass to Healthy Life Research Complex Program, Kobe, Hyogo, Japan

S. Fukuda · H. Kuratsune
Osaka City University Graduate School of Medicine, Osaka, Japan

Kansai University of Welfare Sciences, Osaka, Japan

Y. Nakatomi
Osaka City University Graduate School of Medicine, Osaka, Japan

NAKATOMI Fatigue Care Clinic, Osaka, Japan

Y. Toyama et al. (eds.), *Make Life Visible*,
https://doi.org/10.1007/978-981-13-7908-6_23

discomfort, a desire to rest, and reduced motivation, referred to as fatigue sensation. Acute fatigue is a normal condition or phenomenon that disappears after a period of rest; in contrast, chronic fatigue, lasting at least 6 months, does not disappear after ordinary rest. Chronic fatigue impairs activities and contributes to various medical conditions, such as cardiovascular disease, epileptic seizures, and death. In addition, many people complain of chronic fatigue. For example, in Japan, more than one third of the general adult population complains of chronic fatigue. It would thus be of great value to clarify the mechanisms underlying chronic fatigue and to develop efficient treatment methods to overcome it.

Here, we review the data obtained from molecular imaging and neuroimaging studies related to neural dysfunction as well as autonomic nervous system, sleep, and circadian rhythm disorders in fatigue (Watanabe et al. 2008; Tanaka et al. 2015). These data provide new perspectives on the mechanisms underlying chronic fatigue and on overcoming it.

23.2 Integrated Imaging Studies

Integrated multi-modal imaging technologies with Omics analyses and precise biomarker analyses give us the chance to create Precision Medicine and Precision Health. Especially, PET technologies open up a new era of 4-dimentional analyses of molecular events in human body. In combination with functional and anatomical imaging with MRI and MEG, total understanding of human dysfunction such as fatigue and chronic fatigue could be obtained.

We focused on the multi-modal imaging studies on fatigue and chronic fatigue, even on the patho-physiology of the patients with Myalgic Encephalomyelitis/ Chronic Fatigue Syndrome (ME/CFS). As shown in Fig. 23.1, we especially focused on the correlation studies between neuro-inflammation and serotonergic deterioration maybe intermediated through biological oxidation, and also among autonomic dysfunction (Mizuno et al. 2011; Tanaka et al. 2011), such molecular changes in neurotransmitter systems and cytokine systems, and functional deterioration in the brain.

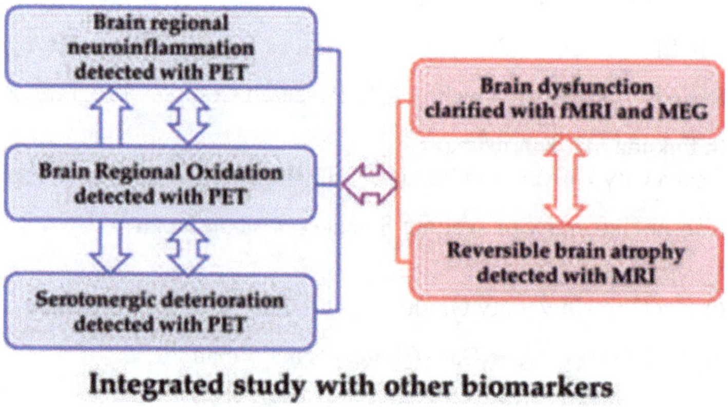

Fig. 23.1 Integrated multi-modal imaging studies on fatigue and chronic fatigue (interactions are the main issues of this chapter supported by The Uehara Memorial Foundation)

23.3 PET Studies

Previously, we found the decrease of the density of serotonin reuptake sites (5-HT transporters) in the rostral subdivision of the anterior cingulate cortex of the patients with ME/CFS by using [^{11}C](+)McN5652 as compared with that in normal volunteers (Yamamoto et al. 2004). This subdivision is different from that in the dorsal anterior cingulate in which binding potential values of individual patient showed a weak negative correlation with self-reported pain score of the patients. Therefore, we thought that an alteration of serotonergic system in the rostral anterior cingulate plays a key role in pathophysiology of ME/CFS. The deterioration of the serotonergic tone in this brain region is related to the autonomic nerve dysfunction, since the autonomic center is close to the region. We recently found with [^{11}C](R)-PK11195 and PET that neuro-inflammation is present in widespread brain areas (in the cingulate cortex, hippocampus, amygdala, thalamus, midbrain, and pons) in ME/CFS patients and was associated with the severity of neuro-psychologic symptoms (Nakatomi et al. 2014). In ME/CFS patients, the BP(ND) values of [^{11}C](R)-PK11195 in the amygdala, thalamus, and midbrain positively correlated with cognitive impairment score, the BP(ND) values in the cingulate cortex and thalamus positively correlated with pain score, and the BP(ND) value in the hippocampus positively correlated with depression score. Evaluation of neuro-inflammation in CFS/ME patients may be essential for understanding the core pathophysiology and for developing objective diagnostic criteria and effective medical treatments.

In the present study, we performed the combination study of autonomic nerve function and other fatigue biomarkers such as biological oxidation (Fukuda et al. 2016), less repair energy (decrease of initial members of TCA cycle) (Yamano et al. 2016), and inflammation biomarkers (highly sensitive CRP etc.), with PET study using [^{11}C]DASB instead of [^{11}C]McN5652 for serotonin transporter density and [^{11}C](R)-PK11195 for extent of neuro-inflammation. So far with 10 ME/CFS patients, we could preliminarily show a positive correlation between autonomic dysfunction and serotonergic tone in the anterior cingulate cortex, and also negative correlation between serotonin transporter density and extent of neuro-inflammation. We are still recruiting more numbers of patients for this study.

For biological oxidation PET study, we developed the novel ^{11}C-labeled PET probe, but this probe is rather rapidly metabolized in chronic fatigue model rats. We are now improving the structure of the probe.

23.4 MRI Morphometry

Previously we found regional gray matter volume reduction in the dorsolateral prefrontal cortices in both hemispheres in the patients with ME/CFS as compared with those of healthy age-matched subjects (Okada et al. 2004). Especially, the extent of volume reduction of right prefrontal cortex was correlated with the severity score of their fatigue. This finding was confirmed by de Lange et al. (2008), and de Lange et al. demonstrated this tentative atrophy recovered in the responders of Cognitive Behavioral Therapy. Then, in the present study, Mizuno et al. tried to see such volume reduction under the subacute-chronic fatigue state, and could demonstrate almost the same results even in the young adult population.

23.5 fMRI Study

In 2006, we reported the over-defense mechanisms of fatigue in ME/CFS patients (Tanaka et al. 2006). Namely, they performed visual tasks resulting in the decrease of visual cortical activity afterward. The healthy volunteers showed almost similar decline in the visual activity, but only the patients with ME/CFS showed the decline of auditory cortical activity, even they just did visual tasks. We hypothesized that the control tower in the brain (might be the prefrontal cortex) is watching the lowered local brain activities and then the control tower ordered the rest in the other brain regions in the case of ME/CFS patients, since the patients should not go into much severer state otherwise could not be recovered. This phenomenon could be confirmed by another angle with resting state fMRI in the subacute-chronic fatigue. Sasaki et al. recently demonstrated particular brain region(s) specific for prolonged fatigue sensation.

23.6 MEG Study

The mechanisms of fatigue sensation were analyzed mostly with MEG. An MEG study related to the mirror system of fatigue sensation has been reported by our group (de Lange et al. 2008). Twelve healthy male volunteers participated in this study and viewed 80 pictures with fatigued facial expressions and those with neutral facial expressions in a randomized order. Since there have been several reports showing that seeing emotional changes in others activates the brain regions involved in experiencing similar emotions, it is hypothesized that the brain regions activated when they viewed the fatigued facial expressions may be candid brain regions related to the neural mechanisms of fatigue sensation. In fact, the equivalent current dipole (ECD) in the posterior cingulate cortex (PCC) was observed in 9 of 12 participants, and the ECD in the insular cortex (IC) was observed in 3 of 12 participants only when they viewed the fatigued facial expressions, suggesting that the PCC and IC are the candid brain regions related to the neural mechanisms of fatigue sensation (Ishii et al. 2012).

Since it has been reported that the PCC is involved in self-reflection or self-monitoring, the neural substrates related to self-evaluation of the level of physical and mental fatigue were examined using MEG. Ten healthy male volunteers participated in a study that examined the neural substrates related to self-evaluation of the level of physical fatigue. When they self-evaluated the level of fatigue of their right hand, the ECD in the PCC was observed in 9 of 10 participants. On the other hand, when they directed their attention to their right hand as a control condition, the ECD in the PCC was observed in 2 of 10 participants. In addition, the intensity of the ECD in the PCC observed in relation to the self-evaluation of the level of physical fatigue was positively associated with the extent to which fatigue of the right hand was successfully evaluated. These results suggest that the activation in the PCC was related to the self-evaluation of the level of physical fatigue (Ishii et al. 2014a).

In the next study, the neural substrates related to self-evaluation of the level of mental fatigue were examined. Fourteen healthy male volunteers participated in this study. They performed 90 evaluation trials and 90 control trials in a randomized order. In the evaluation trials, they were asked to self-evaluate the level of their mental fatigue. The control trials were resting trials in which they were asked to do nothing. The ECD in the PCC was observed in 7 of 14 participants when they self-evaluated the level of their mental fatigue, although it was observed in only 1 of 14 participants when they performed the control trials, suggesting that the activation in the PCC was also related to self-evaluation of the level of mental fatigue (Ishii et al. 2014b). It has been shown that the PCC is not only involved in the neural mechanisms of fatigue sensation but is also involved in the neural mechanisms of making decisions in the presence of fatigue (Ishii et al. 2014c). If individuals do not rest, despite the signs of fatigue, they may experience overwork, which may be a starting point of chronic fatigue as discussed later. Therefore, the decision of whether or not to rest based on the level of fatigue is important. Fifteen healthy male volunteers participated in this study. They performed 1200 reverse Stroop test trials and were intermittently asked whether to take a rest or not to maintain task performance; neural activities related to making decisions to rest were assessed. When they made decisions to rest, a decreased 4–8 Hz band power was observed in the PCC, and this decreased 4–8 Hz band power in the PCC was positively associated with the subjective level of fatigue caused by performing the experiment. As for the IC, it has been reported that the IC is involved in mental effort evaluation in an fMRI study in which the participants rated their mental effort investment required for performing 1-, 2-, and 3-back tests. These findings suggest that the PCC and IC are involved in the neural mechanisms of fatigue sensation to self-evaluate the level of fatigue, and that the PCC plays an important role in making decisions to take a rest in the presence of fatigue.

More recently, we performed the MEG study (Ishii et al. 2018) to examine whether thinking positively about the fatigue sensation would increase motivation to accomplish the workload. Fourteen healthy male volunteers participated in this study and performed a two-back test for 30 min to induce mental fatigue sensation. After their subjective level of fatigue had recovered to the baseline level, they re-experienced the fatigue sensation experienced in the two-back test positively, negatively, and without any modification (i.e., re-experienced the fatigue sensation as it was). The level of motivation to perform another two-back test they felt during the re-experiencing was assessed. The neural activity related to the re-experiencing was recorded using magnetoencephalography. The level of the motivation to perform another two-back test was increased by positively re-experiencing the fatigue sensation. The increase in delta band power in Brodmann area 7 was positively associated with the increase in motivation. These results show that positive thinking about fatigue sensation can enhance motivation and suggest that this enhanced motivation may have some effects on visual attention system.

Finally, we have tried to reveal whether the neural activation level is altered in the patients with ME/CFS. Actually, the subtraction between the resting state with open eyes and that with closed eyes gave a great difference between healthy subjects and the patients with ME/CFS (Tanaka M et al., on-going study).

Acknowledgments We thank The Uehara Memorial Foundation for their support on our recent work described here.

References

de Lange FP, Koers A, Kalkman JS, Bleijenberg G, Hagoort P, van der Meer JW, Toni I (2008) Increase in prefrontal cortical volume following cognitive behavioural therapy in patients with chronic fatigue syndrome. Brain 131:2172–2180

Fukuda S, Nojima J, Motoki Y, Yamaguti K, Nakatomi Y, Okawa N, Fujiwara K, Watanabe Y, Kuratsune H (2016) A potential biomarker for fatigue: oxidative stress and anti-oxidative activity. Biol Psychol 118:88–93

Ishii A, Tanaka M, Yamano E, Watanabe Y (2012) Neural substrates activated by viewing others expressing fatigue: a magnetoencephalography study. Brain Res 1455:68–74

Ishii A, Tanaka M, Yamano E, Watanabe Y (2014a) The neural substrates of physical fatigue sensation to evaluate ourselves: a magnetoencephalography study. Neuroscience 261:60–67

Ishii A, Tanaka M, Watanabe Y (2014b) The neural substrates of self-evaluation of mental fatigue: a magnetoencephalography study. PLoS One 9:e95763

Ishii A, Tanaka M, Watanabe Y (2014c) The neural mechanisms underlying the decision to rest in the presence of fatigue: a magnetoencephalography study. PLoS One 9:e109740

Ishii A, Ishizuka T, Muta Y, Tanaka M, Yamano E, Watanabe Y (2018) The neural effects of positively and negatively re-experiencing mental fatigue sensation: a magnetoencephalography study. Exp Brain Res 1007:s00221

Mizuno K, Tanaka M, Yamaguti K, Kajimoto O, Kuratsune H, Watanabe Y (2011) Mental fatigue caused by prolonged cognitive load associated with sympathetic hyperactivity. Behav Brain Funct 7:17

Nakatomi Y, Mizuno K, Ishii A, Wada Y, Tanaka M, Tazawa S, Onoe K, Fukuda S, Kawabe J, Takahashi K, Kataoka Y, Shiomi S, Yamaguti K, Inaba M, Kuratsune H, Watanabe Y (2014) Neuroinflammation in patients with chronic fatigue syndrome/Myalgic encephalomyelitis: an ^{11}C-(R)-PK11195 PET study. J Nucl Med 55:945–950

Okada T, Tanaka M, Kuratsune H, Watanabe Y, Sadato N (2004) Mechanisms underlying fatigue: a voxel-based morphometric study of chronic fatigue syndrome. BMC Neurol 4:14

Tanaka M, Sadato N, Okada T, Mizuno K, Sasabe T, Tanabe HC, Saito DN, Onoe H, Kuratsune H, Watanabe Y (2006) Reduced responsiveness is an essential feature of chronic fatigue syndrome: a fMRI study. BMC Neurol 6:9

Tanaka M, Mizuno K, Yamaguti K, Kuratsune H, Fujii A, Baba H, Matsuda K, Nishimae A, Takesaka T, Watanabe Y (2011) Autonomic nervous alterations associated with daily level of fatigue. Behav Brain Funct 7:46

Tanaka M, Tajima S, Mizuno K, Ishii A, Konishi Y, Miike T, Watanabe Y (2015) Frontier studies on fatigue, autonomic nerve dysfunction, and sleep-rhythm disorder. J Physiol Sci 65:483–498

Watanabe Y, Evengard B, Natelson BH, Jason LA, Kuratsune H (eds) (2008) Fatigue science for human health. Springer, New York

Yamamoto S, Ouchi Y, Onoe H, Yoshikawa E, Tsukada H, Takahashi H, Iwase M, Yamaguti K, Kuratsune H, Watanabe Y (2004) Reduction of serotonin transporters of patients with chronic fatigue syndrome. Neuroreport 15:2571–2574

Yamano E, Sugimoto M, Hirayama A, Kume S, Yamato M, Jin G, Tajima S, Goda N, Iwai K, Fukuda S, Yamaguti K, Kuratsune H, Soga T, Watanabe Y, Kataoka Y (2016) Index markers of chronic fatigue syndrome with dysfunction of TCA and urea cycles. Sci Rep 6:34990

Chapter 24
Development of Novel Fluorogenic Probes for Realizing Rapid Intraoperative Multi-color Imaging of Tiny Tumors

Yasuteru Urano

24.1 Rational Design of Organic Fluorogenic Probes Based on Unique Spirocyclization of Rhodamines by the Intramolecular Hydroxymethyl Group

Fluorescence imaging is one of the most powerful techniques currently available for continuous observation of dynamic intracellular processes in living cells. In recent years, this technique is not restricted to biological experiments but applicable to clinical fields. Among them, intraoperative fluorescence imaging of lesions or structures that are difficult to identify with the naked eye enable real-time characterization of tumors, thereby aiding clinical decisions on both intra- and postoperative treatments (Stewart and Wild 2014; Hanahan and Weinberg 2000).

Suitable fluorogenic (activatable fluorescence) probes that are initially non-fluorescent and turn to be highly fluorescent upon binding/reaction with target biological molecules of interest, are naturally of critical importance for fluorescence imaging. We have been working for developing novel fluorogenic probes, and succeeded to construct several versatile rational design strategies based on the concept of photoinduced electron transfer (Miura et al. 2003; Urano et al. 2005) and intramolecular spirocyclization (Kamiya et al. 2011; Sakabe et al. 2013). As for the latter design strategy, we have synthesized and evaluated a series of hydroxymethyl rhodamine derivatives and found an intriguing difference of intramolecular spirocyclization behavior: the acetylated derivative of hydroxymethyl rhodamine green

---

Electronic Supplementary Material The online version of this chapter (https://doi.org/10.1007/978-981-13-7908-6_24) contains supplementary material, which is available to authorized users.

Y. Urano (✉)
Graduate School of Pharmaceutical Sciences and of Medicine, The University of Tokyo, Bunkyo, Tokyo, Japan
e-mail: uranokun@m.u-tokyo.ac.jp

Y. Toyama et al. (eds.), *Make Life Visible*,
https://doi.org/10.1007/978-981-13-7908-6_24

(Ac-HMRG) exists as a closed spirocyclic structure in aqueous solution at physiological pH, whereas HMRG itself takes an open non-spirocyclic structure. More precisely, the pK_{cycl} value, the pH at which the absorbance or fluorescence of the compound decreases to a half of the maximum value as a result of spirocyclization, of HMRG was calculated to be 8.1, but that of AcHMRG where one of the amines on the xanthene moiety was amidated, decreased to 5.3. Therefore at the physiological pH of 7.4, HMRG predominantly takes the ring-open form with strong fluorescence at λ_{fl} of 524 nm, but its acetylated derivative AcHMRG would predominantly be the in spirocyclized closed form with reduced absorbance or fluorescence in the visible region.

24.2 Development of Novel Fluorogenic Green Probes for Biological and Medical Purposes, Especially for Intraoperative Rapid Tumor Imaging

Based on the above-mentioned findings, we have established a general design strategy to develop highly sensitive fluorogenic probes for proteases and glycosidases: Converting the acetyl group to different functional groups or peptides that are targeted by proteases and glycosidases would enable a wide range of probes to be developed. Specific cleavage of the substrate moiety in the non-fluorescent probe by the target enzyme generates a strong fluorescence signal. In order to confirm the validity and flexibility of our strategy, we designed and synthesized fluorescence probes for leucine aminopeptidase, fibroblast activation protein, cathepsin B/L, β-galactosidase, and so on (Fig. 24.1a). All these probes were almost non-fluorescent due to the formation of spirocyclic structure, but were converted efficiently to highly fluorescent HMRG by the target enzymes (Fig. 24.1b). We confirmed that the probes can be used in living cells. These probes offer great practical advantages, including high sensitivity and rapid response (owing to regulation of fluorescence at a single reactive site), as well as resistance to photobleaching.

For medical imaging purposes, protease including aminopeptidase activities are known to be important imaging targets, because they play essential roles in many diseases, and some of them show altered expression levels in the pathological context (Hanahan and Weinberg 2011; Weigelt 2005). For endopeptidase, there already developed many fluorogenic or FRET-based probes such as those for MMP and cathepsins, but there were few examples for aminopeptidases, especially those function with visible light irradiation. Therefore, by making use of the above-mentioned strategy based on the spirocyclization, we started to develop many fluorogenic probes for aminopeptidases. For example, gGlu-HMRG, a novel spirocyclized rhodamine-based fluorescence probe for γ-glutamyltranspeptidase (GGT), which is well-known to be upregulated in various cancer cells (Pompella et al. 2006), was successfully developed (Fig. 24.2a). By applying gGlu-HMRG to various cancerous cell lines whose GGT activity is upregulated, fast enzymatic reaction of gGlu-HMRG with GGT occurs on the plasma membrane to yield highly fluorescent

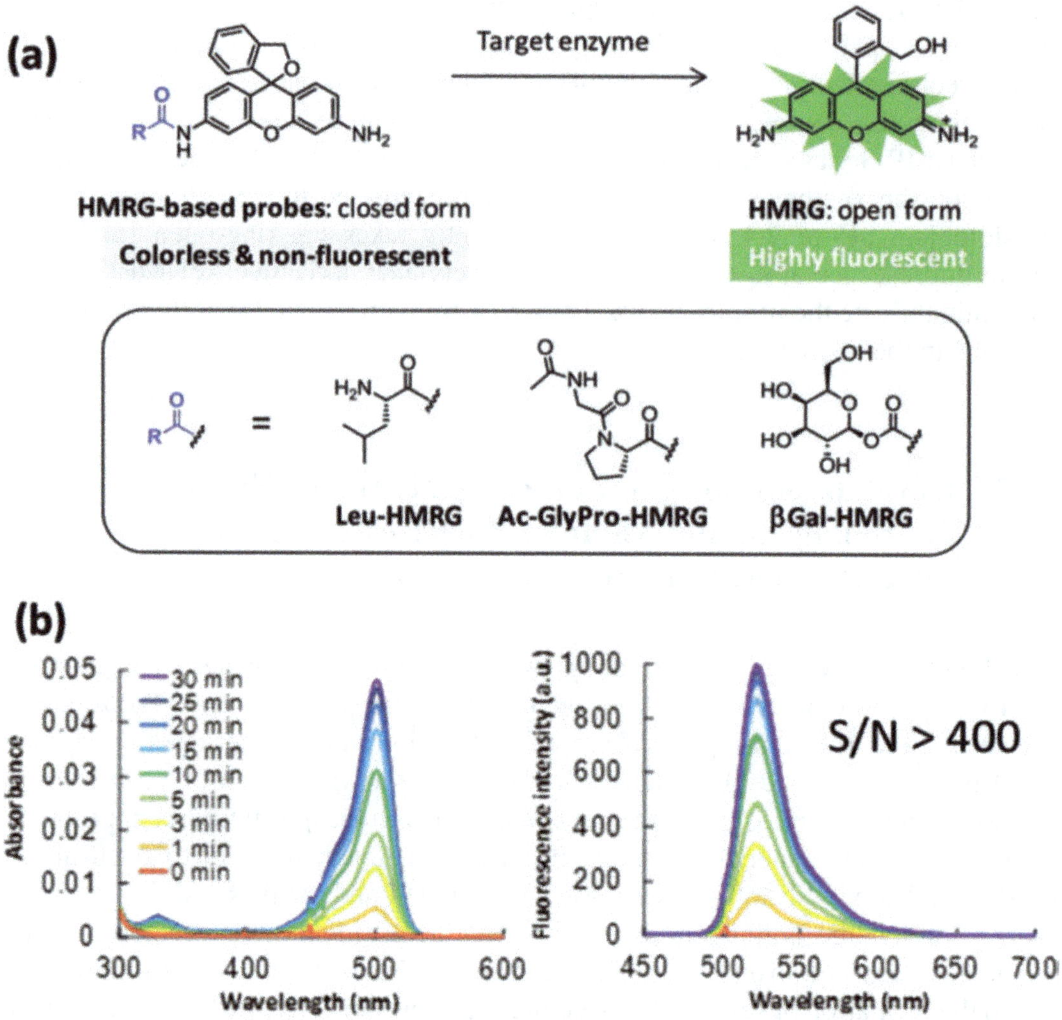

Fig. 24.1 Novel design strategy for various hydrolases-sensitive fluorogenic probes based on HMRG scaffold. (**a**) Enzymatic reaction of HMRG-based probes with the target enzymes. Leu-HMRG for leucine aminopeptidase (LAP), Ac-GlyPo-HMRG for fibroblast activation protein (FAP), βGal-HMRG for β-galactosidase. (**b**) Absorption and emission spectra of 1 μM Leu-HMRG at 0, 1, 3, 5, 10, 15, 20, 25 and 30 min after addition of LAP (0.04 U). Reaction was performed in 0.1 M sodium phosphate buffer (pH 7.4) at 37 °C. Excitation wavelength was 501 nm

product HMRG, which led us to establish a novel and highly activatable strategy for sensitive and fast-responding fluorescence imaging of tiny tumors in vivo. In mouse models of disseminated human peritoneal ovarian cancer, activation of gGlu-HMRG occurred within 1 min of topically spraying onto tissue surfaces that are suspected of harboring tumors, creating high signal contrast between the tumor and the background (Urano et al. 2011) (Fig. 24.2b, c).

Furthermore, not only with tumor mice models, but with freshly resected real human tumor samples, we started to examine the efficacy of gGlu-HMRG as an intraoperative tumor detecting agent by collaborating with many surgeons. Indeed, gGlu-HMRG was proved to be effective for rapid intraoperative imaging of breast (Ueo et al. 2015; Shinden et al. 2016), oral (Shimane et al. 2016), and hepatic

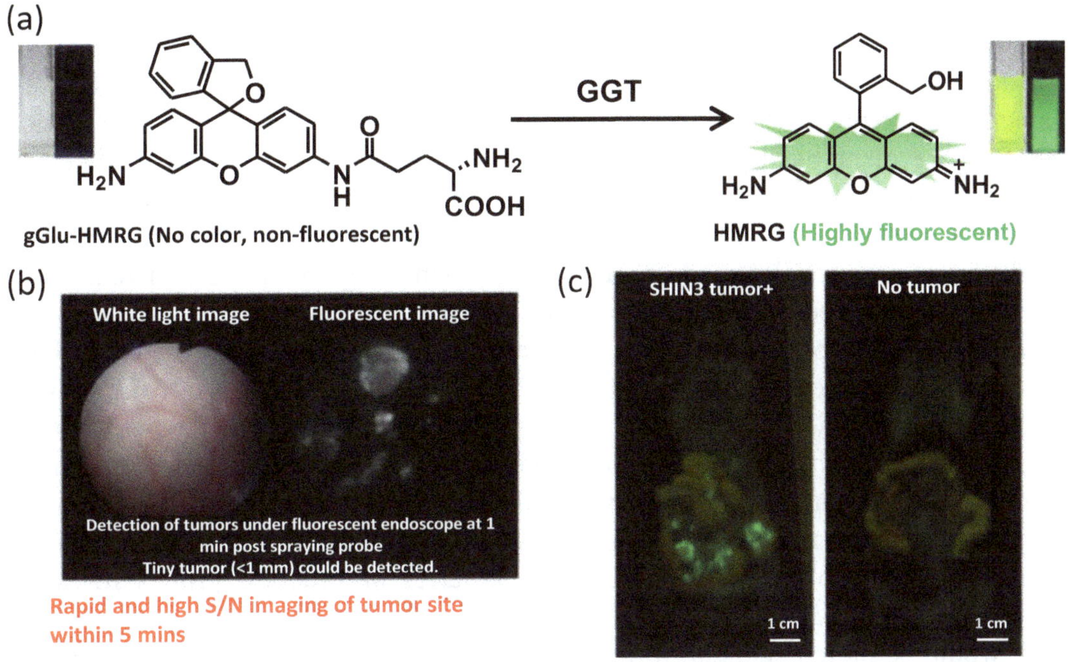

Fig. 24.2 (**a**) Novel HMRG-based fluorescence probe for γ-glutamyl transpeptidase. (**b**) Tiny disseminated tumor sites including those smaller than 1 mm in size could be clearly detected by topically spraying gGlu-HMRG after 1 min in the peritoneal cavity. (**c**) Tumor sites emitted very bright green fluorescence with high selectivity, which could be detected even with our naked eyes, only after 10 min post application of the probe

(Miyata et al. 2017) cancers. For example, breast cancer could be visualized regardless of its types like invasive/non-invasive or ER and HER2(+)/(−) with high specificity and sensitivity, both exceeded 90% (Ueo et al. 2015), and metastases in sentinel lymph nodes could be examined within a few minutes with high negative predictive values (>99%) (Shinden et al. 2016).

24.3 Development of Novel Fluorogenic Scaffold for Detecting Protease Activity in Longer Wavelength by Optimizing the Spirocyclization Properties: Novel Strategy for Fluorescence-Assisted Surgery with Multicolor Protease Imaging (Iwatate et al. 2016)

However, as can be easily imagined, because cancer cells are known to have big heterogeneity, gGlu-HMRG can only image cancer with elevated GGT activity, which accounts for only a small portion of all cancer. Two of the realistic clinical applications of fluorescent probes are preoperative diagnosis by fluorescent endoscopy and intraoperative diagnosis. Yet for fluorescence to be used for these purposes, the fluorescent probe must be able to detect, in principle, all types of cancer.

Although this is difficult to realize with a single probe targeting one protease, by spraying or administering a cocktail of fluorescent probes targeting various proteases that can cover for each other, it would become possible to simultaneously detect multiple proteases. If the cocktail is composed of probes with different fluorescence wavelengths, this would also enable the surgeons to distinguish and characterize the tumors according to the difference in protease activity profiles.

If protease probes that function in a similar manner to gGlu-HMRG but with different target and wavelength were developed, such imaging can be realized. For a protease probe to be used for multicolour imaging with HMRG, the scaffold dye must have a spectroscopic property that can be differentiated from HMRG. If the scaffold was a spirocyclizing rhodamine that bears an amine on xanthene moiety available for peptide conjugation to be the switch for fluorescence activation and retains the hydroxymethyl group on the benzene ring moiety of HMRG for intramolecular spirocyclization to occur, some of the favourable properties of HMRG may also be applicable for the new probes. Thus, modifying parts of HMRG was deemed to be an appropriate strategy to develop a series of protease probes for such purposes.

It would be more beneficial if the scaffolding rhodamine also met the following criteria:

- Has longer λ_{abs} and λ_{fl} than HMRG for better tissue penetration
- Emits fluorescence in the visible region for detection by the naked human eye
- Single reaction point for more sensitive and quantitative detection
- Photobleach-resistant

However, there were no reported rhodamines that met these criteria. Thus, the aim of the research was set to detect a variety of cancer with different protease activity profiles using small molecule based protease probes (Fig. 24.3).

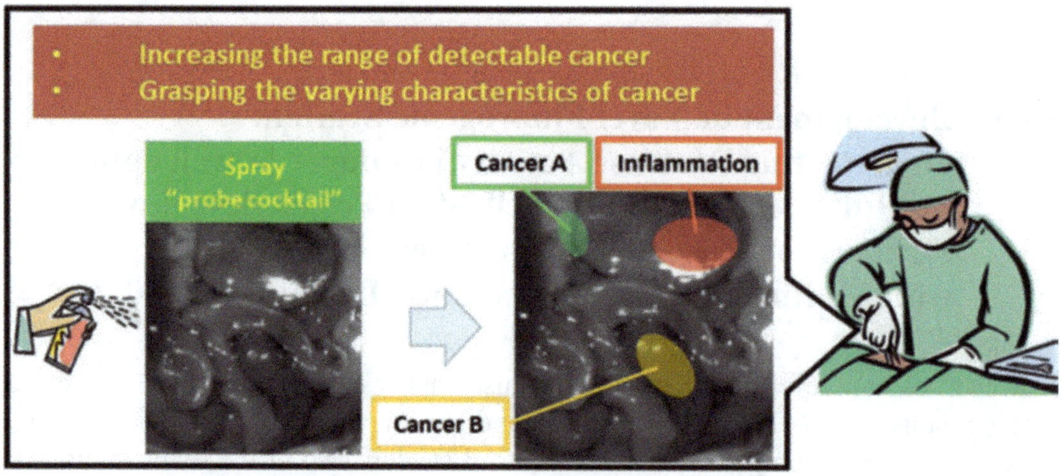

Fig. 24.3 A cartoon showing the outline of the Novel strategy for fluorescence-assisted surgery with multicolor protease imaging

For a rhodamine to function as a scaffold for a protease probe, it must have an unsubstituted amine for peptide conjugation. This meant that only one of the amines on HMRG could be modified, resulting in asymmetrical rhodamines. There were no reports on the synthesis of asymmetrical rhodamines bearing a hydroxymethyl group, therefore a synthetic route based on synthesis of symmetrical rhodamine was developed to prepare three asymmetrical rhodamine derivatives. The carboxyl groups of these asymmetrical rhodamines were then reduced to hydroxymethyl groups to afford three derivatives bearing a hydroxymethyl group: *N,N*-dimethyl derivative (HMDiMeR), *N,N*-diethyl derivative (HMDiEtR) and julolidine-fused derivative (HMJR) (Table 24.1: 1a, 2a, 3a).

Acetylated derivative of a rhodamine has been shown to function as a model compound for protease probes on HMRG. The changes to the absorption and fluorescence spectra matched well and most importantly, the change to pK_{cycl} can be modelled with an easy-to-synthesise compound with a single amidation reaction. Thus, acetylated derivatives of HMDiMeR, HMDiEtR and HMJR were also synthesised (Table 24.1: 1d, 2d, 3d).

Examination of the spectroscopic properties of the synthesised compounds showed that λ_{abs} and λ_{fl} had indeed been extended (Table 24.2). As expected, julolidine-fused HMJR had the biggest red-shift with 46 nm for absorption. All of these rhodamine derivatives exhibited pH dependency by spirocyclization and their absorbance and fluorescence intensities decreased with increasing pH. Correspondingly, the pK_{cycl} values of the acetylated derivatives decreased to acidic values compared with their parental derivatives. The shift was around 2.7 for HMRG, HMDiMeR and HMDiEtR, but it was smaller for HMJR at 2.0. However, the values of pK_{cycl} generally increased to more basic values with the red-shifts. The pK_{cycl} values of acetylated derivatives were turned out to be ranging from 6.2 to 8.3, which were less suitable as scaffolds for protease probes, as protease probes based on them would not preferentially take the closed form at the physiological pH of 7.4. This would result in increased background fluorescence and smaller activation ratio.

As intramolecular spirocyclization occurs through intramolecular nucleophilic attack of the hydroxymethyl group on the 9 position of the xanthene moiety, a hypothesis that making the 9 position less electron-rich would reduce the pK_{cycl} value to the acidic side was contrived. One easy and synthetically-feasible solution was to introduce electron-withdrawing groups such as halogens to the xanthene moiety. Therefore, we started to synthesize three asymmetrical rhodamines with fluorination or chlorination to the 2 position of the xanthene moieties (Table 24.1: 1b, 1c, 2b, 2c, 3b, 3c), together with their acetylated derivatives. (Table 24.1: 1e, 1f, 2e, 2f, 3e, 3f).

The spectroscopic properties of the synthesised compounds supported the hypothesis that halogenation would have no negative effect on the spectroscopic properties such as λ_{abs}, λ_{fl} and Φ_{fl}, but would reduce pK_{cycl} values (Table 24.2). The reduction in pK_{cycl} values was larger for chlorinated compounds.

HMDiMeR derivatives and HMDiEtR derivatives were very dark compared to HMRG with Φ_{fl} of around 0.05, and their λ_{abs} were relatively short at around 530 nm: HMJR derivatives were brighter with Φ_{fl} of around 0.4 and had longer λ_{abs} at around

Table 24.1 Structures of synthesised asymmetrical rhodamines bearing a hydroxymethyl group and their acetylated derivatives

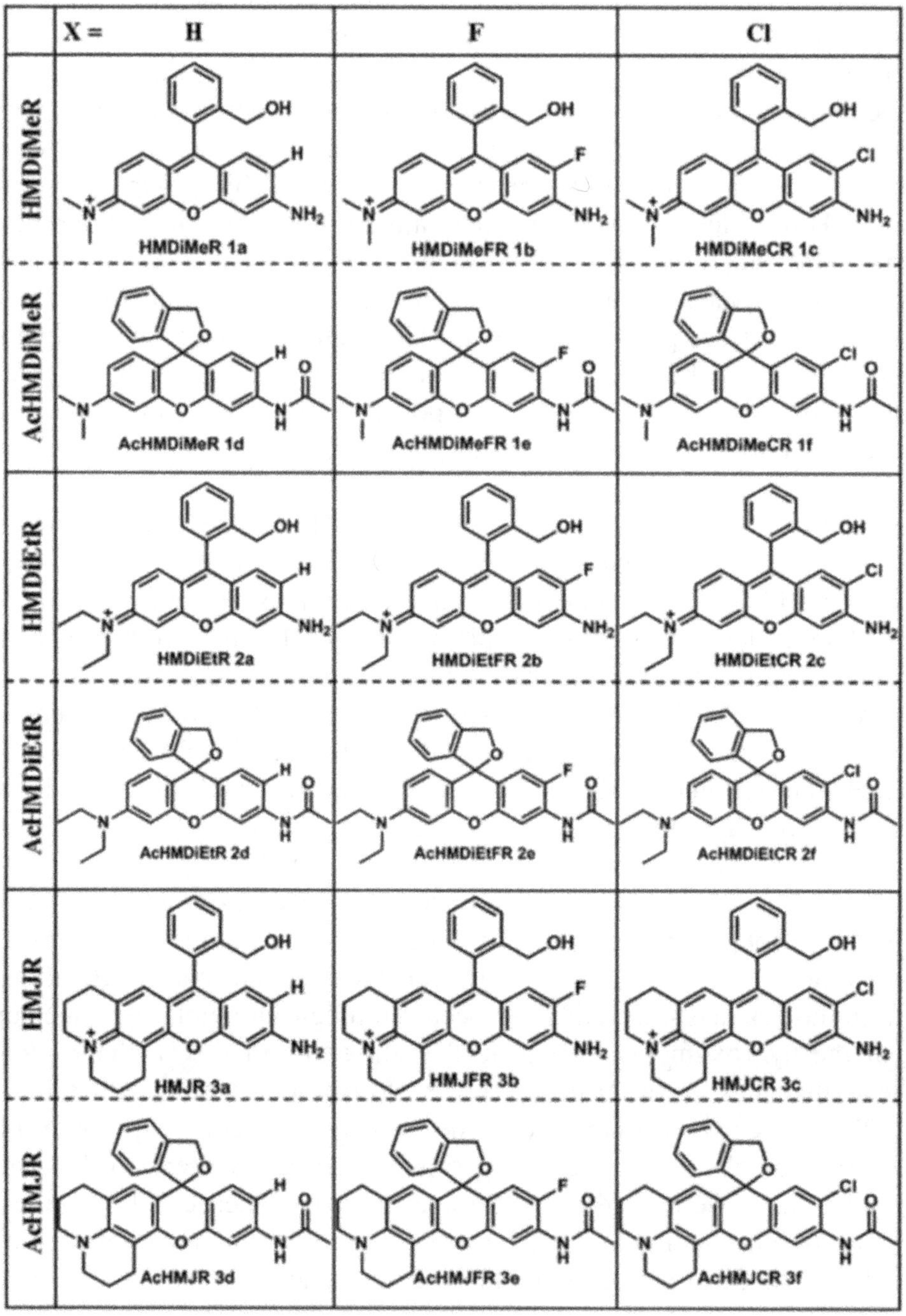

550 nm. The pK_{cycl} value of AcHMJCR was 7.3, which suggests a half of the molecules would take open form under physiological pH, but this increases to 90% after the reaction. Even though these sets of values were not quite optimal in themselves, taking account the changes in Φ_{fl} and ε, fluorescence increase of about 40-fold could have been expected. Therefore HMJCR was chosen as the novel scaffold for a red-shifted protease probe.

Table 24.2 Spectroscopic properties of asymmetric *N*-alkyl rhodamines bearing a hydroxymethyl group

Compound	λ_{abs} (nm)	λ_{fl} (nm)	Φ_{fl}	pK_{cycl}
HMRG	501	524	0.81	8.1
AcHMRG	495	526	0.27	5.3
HMDiMeR **1a**	529	553	0.05	8.9
HMDiMeFR **1b**	532	559	0.06	8.2
HMDiMeCR **1c**	536	559	0.04	7.7
AcHMDiMeR **1d**	499	571	0.02	6.2
AcHMDiMeFR **1e**	507	582	<0.01	5.7
AcHMDiMeCR **1f**	505	581	0.01	5.2
HMDiEtR **2a**	532	555	0.05	9.3
HMDiEtFR **2b**	538	566	0.02	8.6
HMDiEtCR **2c**	541	568	0.02	8.1
AcHMDiEtR **2d**	501	573	0.01	6.7
AcHMDiEtFR **2e**	508	583	0.01	6.1
AcHMDiEtCR **2f**	507	578	0.01	5.5
HMJR **3a**	547	569	0.50	10.3
HMJFR **3b**	553	582	0.37	9.8
HMJCR **3c**	555	582	0.42	9.1
AcHMJR **3d**	513	589	0.11	8.3
AcHMJFR **3e**	519	599	0.06	7.9
AcHMJCR **3f**	517	592	0.07	7.3

The Φ_{fl} values were measured in 0.2 M sodium phosphate buffer at pH 7.4 for rhodamines or pH 2.0 for acetylated derivatives

As a proof of concept, HMJCR was used as the scaffold for a probe designed to target GGT, by replacing the acetyl group of AcHMJCR with a gamma-glutamyl group (Fig. 24.4).

The pK_{cycl} value of gGlu-HMJCR was calculated to be 7.7, suggesting that approximately 33% of the probe exists in non-fluorescent spirocyclized form at the physiological pH of 7.4, whereas the putative hydrolysis product HMJCR with pK_{cycl} of 8.9 exists predominantly in the fluorescent open form. In addition, the open form of gGlu-HMJCR was found to have remarkably reduced Φ_{fl} (0.06) and ε (20,000) compared to those of HMJCR (0.42 and 50,000, respectively). The combination of the diminutions in pK_{cycl}, Φ_{fl} and ε resulted in efficient quenching of the fluorescence of gGlu-HMJCR.

Then, gGlu-HMJCR was examined if it reacted with GGT *in vitro*. gGlu-HMJCR in aqueous solution was added commercially available purified GGT enzyme. A dramatic increase in fluorescence intensity of more than 30-fold was observed as a result (Fig. 24.5). gGlu-HMJCR was also proven to be stable in aqueous buffer at physiological pH. The product of the reaction between gGlu-HMJCR and GGT was analyzed by HPLC. The results confirmed that the putative hydrolysis product of reaction was indeed HMJCR. The above results suggested that gGlu-HMJCR could be recognised by GGT to be converted into HMJCR.

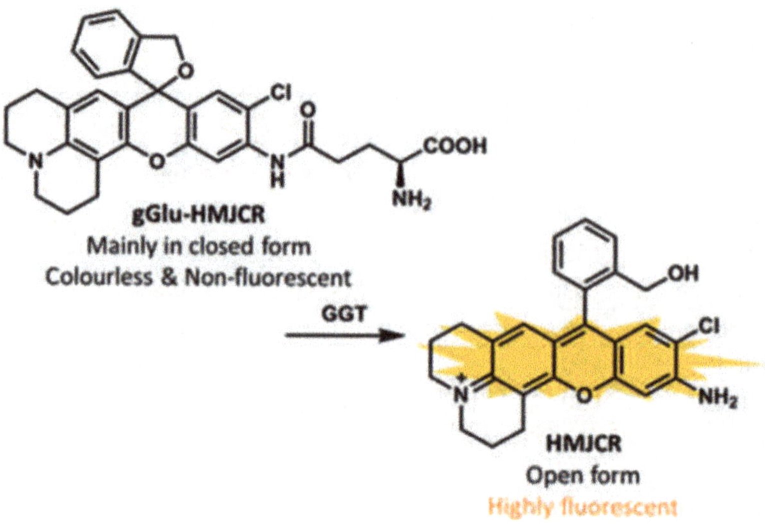

Fig. 24.4 Reaction scheme of gGlu-HMJCR

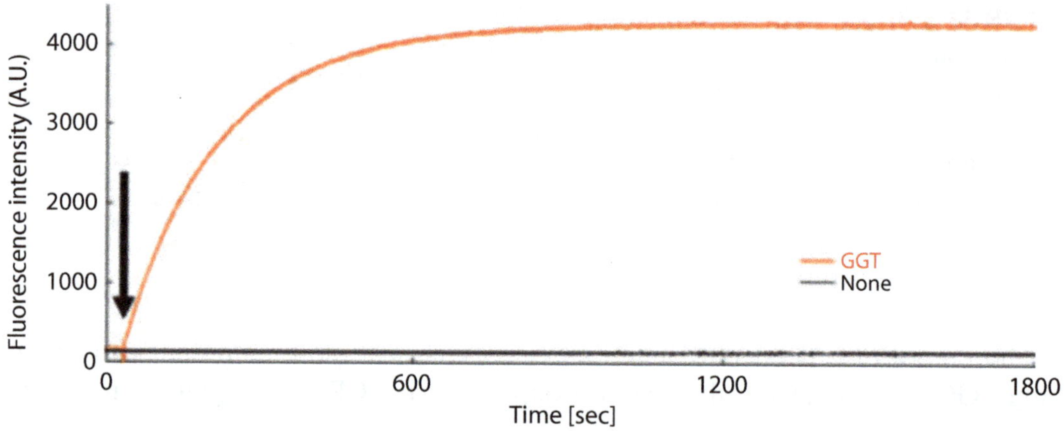

Fig. 24.5 Time course of enzymatic reaction of gGlu-HMJCR with GGT. Arrow indicates the time of GGT addition

Finally, an experiment was set up to discriminate two types of tumors by variation in protease activity profiles *in vivo*, using a cocktail of gGlu-HMJCR and previously reported Z-Phe-Arg-HMRG for cathepsins (Fig. 24.6) (Fujii et al. 2014).

Z-Phe-Arg-HMRG reacts with cysteine proteases in the cathepsins family such as cathepsin B and L, which are lysosomal endopeptidases with the increase in fluorescence of over 800-fold. As both cathepsins play a variety of roles in maintaining normal cellular metabolism, they are also naturally upregulated, secreted and show changes in localisation in various diseases, including breast, colorectal, gastric, lung, prostate, and ovarian cancers. These cathepsins are also known to contribute to the invasion of tumor cells to basal membrane, by degrading extracellular matrix components such as collagen I, collagen IV, laminin, fibronectin and elastin.

Mouse models of dual tumour implant were developed using two ovarian cancer cell lines with differing protease activities: SKOV-3/RFP and SHIN3. SHIN3 cells

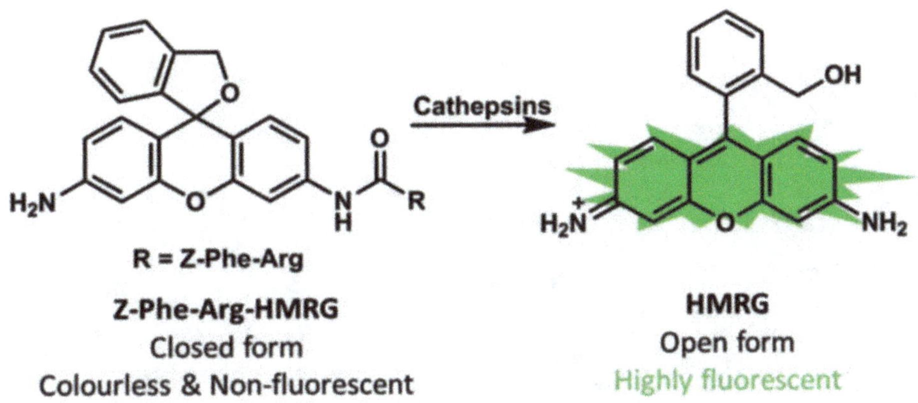

Fig. 24.6 Reaction scheme of Z-Phe-Arg-HMRG

exhibit both cathepsins and GGT activities, while SKOV-3/RFP cells only show cathepsins activity. Thus, whereas Z-Phe-Arg-HMRG should label both SHIN3 and SKOV-3/RFP derived tumors, gGlu-HMJCR should only label SHIN3 derived tumors.

Mice were injected intraperitoneally with 300 μl of PBS(−) containing 100 μM Z-Phe-Arg-HMRG and 1 mM gGlu-HMJCR, and sacrificed after 60 min incubation for fluorescence imaging with a Maestro. By unmixing the obtained images by HMJCR, HMRG, RFP and autofluorescence spectra, clear discrimination of two types of tumors with varying levels of protease activities by color *in vivo* was achieved (Figs. 24.7 and 24.8).

This was the first example known to date of such discrimination, and would serve as a guide for real-time and accurate characterization of tumor. The relationship between protease activity and therapeutic effect or prognosis are largely yet to be discovered, but such knowledge could be beneficial for aiding clinical decisions on intra- and postoperative treatments, leading to personalised medicine.

24.4 Conclusion

We have succeeded to construct a new fluorogenic scaffold HMJCR by optimizing its color, brightness, and spirocyclization property. HMJCR-based probes are capable of detecting various aminopeptidase activities in different color from so far-developed HMRG-based green probes. Thus, simultaneous live imaging of different protease activities in living cells, clinical specimen, and preferably in human patients in the future, are doable by the cocktail of HMRG- and HMJCR-probes.

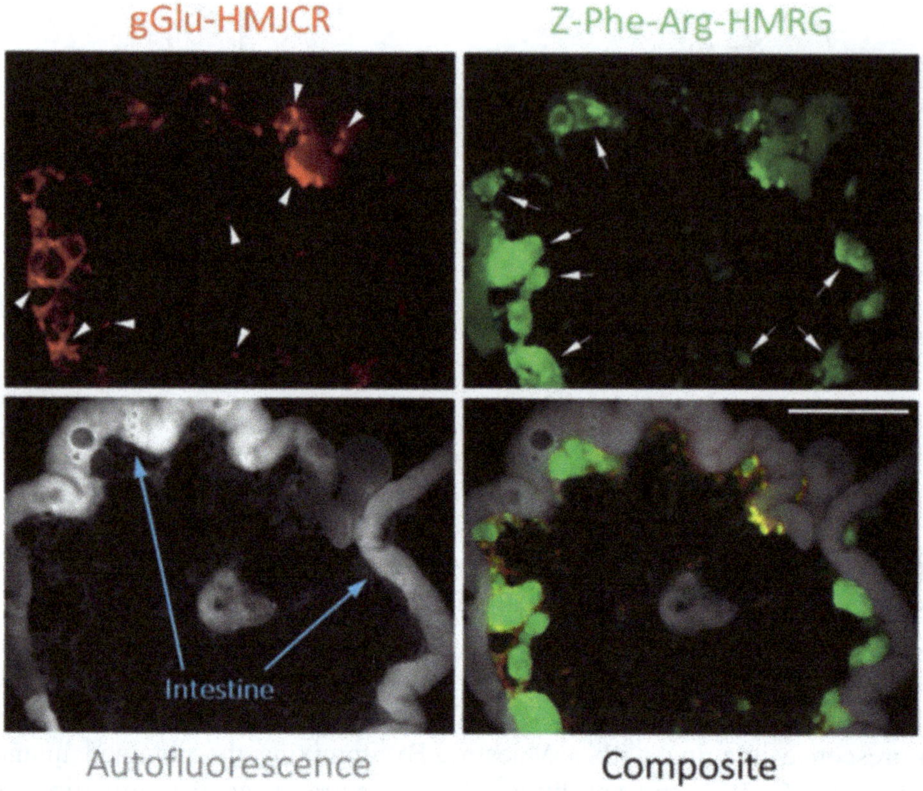

Fig. 24.7 Unmixed fluorescence images of a mouse model of dual peritoneal metastasis, at 60 min after combined intraperitoneal injection of Z-Phe-Arg-HMRG (100 μM) and gGlu-HMJCR (1 mM). Arrowheads indicate SHIN3-derived tumour locations and arrows indicate SKOV-3/RFP-derived tumour locations. Exposure time was 100 ms for the blue-filter setting and 35 ms for the yellow-filter setting. Scale bar represents 1 cm

Advantages of multicolor imaging *in vivo* using more than one of the synthesised protease probes are:

1. Wide range of tumors that cannot be detected and characterised with a single protease activity can be captured simultaneously.
2. Tumors with a difference in protease activity profiles can be distinguished intraoperatively.
3. Some of the probes emit fluorescence in the visible region and are detectable and distinguishable from each other by the naked human eye, suggesting good translatability to clinical purposes such as intraoperative imaging.

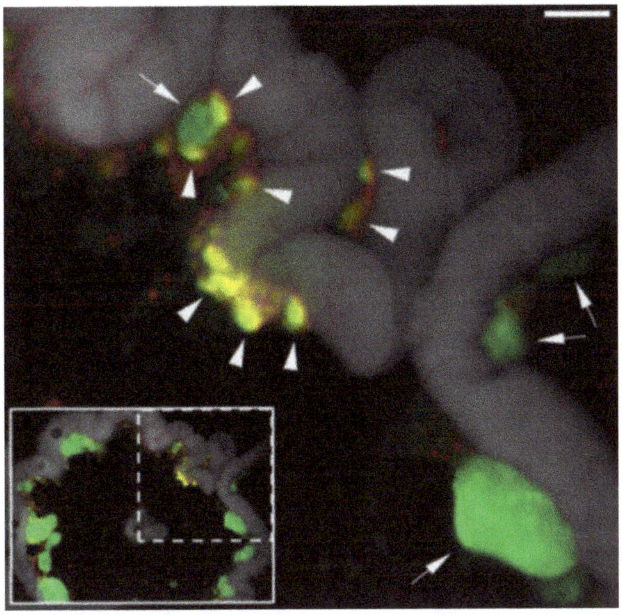

Fig. 24.8 Unmixed fluorescence images of a mouse model of dual peritoneal metastasis, at 60 min after combined intraperitoneal injection of Z-Phe-Arg-HMRG (green) and gGlu-HMJCR (red). Arrowheads indicate SHIN3-derived tumour locations and arrows indicate SKOV-3/RFP-derived tumour locations. Exposure time was 100 ms for the blue-filter setting and 35 ms for the yellow-filter setting. Scale bar represents 1 mm. Image enlarged from the dotted region of the original (inset, Fig. 24.7)

References

Fujii T, Kamiya M, Urano Y (2014) In vivo imaging of intraperitoneally disseminated tumors in model mice by using activatable fluorescent small-molecular probes for activity of cathepsins. Bioconjug Chem 25:1838–1846

Hanahan D, Weinberg RA (2000) The hallmarks of cancer. Cell 100:57–70

Hanahan D, Weinberg RA (2011) Hallmarks of cancer: the next generation. Cell 144:646–674

Iwatate RJ, Kamiya M, Urano Y (2016) Asymmetric rhodamine-based fluorescence probes for multi-colour in vivo imaging. Chem Eur J 22:1696–1703

Kamiya M et al (2011) β-galactosidase fluorescence probe with improved cellular accumulation based on spirocyclized rhodol scaffold. J Am Chem Soc 133:12960–12963

Miura T et al (2003) Rational design principle for modulating fluorescence properties of fluorescein-based probes by photoinduced electron transfer. J Am Chem Soc 125:8666–8671

Miyata Y et al (2017) Intraoperative imaging of hepatic cancers using γ-glutamyltranspeptidase-specific fluorophore enabling real-time identification and estimation of recurrence. Sci Rep 7:3542

Pompella A, De Tata V, Paolicchi A, Zunino F (2006) Expression of gamma-glutamyltransferase in cancer cells and its significance in drug resistance. Biochem Pharmacol 71:231–238

Sakabe M et al (2013) Rational design of highly sensitive fluorescence probes for protease and glycosidase based on precisely controlled spirocyclization. J Am Chem Soc 135:409–414

Shimane T et al (2016) Oral cancer intraoperative detection by topically spraying a γ-glutamyl transpeptidase-activated fluorescent probe. Oral Oncol 54:e16–e18

Shinden Y et al (2016) Rapid diagnosis of lymph node metastasis in breast cancer using a new fluorescent method with γ-glutamyl hydroxymethyl rhodamine green. Sci Rep 6:27525

Stewart BW, Wild CP (2014) World cancer report 2014. IARC Press, Lyon

Ueo H et al (2015) Rapid intraoperative visualization of breast lesions with γ-glutamyl hydroxymethyl rhodamine green. Sci Rep 5:12080

Urano Y et al (2005) Evolution of fluorescein as a platform for finely tunable fluorescence probes. J Am Chem Soc 127:4888–4894

Urano Y et al (2011) Rapid cancer detection by topically spraying a gamma-glutamyltranspeptidase-activated fluorescent probe. Sci Transl Med 3:110ra119

Weigelt B, Peterse JL, van't Veer LJ (2005) Breast cancer metastasis: markers and models. Nat Rev Cancer 5:591–602

Chapter 25
Coronary Heart Disease Diagnosis by FFR_{CT}: Engineering Triumphs and Value Chain Analysis

Geoffrey D. Rubin

Coronary heart disease is the leading cause of death throughout the developed world, yet the symptoms that patients experience as a result of coronary disease are often not specific. Determining who are the minority of patients with myocardial ischemia necessitating revascularization is a major activity of many medical centers. This task has traditionally fallen to coronary angiography, which is an expensive and invasive approach to identifying coronary artery lesions necessitating treatment through revascularization with stents or bypass grafts. Recently, computational fluid dynamic methods have been developed for cardiac CT that have been shown to effectively exclude patients from an invasive test when they do not have significant coronary artery disease. This manuscript reviews the technique of CTFFR and discusses some of the challenges of widespread clinical implementation through value chain analysis.

25.1 Coronary Heart Disease Pathophysiology

Development of coronary heart disease occurs over many years with atherosclerotic plaque deposition beginning in childhood and gradually progressing to a stage that can result in narrowing of the coronary arteries that may restrict blood flow to the heart muscle, particularly during high demand such as during exercise. Diminished

---

Electronic Supplementary Material The online version of this chapter (https://doi.org/10.1007/978-981-13-7908-6_25) contains supplementary material, which is available to authorized users.

G. D. Rubin (✉)
Duke University School of Medicine, Durham, NC, USA
e-mail: grubin@duke.edu

Y. Toyama et al. (eds.), *Make Life Visible*,
https://doi.org/10.1007/978-981-13-7908-6_25

oxygen delivery to the heart muscle causes tissue injury and death. Dead myocardium leads to fatal arrhythmia, pump failure, or in rare instances cardiac rupture.

Common and low-cost testing for coronary heart disease performed with electrocardiography or blood testing are often of limited accuracy. The definitive diagnosis of coronary heart disease rests upon imaging. Imaging is typically performed in two phases. In the first phase, a non-invasive imaging test is typically performed to determine if the patient should proceed to invasive imaging for definitive characterization and management.

Three non-invasive tests are available to assess for coronary heart disease. Two tests center on visualizing functional impairment in the myocardium, whereas one of these tests is capable of direct visualization of coronary artery lesions. The functional tests are radionuclide perfusion imaging (Sabharwal 2017) and stress echocardiography (Elhendy 2018). Both exams are performed during physical or pharmacologic stress and periods of rest to assess for reversible changes in myocardial perfusion or wall motion, respectively. Computed tomography angiography (CTA) is a newer entrance into the field of noninvasive coronary heart disease imaging (Rubin et al. 2014). It has undergone rapid refinement with technological improvement in CT scanners, overcoming limitations related to motion induced blurring to provide three dimensional representations of the coronary artery tree.

In distinction to radionuclide perfusion imaging and echocardiography, CTA allows direct visualization of the coronary artery tree and localization of atherosclerotic plaque, demonstrating both degree of arterial stenosis as well as character of the plaque. These features of CTA provided with the potential to plan therapeutic intervention through transluminal stent-based revascularization or coronary artery bypass grafting. In the absence of an anatomic delineation of coronary artery lesions, radionuclide perfusion imaging and echocardiography require a secondary test to identify treatable coronary artery lesions prior to initiating definitive therapy.

The anatomic mapping required in these latter instances is performed using invasive coronary angiography (ICA). ICA has been the reference standard for coronary artery anatomic visualization since the 1960s when it first became a mainstream clinical test. ICA requires the placement of a catheter into the arterial system with entry point most commonly through the femoral artery located in the groin. A catheter is then advanced in a direction opposite of blood flow until it reaches the heart, whereupon the operator engages the origins of the coronary arteries and directly injects a radio-opaque iodine solution into the coronary arteries while high frequency video is acquired using projectional radiography. Because ICA is a projectional technique, it is susceptible to a number of geometric limitations that hinder detailed evaluation of the coronary artery lumen. In particular, it is incapable of demonstrating discreet arterial cross sections. Its advantage is that it offers a high degree of spatial resolution when compared to noninvasive imaging modalities. Although CTA has substantially lower spatial resolution than ICA, its volumetric acquisition offers substantial advantages by allowing the anatomy to be reconstructed through innumerable projectional view angles and cross sections from a single volumetric acquisition.

An additional and often valuable characteristic of ICA, is that coronary artery access required for coronary angiography is identical to that required for revascularization using transluminal stent deployment. Consequently, patients with significant coronary artery lesions that are amenable to stenting can be treated immediately following their diagnosis as part of a single setting integrated procedure.

On the other hand, ICA is expensive. It requires multiple skilled personnel to perform a procedure that lasts between 1 and 3 h. It requires a patient to take a full day from work. There is discomfort associated with having a catheter inserted into the groin and manipulated during the procedure as well as pressure being applied for hemostasis over several hours after the procedure. Finally, there is a small but measurable risk of coronary artery injury due to the insertion of the catheter which can result in myocardial infarction or cardiac rhythm disturbances.

25.2 Invasive Coronary Angiography Is Inefficient

Because ICA is the reference standard for depicting coronary artery lesions and is a prerequisite for performing revascularization in patients with suspected coronary heart disease characterized with either SPECT or echocardiography, it has been a critical path for the management or coronary heart disease for many years. Because it is an invasive examination, ICA is more expensive than non-invasive imaging tests owing to the greater intensity of personnel required to perform an ICA, the overhead costs associated with a catheterization laboratory, and requirements for pre and post procedural care. In addition to financial expense, ICA exposes patients to greater risk owing to its invasive nature. While in experienced hands, the likelihood of complications from ICA is very low, it is still substantially higher than for non-invasive examinations.

In 2010, an analysis of almost 400,000 elective ICAs performed at 663 United States hospitals between 2004 and 2008 revealed that only 38% of subjects had obstructive coronary lesions and thus warranted intervention (Patel et al. 2010). Characterized based upon a visual assessment of at least 50% luminal narrowing, significant coronary artery lesions were found in only 38% of subjects.

While a positivity rate of only 38% is seen to represent an inefficient use of invasive testing for treatment planning, the value of visually assessed luminal stenosis at ICA is further degraded when considering the results of multiple studies reported in a meta-analysis (Stergiopoulos et al. 2014), which revealed that patients with stable chest pain who were re-vascularized based upon ICA did not have better health outcomes than patients who were managed with non-operative medical (pharmacologic) therapy. Suggesting that the appearance of a "significant" narrowing at ICA was not a reasonable determinant of the need for re-vascularization.

25.3 Fractional Flow Reserve

Until recently, the assessment of coronary artery disease using ICA was restricted to an image-based assessment of variations in coronary artery diameter. Particularly given the fact that conventional angiography is a projectional technique obtained using fluoroscopy, the ability to accurately represent flow-limiting arterial stenosis is limited. The introduction of the physiologic measurement, fractional flow reserve (FFR), has been revolutionary for the characterization of patients being assessed with ICA.

Obtained during infusion of the vasodilator adenosine to maximize coronary flow, FFR represents the ratio of the mean arterial pressure obtained immediately beyond a region of arterial narrowing to the mean arterial pressure within the root of the aorta (Pijls et al. 1996). These measurements provide an indication of the pressure drop along the length of the coronary artery. An FFR of 0.8 or lower is the most common threshold for considering a coronary lesion to be flow limiting.

The value of FFR guided coronary revascularization was established with publication of 2-year outcomes from the FAME trial in 2010 (Pijls et al. 2010). In FAME patients with multi-vessel coronary artery disease, defied as coronary artery stenosis with greater than 50% diameter reduction in at least two of the three major coronary arteries, were randomized to one of two treatment planning approaches. Half the 1205 subjects underwent percutaneous coronary revascularization based upon the visual appearance of the coronary angiogram while the other half underwent percutaneous coronary intervention based upon the FFR measurement.

Two years following treatment, there was a 33% reduction in the risk of death or major cardiac events amongst the patients who were treated based upon FFR guidance vs appearance guided coronary artery revascularization. Amongst the patients in whom FFR measurements were made, only 38% of lesions suspected to be significant based upon their appearance were positive by FFR criteria, this explains the result that despite a greater frequency of death or mild myocardial infarction, 42% more stents were placed on average in patients with appearance guided revascularization when compared to FFR guided revascularization.

As a result of the FAME trial and other subsequent clinical investigations, FFR has become the established standard for determining which coronary lesions merit revascularization. Moreover, when considering that only 38% of patients referred to US hospitals have obstructive coronary artery disease, multiplied by the observations through FAME that 30% of those lesions are FFR positive, it is possible to extrapolate a prevalence of 11% of patients referred to ICA having disease necessitating revascularization.

These results underscore the inefficient and ultimately expensive practice of using ICA as a means of determining which patients will need revascularization. Thus, a gate-keeper to inter-coronary angiography is needed. A noninvasive gatekeeper that reliably predicts FFR positive coronary artery lesions with a minimum of false positive results should have a substantial impact on the quality and cost of care for patients suspected of having significant coronary artery disease.

25.4 CT Angiography

CT scanners provide an opportunity to acquire volumetric coronary angiograms following a single injection of an iodine solution into a peripheral vein. With recent generation scanners CTAs encompassing the entirety of the heart frequently require less than 5 s to acquire and offer a temporal resolution as low as 70 ms (Rubin et al. 2014).

Multiple clinical studies have established the diagnostic performance of CT angiography with a very high negative predictive value of between 0.97 and 0.99. However, the positive predictive value of CT angiography when interpreted using a visual assessment akin to that of conventional angiography suffers from false positive results that provide a positive predictive value of 0.64–0.86 (Budoff et al. 2008; Miller et al. 2008; Meijboom et al. 2008a). While this diagnostic performance is fair, it falls off substantially when the reference standard for coronary artery disease is FFR rather than the visual assessment of the coronary lesion at ICA. In fact, when using an FFR greater than 0.8 as the reference standard for significant coronary lesions, 75% of lesions that appear to be narrowed by at least 50% on CT angiography are falsely positive, resulting in a positive predictive value of only 0.25 (Meijboom et al. 2008b). If CT angiography is to serve as an effective gatekeeper for ICA, an additional technology is needed to determine which of the apparently significant coronary lesions on CTA are actually flow limiting. That technology has recently become available based upon the use of computational fluid dynamics applied to the CT scan data resulting in the modeling of FFR from the CT data, referred to as FFR_{CT}.

Relying upon a painstakingly segmented anatomic model of the coronary arteries and the aggregate myocardial mass, the application of computational fluid dynamics has provided the basis for predicting FFR values along the length of the coronary arteries, both at baseline and maximal flow conditions, simulating the intra-arterial injection of adenosine that is used with invasive FFR measurement. This is accomplished by solving Navier–Stokes equations of blood flow where mass and momentum are conserved as they are applied to the movement of viscous fluid. Mean coronary artery pressure is thus derived along the length of the coronary arteries allowing for the calculation of FFR by dividing mean coronary pressures by the aortic pressure (Taylor et al. 2013). When compared to invasive FFR, FFR_{CT} slightly underestimates the FFR value with a mean difference of 0.03 but correlates with FFR with a Pearson's correlation coefficient of 0.82 (P-0.001) (Norgaard et al. 2014).

When applied to a cohort of 103 patients with stable chest pain, FFR_{CT} results improved the specificity of coronary CT angiographic evaluation from 25% to 82%, raised the positive predictive value from 58% to 85%, and overall improved the accuracy of the exam by 26%. In aggregate, the frequency of false positive results was reduced by 70% with FFR_{CT} when compared to visual interpretation of the coronary CT angiograms with reclassification of those false positive results as true negatives (Koo et al. 2011). In a subsequent clinical trial focused on characterizing visually equivocal 30–70% arterial narrowing observed at CT angiography, FFR_{CT} similarly improved specificity from 32% to 85% and positive predictive value from 37% to 63% (Norgaard et al. 2014). Figures 25.1 and 25.2 illustrate coronary CT angiograms and associated FFR_{CT} calculations.

Most recently, a prospective cohort of patients deemed to have an intermediate likelihood of significant coronary artery disease but without known disease was assembled across 11 European sites. Patients were enrolled into two testing arms, one receiving usual care and testing and the other receiving CTA/FFR_{CT} testing.

Amongst the 187 patients with usual care testing who then went on for ICA, 32% underwent coronary revascularization either with coronary artery stenting performed in the catheterization lab (42 patients) or surgical coronary bypass grafting (17 patients). Consequently, 68% of patients undergoing ICA in the usual care cohort were determined not to have significant disease (Douglas et al. 2015).

In comparison, 193 patients assigned to undergo ICA first underwent FFR_{CT} measurement. Based upon the FFR_{CT} value, catheterization was not performed in 61%. Amongst the remaining 39% that went on to ICA, 70% of subjects had

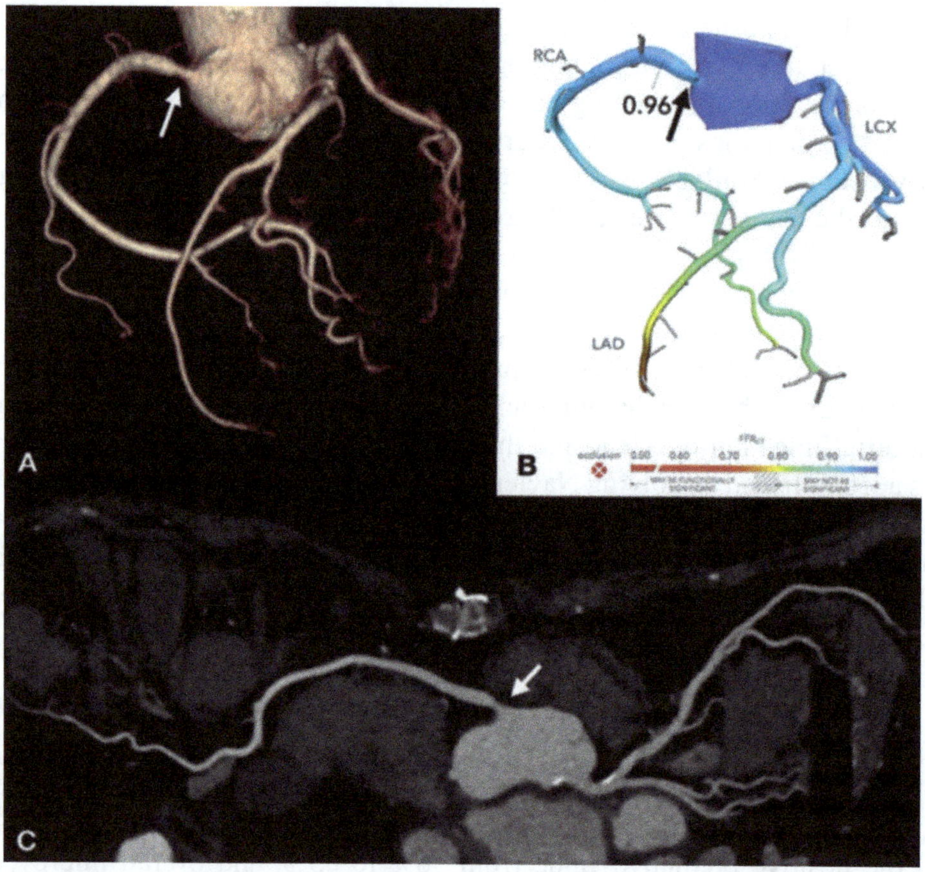

Fig. 25.1 CT angiogram from a patient with chest pain. (**a**) Three-dimensional volume rendering and (**c**) curved reformation shows narrowing at the origin of the right coronary artery (arrow). (**b**) Three-dimensional surface representation uses color overlay to indicate FFR_{CT} values along the length of the major coronary arteries. A value of 0.96 just distal to the right coronary artery origin indicates that it is not hemodynamically significant. No further testing was required

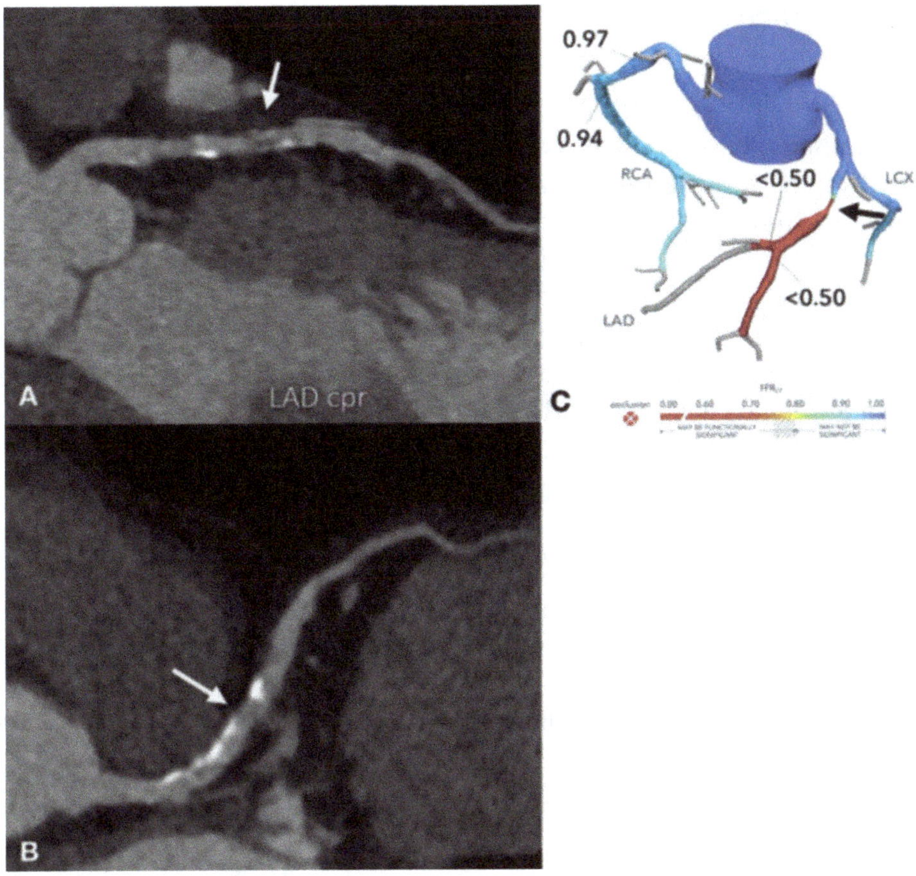

Fig. 25.2 CT angiogram from a different patient with chest pain. (**a**, **b**) Curved reformations through the centerline of the left anterior descending coronary artery and oriented 90° to one another reveal an area of heterogeneity in the artery which is not clearly represented as a significant narrowing (arrow). (**c**) The same region is associated with a significant drop in FFRCT to <0.50 (arrow), indicating an area of significant flow limitation

obstructive coronary artery disease necessitating revascularization while only 30% of patients referred to ICA based upon FFR_{CT} measurements or 12% of all patients undergoing FFR_{CT} underwent ICA without demonstration of a significant coronary lesion. These results correspond to a six-fold reduction in negative ICAs when FFR_{CT} served as gatekeeper to the angiography suite, while the percentage of significant obstructive disease was identical to the patients referred to ICA following the usual care. Moreover, when assessed after 1 year and despite a sixfold reduction in the number of patients undergoing invasive catheterization within the FFR_{CT} arm of the study, there was no difference in the frequency of major cardiac events (1% for both usual and CT groups) nor was there a difference in quality of life measure or in aggregate risk for future events (11, 12).

25.5 Comparing Costs

The reduction in invasive catheterization associated with CT use has been shown to impact the future cost of care as well. When considering 2015 United States Medicare Reimbursement Rates as a proxy for costs, a standard ICA costs $2838 or more than nine times that of a CT angiogram ($301). Without accommodating for the costs of performing FFR_{CT}, this suggests that if only one negative coronary artery angiogram were avoided for every nine CTs performed, then the aggregate cost of diagnosis would be less when FFR_{CT} serves as gatekeeper to ICA (Douglas et al. 2016). However, this analysis oversimplifies the issue of cost measurement as it does not address downstream utilization of medical resources, which may vary following diagnosis with CT versus ICA.

The PLATFORM trial provides a basis for understanding the potential impact of FFR_{CT} on acute and downstream costs. One year following diagnostic testing, the average cost of cardiac care was 33% lower for FFR_{CT} ($8127) versus ICA ($12,145). However, when examining median costs, which avoid the skew associated with the high cost of treating patients with coronary artery disease, the FFR_{CT} pathway cost 12 times less than the ICA pathway ($546 versus $6472). As long as the cost of FFRCT is limited to less than 15 times that of performing and interpreting the CT scan, the use of FFR_{CT} as a gateway to ICA would still result in diminished cost of care when compared to the standard approach of today (Douglas et al. 2016).

25.6 Economic Considerations for Translation to Routine Care

Based upon the aforementioned results, it appears that the use of FFR_{CT} as a determinant of who should undergo ICA is a compelling application that should reduce costs and improve care of patients with coronary heart disease. Nevertheless, the practicality of transitioning current medical practice to a future state based upon FFR_{CT} is fraught with barriers. In order to understand where these barriers might appear, it is useful to consider value chain analysis for FFR_{CT}. Specifically, value chain analysis (Rubin 2017) examines all industry participants in the production of FFR_{CT} as it provides its ultimate impact on individual patients and society as a whole.

As a first step, when considering value to the patient, where value is conceptualized as benefit divided by costs, the patient benefits from the availability of a quicker and less invasive diagnostic test that should result in the same clinical outcomes and quality of life downstream. Assuming that the lower cost of performing FFR_{CT} compared to ICA are passed on to the patient in the form of lower pricing, patients costs are diminished while benefits increase, resulting in substantial increase in value.

When aggregating this value across many patients, society stands to gain from a lower cost of care for coronary heart disease resulting in savings that might be used to support other healthcare priorities or reduce taxes required to support healthcare. Thus, societal value appears to be enhanced as well.

It is the interaction between four distinct entities upstream from the patient in the value chain that lend complexity to our economic considerations. These four entities represent the diagnostic imager, the cardiac interventionalist who performs ICA and coronary stenting, the hospital facility where catheterization laboratories represent an important capital asset, and healthcare payers, both private and public.

For the imager, the performance of FFR_{CT} requires extra effort which diminishes time available for other activities. Incremental support should be provided to accommodate the added work of FFR_{CT}. When physicians are compensated based upon a fee-for-service model, uncompensated additional work associated with FFR_{CT} analysis may reduce net revenue to imaging providers unless their efforts are mitigated by an overall increase in CT referrals and the allocation of revenue from those CT referrals provided to offset the added effort required to perform the FFR_{CT} analysis.

The interventionalist stands to lose substantial revenue by performing fewer diagnostic ICAs. In order to offset this loss of activity and revenue, interventionalists will need to identify other activities to compensate and backfill their new-found availability. Paradoxically, over time there may be an increase in the need for diagnostic ICA if FFR_{CT} is applied widely to the population identifying patients at risk, allowing detection of patients at a treatable stage, prior to their suffering from a serious cardiac event such as sudden death.

The hospital faces similar pressures as does the interventionalist. There is the risk of an empty cardiac catheterization lab challenging the institution to support the fixed costs of the laboratory and its supporting personnel with lower payment from payers in response to the lower ICA volumes. The hospital will not be motivated to support FFR_{CT} adoption unless they can find other procedures to backfill the volume within the catheterization lab as a basis for generating revenue to cover their costs.

Finally, the payer stands to gain substantially from the introduction of FFR_{CT}. When considering the prevalence of coronary heart disease across a payers' pool of beneficiaries, the reduction in ICA represents a basis for substantial cost reductions across the pool of beneficiaries. These cost reductions may translate into greater overall profit for shareholders, and an opportunity to lower insurance premiums to enhance competitiveness, or the application of excess revenue to other expense-generating priorities.

When considered across the whole of the value chain, the aggregate reduction in costs with what is assumed to be minimal change in healthcare outcomes provides a basis for substantial value to the patient, the payer, and society as a whole. While the imager is most likely to experience a net increase in value as well, the interventionalist and the hospital are positioned to potentially experience a reduction in value which, without mitigating economic intervention, might hinder the adoption of FFR_{CT}. Consequently, a value chain based examination of FFR_{CT} delivery and its economic impact suggests that payers may need to incent interventionalists and hospitals to adopt FFR_{CT} by sharing some of their cost savings with the interventionalists and the hospitals in order to help them transition to a value preserving state (Fig. 25.3).

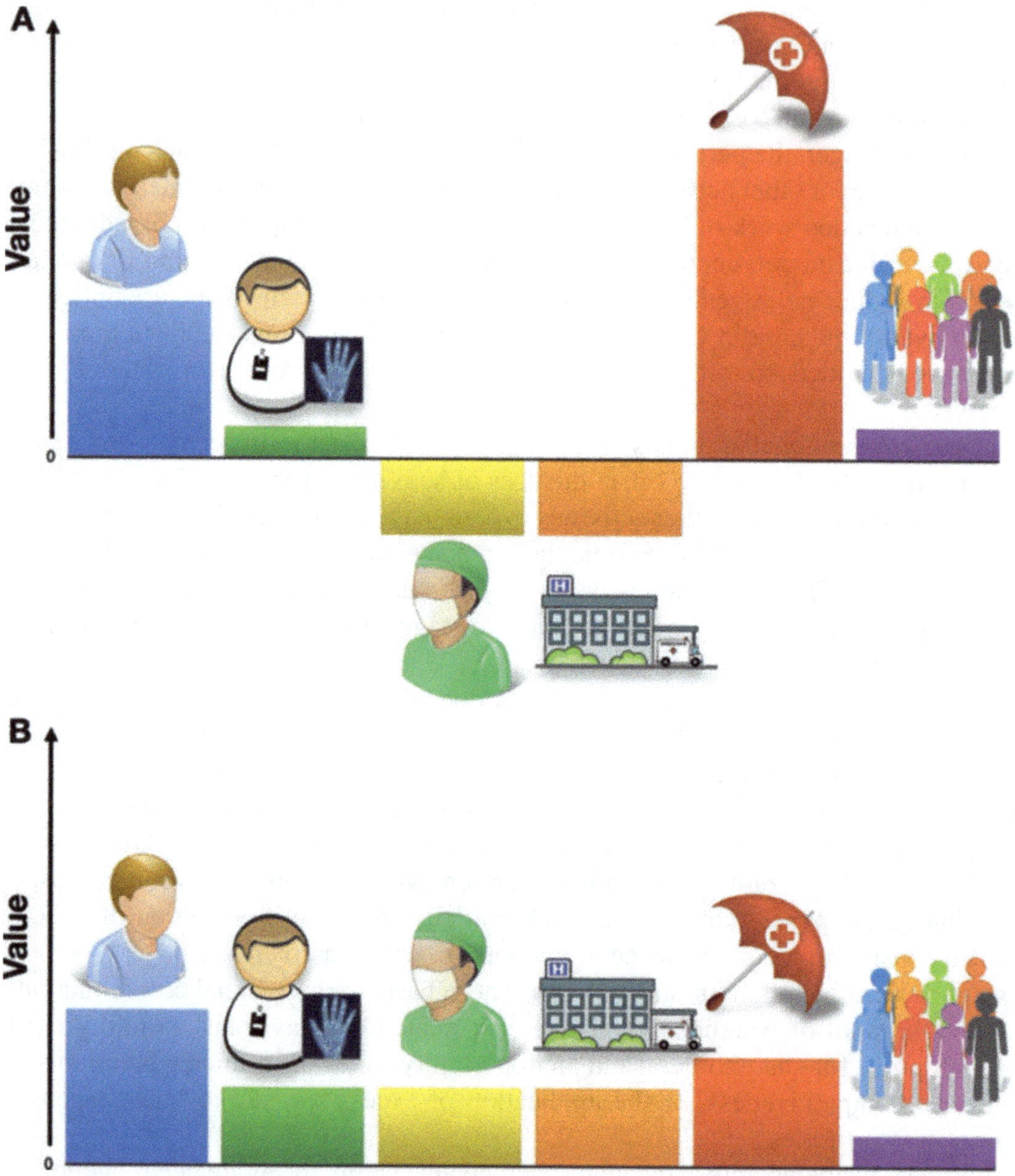

Fig. 25.3 (**a**) Graphical representation of relative value changes resulting from a transition from current diagnostic patterns that result in many non-actionable ICAs to the use of FFR_{CT} as a determinant of referral to ICA. The stakeholders from left to right respectively are the patient, the imager, the interventionalist, the ICA facility, the insurer, and society as a whole. Relative value is representational and not quantitative. The reduction in value experienced by interventionalists and facilities might block the realization of value for other participants in the value chain. A redistribution of value as represented in (**b**) would substantially reduce economic barriers and align interests for adoption

25.7 Conclusion

As a leading cause of death across the developed world, coronary heart disease is a major public health problem. The traditional methods for diagnosis leading to therapy are inefficient and expensive. The development of computational fluid dynamic methods applied to high resolution volumetric CT data provide a means for estimating the physiologic impact of coronary artery narrowing by quantifying FFR_{CT} values. Preliminary clinical testing supports the idea that FFR_{CT} should be an excellent gatekeeper for entry into catheterization laboratories so that fewer negative ICAs are performed. In this scenario, ICA would be largely used as a prelude to needed coronary revascularization while patients who do not undergo ICA are safely managed with medical therapy. Despite the remarkable technical and clinical advances that would seem to compel the widespread adoption of FFR_{CT}, economic drivers must be understood and addressed to assure that patients and society will receive whatever benefits might be achieved through the widespread adoptions of this technology.

References

Budoff MJ, Dowe D, Jollis JG et al (2008) Diagnostic performance of 64-multidetector row coronary computed tomographic angiography for evaluation of coronary artery stenosis in individuals without known coronary artery disease: results from the prospective multicenter ACCURACY (Assessment by Coronary Computed Tomographic Angiography of Individuals Undergoing Invasive Coronary Angiography) trial. J Am Coll Cardiol 52:1724–1732. https://doi.org/10.1016/j.jacc.2008.07.031

Douglas PS, Pontone G, Hlatky MA et al (2015) Clinical outcomes of fractional flow reserve by computed tomographic angiography-guided diagnostic strategies vs. usual care in patients with suspected coronary artery disease: the prospective longitudinal trial of FFRct: outcome and resource impacts study. Eur Heart J 36:ehv444–ehv449. https://doi.org/10.1093/eurheartj/ehv444

Douglas PS, De Bruyne B, Pontone G et al (2016) 1-year outcomes of FFRCT-guided care in patients with suspected coronary disease: the PLATFORM study. J Am Coll Cardiol 68:435–445. https://doi.org/10.1016/j.jacc.2016.05.057

Elhendy A (2018) The power of stress echocardiography and myocardial perfusion scintigraphy in predicting long-term outcome. Nothing lasts forever. J Nucl Cardiol 25:480–482. https://doi.org/10.1007/s12350-016-0621-1

Koo B-K, Erglis A, Doh J-H et al (2011) Diagnosis of ischemia-causing coronary stenoses by noninvasive fractional flow reserve computed from coronary computed tomographic angiograms results from the prospective multicenter DISCOVER-FLOW (Diagnosis of Ischemia-Causing Stenoses Obtained Via Noninvasive Fractional Flow Reserve) study. J Am Coll Cardiol 58:1989–1997. https://doi.org/10.1016/j.jacc.2011.06.066

Meijboom WB, Meijs MFL, Schuijf JD et al (2008a) Diagnostic accuracy of 64-slice computed tomography coronary angiography: a prospective, multicenter, multivendor study. J Am Coll Cardiol 52:2135–2144. https://doi.org/10.1016/j.jacc.2008.08.058

Meijboom WB, van Mieghem CAG, van Pelt N et al (2008b) Comprehensive assessment of coronary artery stenoses: computed tomography coronary angiography versus conventional coronary angiography and correlation with fractional flow reserve in patients with stable angina. J Am Coll Cardiol 52:636–643. https://doi.org/10.1016/j.jacc.2008.05.024

Miller JM, Rochitte CE, Dewey M et al (2008) Diagnostic performance of coronary angiography by 64-row CT. N Engl J Med 359:2324–2336. https://doi.org/10.1056/NEJMoa0806576

Norgaard BL, Gaur S, Leipsic J et al (2014) Diagnostic performance of noninvasive fractional flow reserve derived from coronary computed tomography angiography in suspected coronary artery disease: the NXT trial (Analysis of Coronary Blood Flow Using CT Angiography: Next Steps). J Am Coll Cardiol 63:1145–1155. https://doi.org/10.1016/j.jacc.2013.11.043

Patel MR, Peterson ED, Dai D et al (2010) Low diagnostic yield of elective coronary angiography. N Engl J Med 362:886–895. https://doi.org/10.1056/NEJMoa0907272

Pijls NH, De Bruyne B, Peels K et al (1996) Measurement of fractional flow reserve to assess the functional severity of coronary-artery stenoses. N Engl J Med 334:1703–1708. https://doi.org/10.1056/NEJM199606273342604

Pijls NHJ, Fearon WF, Tonino PAL et al (2010) Fractional flow reserve versus angiography for guiding percutaneous coronary intervention in patients with multivessel coronary artery disease: 2-year follow-up of the FAME (Fractional Flow Reserve Versus Angiography for Multivessel Evaluation) study. J Am Coll Cardiol 56:177–184. https://doi.org/10.1016/j.jacc.2010.04.012

Rubin GD (2017) Costing in radiology and health care: rationale, relativity, rudiments, and realities. Radiology 282:333–347. https://doi.org/10.1148/radiol.2016160749

Rubin GD, Leipsic J, Joseph Schoepf U et al (2014) CT angiography after 20 years: a transformation in cardiovascular disease characterization continues to advance. Radiology 271:633–652. https://doi.org/10.1148/radiol.14132232

Sabharwal NK (2017) State of the art in nuclear cardiology. Heart 103:790–799. https://doi.org/10.1136/heartjnl-2015-308670

Stergiopoulos K, Boden WE, Hartigan P et al (2014) Percutaneous coronary intervention outcomes in patients with stable obstructive coronary artery disease and myocardial ischemia: a collaborative meta-analysis of contemporary randomized clinical trials. JAMA Intern Med 174:232–240. https://doi.org/10.1001/jamainternmed.2013.12855

Taylor CA, Fonte TA, Min JK (2013) Computational fluid dynamics applied to cardiac computed tomography for noninvasive quantification of fractional flow reserve: scientific basis. J Am Coll Cardiol 61:2233–2241. https://doi.org/10.1016/j.jacc.2012.11.083

Chapter 26
Live Imaging of the Skin Immune Responses

Zachary Chow, Gyohei Egawa, and Kenji Kabashima

26.1 Introduction

Amongst the various organs in the human body, the skin is particularly unique due to its diverse set of roles. From physical to immune protection, thermoregulation for homeostasis and sensory functions, the skin can do it all. This can, however, sometimes be a double-edged sword. Although skin immune cells can confer protection against invading pathogens, they can also become aberrant, leading to autoimmune diseases such as alopecia areata and vitiligo. Histology, flow cytometry and RNA sequencing have been useful tools in the analysis and understanding of immune cell function in the skin in normal and diseased states. These techniques are, however, unable to reveal the dynamics of immune cell migration and cellular interaction in these states in real-time. The technique most suitable for this is the *in vivo* imaging of the skin. In this chapter, we will cover some tools that are utilized for this, and examine key studies that have advanced our understanding of immune responses in the skin.

Z. Chow · G. Egawa
Department of Dermatology, Graduate School of Medicine, Kyoto University, Kyoto, Japan

K. Kabashima (✉)
Department of Dermatology, Graduate School of Medicine, Kyoto University, Kyoto, Japan

Singapore Immunology Network (SIgN) and Institute of Medical Biology (IMB), Agency for Science, Technology and Research (A∗STAR), Biopolis, Singapore
e-mail: kaba@kuhp.kyoto-u.ac.jp

Y. Toyama et al. (eds.), *Make Life Visible*,
https://doi.org/10.1007/978-981-13-7908-6_26

26.2 The Skin and Its Key Immune Cells

Histologically, the skin can be divided into two distinct sections, each with their own set of immune cells that function to keep the skin healthy. The upper layer, known as the epidermis, contains keratinocytes and Langerhans cells (LCs), whereas the dermis contains innate immune cells, including macrophages, neutrophils, mast cells, as well as cells for adaptive immune responses, such as dermal dendritic cells (DCs) and T cells (Fig. 26.1).

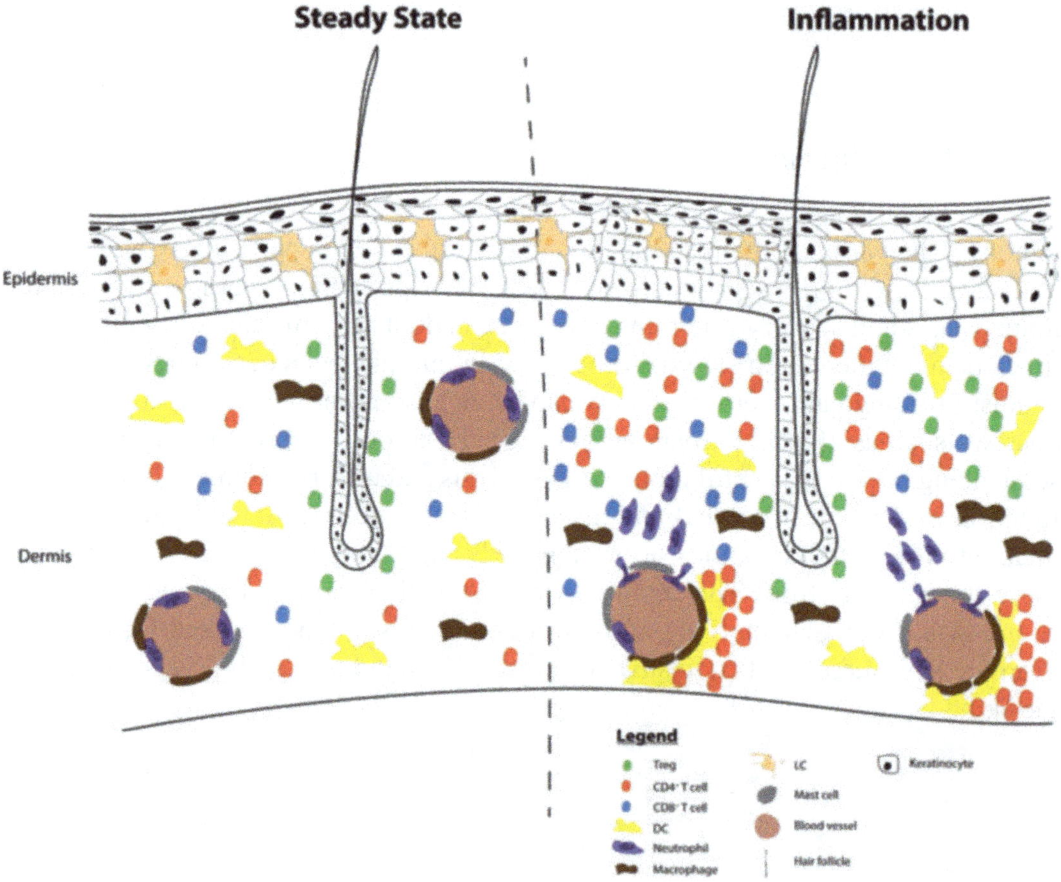

Fig. 26.1 A brief schematic of skin immune cells under steady state and inflammatory conditions

In the steady state, resident populations of LCs, dermal DCs, macrophages, mast cells and T cells exist within the skin. LCs are immobilized between keratinocytes in the epidermis whereas dermal DCs actively migrate around the dermis (Ng et al. 2008). Dermal macrophages are present throughout the dermis as well as around the dermal vasculature where mast cells also typically reside. Resident $CD4^+$ and $CD8^+$ T cells are also present throughout the dermal regions (Carbone 2015; Clark et al. 2006) whereas Tregs preferentially localize around the hair follicles (Ali et al. 2017; Chow et al. 2013)

During inflammation, neutrophils are swiftly mobilized and recruited to the site of inflammation (Goh et al. 2015). T cells are also recruited to the inflamed site albeit at a slower rate. Perivascular macrophages induce the recruitment and formation of DC clusters around dermal vessels that also contain T cells for efficient antigen presentation and activation (Natsuaki et al. 2014)

26.2.1 Dendritic Cells

DCs are specialized antigen-presenting cells (APCs) that are key to the development of immune responses. DCs are a heterogeneous population and, in steady-state skin, exist as LCs in the epidermis (Romani et al. 2010), and as dermal DCs in the dermis (Ginhoux et al. 2009). During inflammation, more DC subsets are recruited and can be found in the skin— these are the monocyte-derived DCs (Leon and Ardavin 2008) and plasmacytoid DCs (Nestle et al. 2009; Wollenberg et al. 2002). Emerging evidence in the field of LC biology highlights the similarities between LC and macrophage ontogeny, leading to the idea that LCs may be a specialized subset of tissue-resident macrophages with the capabilities of DCs (Doebel et al. 2017; Kaplan 2017).

26.2.2 Neutrophils

Neutrophils are short-lived, multi-nucleated leukocytes whose key role is to engulf pathogens. In a human adult, approximately 10^{11} neutrophils are produced in the bone marrow daily, though only 1–2% of these cells are present within the blood circulation (Borregaard 2010; Dancey et al. 1976). A small population of neutrophils has been reported to actively survey uninflamed dermis, a phenomenon that possibly allows for an immediate response to tissue damage (Li and Ng 2012; Ng et al. 2011). Upon initiation of cutaneous inflammation, neutrophils are rapidly recruited to the inflamed site (Phillipson and Kubes 2011). Upon entering the site of inflammation, neutrophils neutralize invading pathogens via phagocytosis and degranulation (Amulic et al. 2012).

26.2.3 Macrophages

Macrophages are important innate immune cells that are capable of a wide array of functions in response to the local microenvironment. Dermal macrophages are derived from blood-circulating monocytes that migrate into the skin (Geissmann et al. 2010; Jakubzick et al. 2013). In addition to phagocytosing invading pathogens, macrophages also play a role in the resolution of inflammation and subsequent wound repair (Lucas et al. 2010; Mirza et al. 2009). These differing abilities are observed with the different macrophage activation states, known as M1 and M2 macrophages or the classically activated macrophage and alternatively activated macrophage, respectively (Sica and Mantovani 2012). During wound repair, the initial pro-inflammatory phase involves M1 macrophages scavenging for, and killing, invading pathogens in the inflamed tissue. The subsequent phase of tissue regeneration involves M2 macrophages producing anti-inflammatory cytokines and growth factors to activate epithelial cells and fibroblasts.

26.2.4 Mast Cells

Deriving from hematopoietic stem cells, mast cells only differentiate to maturity upon entering peripheral tissues (Galli et al. 2005). Mast cells are long-lived immune cells that are particularly present in tissues exposed to the environment, enabling them to be first responders against environmental allergens and antigens (Galli and Tsai 2010). In the skin, mast cells localize around dermal blood vessels in an immotile state (Dudeck et al. 2011). With a spindle-like morphology in the steady state, inflammation results in mast cells taking on a more globular shape. During inflammation, mast cells secrete histamines to increase vascular permeability and promote neutrophil and effector T cell infiltration into the inflamed tissue (Biedermann et al. 2000).

26.2.5 T Cells

T cells are key players in the adaptive immune response, and can be classified into CD4- or CD8-expressing T cells, and natural killer (NK) T cells. CD4 T cells can be further subdivided into helper T cells (Th1, Th2, Th17) and regulatory T cells (Tregs). In a simplistic sense, helper T cells aid other immune cells in mounting an adaptable immune response to a wide variety of pathogens. Th1 cells protect against intracellular pathogens. Th2 cells promote the humoral immune response, stimulating B cells to produce antibodies. Th17 cells help with the recruitment of neutrophils. Tregs, as their name suggests, have a regulatory role and dampen inflammatory responses. CD8 T cells are also known as cytotoxic T cells for their ability to recognize and kill infected host cells.

Normal human skin contains approximately one million T cells per square centimeter of skin, which extrapolates to around 20 billion T cells, close to double the amount present in the blood (Clark et al. 2006). The majority of these T cells express the T cell receptor α and β chains (αβ T cells), and preferentially home to skin with CCR4 and cutaneous lymphocyte antigen (CLA). Most skin-homing T cells consist of CD4 memory T cells, and reside in the dermis. The epidermis, on the other hand, contains a minor population of tissue-resident CD8 memory T cells (Trm) (Carbone 2015). Resident Tregs in the skin preferentially localize around hair follicles (Chow et al. 2013; Gratz et al. 2013; Sanchez Rodriguez et al. 2014), and it has been reported that Treg-expressed Jag1 facilitates the hair follicular stem cell function for hair follicle regeneration (Ali et al. 2017).

The skin houses a special minor population of T cells that expresses the T cell receptor γ and δ chains (γδ T cells). In mice, γδ T cells exist in abundant numbers and are termed dendritic epidermal T cells (DETCs) (Witherden and Havran 2011). The human epidermis, however, does not have γδ T cells such as DETCs, but does have resident γδ T cells in the dermis (Ebert et al. 2006). Unlike the diverse T cell receptor repertoire of αβ T cells, γδ T cells express tissue-specific invariant T cell receptors and possess innate-like functions.

26.3 Tools for *In Vivo* Imaging

26.3.1 Microscopy

Previously, intravital imaging was limited to either the bright-field illumination of transparent tissues (Hickey et al. 1999), epifluorescence imaging of exposed dermal microvasculature (Hickey et al. 2002), or immune responses in the surface layer of the skin, the epidermis (Kissenpfennig et al. 2005). This was due to the poor penetrative ability of visible light. Technological advances led to the use of lasers, making way for a form of microscopy known as multiphoton (MP) microscopy. Also known as two-photon excitation microscopy, this is a process whereby a fluorescent molecule simultaneously absorbs two photons from rapid laser pulses. The benefit of this over conventional single-photon excitation is the deeper penetration into the tissue coupled with the reduced photodamage due to the lower energy transfer. This allows for a greater imaging depth as well as the maintenance of tissue health and viability over long imaging periods. These developments enabled the examination of a variety of fluorescently labelled leukocytes in various tissues in four dimensions (Devi et al. 2010; Gebhardt et al. 2011; Li et al. 2012; Mempel et al. 2006).

26.3.2 Animal Systems and Fluorescent-Cell Labelling Techniques

When using MP microscopy on the skin, structures such as hair shafts and elastic fibers, and collagen fibers, can be visualized due to their intrinsic autofluorescence or second harmonic generation, respectively. The visualization of collagen fibers in the skin distinguishes the epidermal and dermal layers in the skin. The conjugation of quantum dots to antibodies against lymphatic vessel endothelial hyaluronan receptor 1 (LYVE-1) can be used to visualize the peripheral lymphatic vessels (Sen et al. 2010). To observe the skin vasculature in the dermis, fluorescently labelled dextran can be used as it is retained within blood vessels for several hours (Egawa et al. 2013). The disadvantage to using fluorescently labelled dextran, however, is leakage due to vascular permeability as a result of inflammation. To circumvent this, a fluorescently labelled antibody against the endothelial cell surface marker CD31 (PECAM-1) can be used (Runnels et al. 2006). Runnels et al. demonstrated that a single administration of anti-CD31 antibody can stain the vasculature for 3–4 days after injection.

To visualize leukocytes endogenously, one can either fluorescently label leukocytes *in vitro* and adoptively transfer them into the animal, or undertake it *in situ* via intravenous injections of fluorescently labelled cell surface markers (Abeynaike et al. 2014; Deane et al. 2012). An alternative, which is currently the gold standard and essential to intravital imaging, is the use of transgenic animals that express fluorescent proteins in specific cells. In the field of immunology, there exists a variety

Table 26.1 List of transgenic mice utilized in *in vivo* imaging

Target cell	Promoter	Reporter	References
Neutrophils	Lysozyme M	eGFP	Goh et al. (2015)
Langerhans cells, Langerin+ dermal DCs	Langerin	GFP	Kissenpfennig et al. (2005)
DCs	CD11c	eYFP	Goh et al. (2015) and Ng et al. (2008)
Tregs	Foxp3	GFP	Chow et al. (2013)
T cells	T cell-specific enhancer	eGFP DsRed	Bauer et al. (2014), Manjunath et al. (1999), and Mempel et al. (2006)
Mast cells	Mcpt5	eYFP	Dudeck et al. (2011)
Ubiquitous (Photoconvertible)	CAG	Kaede	Tomura et al. (2010)
		KikGR	Nowotschin and Hadjantonakis (2009)

of transgenic fluorescent reporter mice (Table 26.1), and their use has contributed significantly to the knowledge of immune responses in the skin (Chow et al. 2013; Egawa et al. 2011; Gebhardt et al. 2011; Goh et al. 2015; Li et al. 2012; Ng et al. 2008; Overstreet et al. 2013). In addition, unique fluorescent proteins, such as KikGR and Kaede have the ability to change their fluorescence via photoconversion by ultraviolet irradiation. These proteins allow researchers to trace cell migration endogenously between peripheral tissues and lymphoid organs (Nowotschin and Hadjantonakis 2009; Tomura et al. 2010).

26.4 *In vivo* Imaging of Skin Immune Responses

In the past decade, intravital MP microscopy has become a vital tool in understanding the behavior of leukocytes in the development and resolution of various skin immune responses.

26.4.1 Sterile Injury

Goh et al. recently employed intravital MP microscopy to investigate dermal DC migration in the skin. Their study was unique in that the transgenic mice they used had two fluorescent cell populations. These LysM-eGFP x CD11c-EYFP mice contained LysM+ neutrophils expressing enhanced green fluorescent protein (eGFP), and CD11c+ DCs expressing enhanced yellow fluorescent protein (EYFP). This allowed Goh et al. to investigate the dynamic responses of the two cell types during sterile injury of the skin (Goh et al. 2015). Their findings demonstrated that the onset of sterile injury to ear skin resulted in a transition in dermal DC motility from a random probing behavior to a highly directional one. This directional motility occurred towards the site of injury with an increase in cell velocity. This transition occurred over a span of 50 min, the outcome of which saw dermal DCs surrounding the periphery of the injury and a cessation in motility upon arrival. Conversely, neutrophils responded much quicker, arriving at the site of injury within 20 min and infiltrating to the core.

26.4.2 Contact Hypersensitivity

Contact hypersensitivity (CHS) is a commonly used mouse model of contact dermatitis, involving a type IV delayed-type hypersensitivity response. CHS is induced by small chemical compounds known as haptens that, upon binding to self-proteins, form immunogenic structures (Kaplan et al. 2012). CHS is a biphasic response, with the initial sensitization phase composed of these new immunogens activating innate immune cells, such as mast cells, macrophages, and keratinocytes. These innate cells secrete inflammatory mediators that activate resident DCs to capture the haptenated proteins. Following antigen uptake, skin DCs transiently increase their motility (Sawada et al. 2015; Sen et al. 2010) and migrate to the draining lymph nodes for presentation to, and activation of, T cells. Some skin DCs however remain, forming clusters after hapten introduction (Natsuaki et al. 2014). A subsequent exposure to the hapten initiates the second phase of CHS, which is the elicitation phase. Similar to the sensitization phase, innate immune cells are activated and skin DCs take up haptenated proteins. The presence of antigen-specific T cells in the skin generated during the sensitization phase, however, brings about a more robust inflammatory response in the skin.

Using MP microscopy, Natsuaki et al. highlighted the importance of dermal DC clusters for efficient T cell activation in the skin (Natsuaki et al. 2014). Their study showed that dermal DCs localize around perivascular macrophages that are situated on post-capillary venules. Following this, recruited T cells accumulate around these clusters, allowing for activation by proximal antigen-bearing dermal DCs. As these clusters only appear during inflammation, they have been termed "inducible skin-associated lymphoid tissues (iSALT)" (Ono and Kabashima 2015).

MP microscopy in conjunction with the CHS model has also been used to study T cell dynamics in cutaneous inflammation. Honda et al. demonstrated that effector T cells become sessile and form stable contacts with DCs within 10 min of antigen recognition (Honda et al. 2014). These effector T cells successively regain their motility within 6–8 h. Interestingly, Honda et al. discovered an inverse correlation between cytokine production and cell motility whereby these effector T cells only produce cytokines while immobile. Another study by Chow et al. investigated the dynamics of skin regulatory T cells (Tregs) during a CHS response via MP microscopy (Chow et al. 2013). They reported that, unlike the high motility of effector $CD4^+$ T cells, most Tregs were sessile in steady state skin. During the elicitation phase of CHS, however, approximately 40% of Tregs increased their motility. It is possible that migratory Tregs are either increasing their area of regulatory influence via cytokine secretion (Vignali et al. 2008), or are in the process of migrating to draining lymph nodes (Tomura et al. 2010). Sessile Tregs on the other hand, could be interacting with DC-effector T cell clusters to exert their regulatory control (Onishi et al. 2008).

26.4.3 Infection

Using intravital MP microscopy, Ng et al. investigated the behavior of dermal DCs in ear skin in response to *Leishmania major* injection (Ng et al. 2008). Their study revealed that dermal DCs continuously surveyed the dermis in a highly motile, and G protein-coupled receptor-dependent manner under homeostatic conditions. Upon the introduction of *L. major* parasites to the dermis, local dermal DCs became immotile, initiating parasite uptake into cytosolic vacuoles. These changes in migration suggest that dermal DCs are constantly probing the microenvironment for foreign antigens, and may undergo arrest to process and present these antigens to cells.

Gebhardt et al. utilized MP microscopy to demonstrate the localization and distinct migratory behavior of herpes virus-specific $CD4^+$ (gDT-II) and $CD8^+$ (gBT-I) effector memory T (T_{EM}) cells in mouse skin following resolution of a cutaneous herpes simplex virus (HSV) infection (Gebhardt et al. 2011). Their study describes a slow-moving population of $CD8^+$ T_{EM} cells during the memory phase (30 days post-infection) that were resident in the epidermis, and in close proximity to the site of HSV infection. On the other hand, $CD4^+$ T_{EM} cells were observed to be migrating extensively in a recirculating pattern that was limited to the dermis.

26.4.4 Cancer

Of clinical importance is the role of Tregs in tumor immunology. With the potential to restrict the hosts' anti-tumor immune response, a copious amount of Tregs surrounding the tumor can be a negative prognostic indicator (Tanaka and Sakaguchi 2017). To understand the actions of Tregs in the tumor microenvironment, studies have been conducted using MP microscopy to observe Treg behavior *in vivo*.

Using a mouse model in which influenza HA-expressing tumors were implanted under the flank skin, Bauer et al. documented the interactions of $CD8^+$ T cells and Tregs via MP microscopy (Bauer et al. 2014). By adoptively transferring HA-specific Tregs, tumor-infiltrating $CD8^+$ T cells transitioned to a state resembling T cell exhaustion. Further analysis using MP microscopy revealed that Tregs in the tumor microenvironment were migratory, which was in stark contrast to the surrounding $CD8^+$ T cells. Interestingly, the migratory behavior of the Tregs included moments of arrests to form unstable contacts with $CD11c^+$ APCs. These interacting APCs had a marked reduction in their expression of costimulatory molecules CD80/86, and $CD8^+$ T cell activation by these incapacitated APCs resulted in the expression of inhibitory receptors programmed cell death protein 1 (PD-1) and T cell immunoglobulin- and mucin-domain-containing-3 (TIM-3) on $CD8^+$ T cells. These findings emphasize the capability of MP microscopy in revealing the mechanism by which Tregs can promote tumor survival.

26.5 Concluding Remarks – Looking Ahead to the Future

Over the last two decades, intravital imaging has proved to be a useful tool in expanding our knowledge on cellular behavior in their native environment. Although techniques such as flow cytometry, immunohistochemistry and RNA sequencing are able to provide insight into cellular function, they are but snapshots. The way in which an immune cell changes shape, moves, and interacts with neighboring cells during various types of immune responses can only be visualized via intravital imaging. Together, these techniques complement each other to not only help us build upon our current understanding of skin immunology, but also potentially discover new facets of leukocyte behavior in the skin.

Currently, MP microscopy is heavily utilized in animal studies, but not in human studies. One key limitation is the thickness of human skin compared to mouse skin, which reduces the penetrative ability of the laser. MP microscopy has been used on humans to evaluate skin tumors, skin aging, and epidermal cells in skin diseases (Klemp et al. 2016; Koehler et al. 2011; Murata et al. 2013; Tsai et al. 2009). For further use on humans, advancements in MP microscopy are necessary. Until then, the development of better cell-labelling systems, novel transgenic mouse systems and optical microscopic systems will drive our continual discovery of skin immunology.

References

Abeynaike LD, Deane JA, Westhorpe CL, Chow Z, Alikhan MA, Kitching AR, Issekutz A, Hickey MJ (2014) Regulatory T cells dynamically regulate selectin ligand function during multiple challenge contact hypersensitivity. J Immunol 193:4934–4944

Ali N, Zirak B, Rodriguez RS, Pauli ML, Truong HA, Lai K, Ahn R, Corbin K, Lowe MM, Scharschmidt TC et al (2017) Regulatory T cells in skin facilitate epithelial stem cell differentiation. Cell 169:1119–1129 e1111

Amulic B, Cazalet C, Hayes GL, Metzler KD, Zychlinsky A (2012) Neutrophil function: from mechanisms to disease. Annu Rev Immunol 30:459–489

Bauer CA, Kim EY, Marangoni F, Carrizosa E, Claudio NM, Mempel TR (2014) Dynamic treg interactions with intratumoral APCs promote local CTL dysfunction. J Clin Invest 124:2425–2440

Biedermann T, Kneilling M, Mailhammer R, Maier K, Sander CA, Kollias G, Kunkel SL, Hultner L, Rocken M (2000) Mast cells control neutrophil recruitment during T cell-mediated delayed-type hypersensitivity reactions through tumor necrosis factor and macrophage inflammatory protein 2. J Exp Med 192:1441–1452

Borregaard N (2010) Neutrophils, from marrow to microbes. Immunity 33:657–670

Carbone FR (2015) Tissue-resident memory T cells and fixed immune surveillance in nonlymphoid organs. J Immunol 195:17–22

Chow Z, Mueller SN, Deane JA, Hickey MJ (2013) Dermal regulatory T cells display distinct migratory behavior that is modulated during adaptive and innate inflammation. J Immunol 191:3049–3056

Clark RA, Chong B, Mirchandani N, Brinster NK, Yamanaka K, Dowgiert RK, Kupper TS (2006) The vast majority of CLA+ T cells are resident in normal skin. J Immunol 176:4431–4439

Dancey JT, Deubelbeiss KA, Harker LA, Finch CA (1976) Neutrophil kinetics in man. J Clin Invest 58:705–715

Deane JA, Abeynaike LD, Norman MU, Wee JL, Kitching AR, Kubes P, Hickey MJ (2012) Endogenous regulatory T cells adhere in inflamed dermal vessels via ICAM-1: association with regulation of effector leukocyte adhesion. J Immunol 188:2179–2188

Devi S, Kuligowski MP, Kwan RY, Westein E, Jackson SP, Kitching AR, Hickey MJ (2010) Platelet recruitment to the inflamed glomerulus occurs via an alphaIIbbeta3/GPVI-dependent pathway. Am J Pathol 177:1131–1142

Doebel T, Voisin B, Nagao K (2017) Langerhans cells – the macrophage in dendritic cell clothing. Trends Immunol 38:817–828

Dudeck A, Dudeck J, Scholten J, Petzold A, Surianarayanan S, Kohler A, Peschke K, Vohringer D, Waskow C, Krieg T et al (2011) Mast cells are key promoters of contact allergy that mediate the adjuvant effects of haptens. Immunity 34:973–984

Ebert LM, Meuter S, Moser B (2006) Homing and function of human skin gammadelta T cells and NK cells: relevance for tumor surveillance. J Immunol 176:4331–4336

Egawa G, Honda T, Tanizaki H, Doi H, Miyachi Y, Kabashima K (2011) In vivo imaging of T-cell motility in the elicitation phase of contact hypersensitivity using two-photon microscopy. J Invest Dermatol 131:977–979

Egawa G, Nakamizo S, Natsuaki Y, Doi H, Miyachi Y, Kabashima K (2013) Intravital analysis of vascular permeability in mice using two-photon microscopy. Sci Rep 3:1932

Galli SJ, Tsai M (2010) Mast cells in allergy and infection: versatile effector and regulatory cells in innate and adaptive immunity. Eur J Immunol 40:1843–1851

Galli SJ, Kalesnikoff J, Grimbaldeston MA, Piliponsky AM, Williams CM, Tsai M (2005) Mast cells as "tunable" effector and immunoregulatory cells: recent advances. Annu Rev Immunol 23:749–786

Gebhardt T, Whitney PG, Zaid A, Mackay LK, Brooks AG, Heath WR, Carbone FR, Mueller SN (2011) Different patterns of peripheral migration by memory CD4+ and CD8+ T cells. Nature 477:216–219

Geissmann F, Manz MG, Jung S, Sieweke MH, Merad M, Ley K (2010) Development of monocytes, macrophages, and dendritic cells. Science 327:656–661

Ginhoux F, Liu K, Helft J, Bogunovic M, Greter M, Hashimoto D, Price J, Yin N, Bromberg J, Lira SA et al (2009) The origin and development of nonlymphoid tissue CD103+ DCs. J Exp Med 206:3115–3130

Goh CC, Li JL, Devi S, Bakocevic N, See P, Larbi A, Weninger W, Ginhoux F, Angeli V, Ng LG (2015) Real-time imaging of dendritic cell responses to sterile tissue injury. J Invest Dermatol 135:1181–1184

Gratz IK, Truong HA, Yang SH, Maurano MM, Lee K, Abbas AK, Rosenblum MD (2013) Cutting edge: memory regulatory t cells require IL-7 and not IL-2 for their maintenance in peripheral tissues. J Immunol 190:4483–4487

Hickey MJ, Kanwar S, McCafferty DM, Granger DN, Eppihimer MJ, Kubes P (1999) Varying roles of E-selectin and P-selectin in different microvascular beds in response to antigen. J Immunol 162:1137–1143

Hickey MJ, Bullard DC, Issekutz A, James WG (2002) Leukocyte-endothelial cell interactions are enhanced in dermal postcapillary venules of MRL/fas(lpr) (lupus-prone) mice: roles of P- and E-selectin. J Immunol 168:4728–4736

Honda T, Egen JG, Lammermann T, Kastenmuller W, Torabi-Parizi P, Germain RN (2014) Tuning of antigen sensitivity by T cell receptor-dependent negative feedback controls T cell effector function in inflamed tissues. Immunity 40:235–247

Jakubzick C, Gautier EL, Gibbings SL, Sojka DK, Schlitzer A, Johnson TE, Ivanov S, Duan Q, Bala S, Condon T et al (2013) Minimal differentiation of classical monocytes as they survey steady-state tissues and transport antigen to lymph nodes. Immunity 39:599–610

Kaplan DH (2017) Ontogeny and function of murine epidermal Langerhans cells. Nat Immunol 18:1068–1075

Kaplan DH, Igyarto BZ, Gaspari AA (2012) Early immune events in the induction of allergic contact dermatitis. Nat Rev Immunol 12:114–124

Kissenpfennig A, Henri S, Dubois B, Laplace-Builhe C, Perrin P, Romani N, Tripp CH, Douillard P, Leserman L, Kaiserlian D et al (2005) Dynamics and function of Langerhans cells in vivo: dermal dendritic cells colonize lymph node areas distinct from slower migrating Langerhans cells. Immunity 22:643–654

Klemp M, Meinke MC, Weinigel M, Rowert-Huber HJ, Konig K, Ulrich M, Lademann J, Darvin ME (2016) Comparison of morphologic criteria for actinic keratosis and squamous cell carcinoma using in vivo multiphoton tomography. Exp Dermatol 25:218–222

Koehler MJ, Zimmermann S, Springer S, Elsner P, Konig K, Kaatz M (2011) Keratinocyte morphology of human skin evaluated by in vivo multiphoton laser tomography. Skin Res Technol 17:479–486

Leon B, Ardavin C (2008) Monocyte-derived dendritic cells in innate and adaptive immunity. Immunol Cell Biol 86:320–324

Li JL, Ng LG (2012) Peeking into the secret life of neutrophils. Immunol Res 53:168–181

Li JL, Goh CC, Keeble JL, Qin JS, Roediger B, Jain R, Wang Y, Chew WK, Weninger W, Ng LG (2012) Intravital multiphoton imaging of immune responses in the mouse ear skin. Nat Protoc 7:221–234

Lucas T, Waisman A, Ranjan R, Roes J, Krieg T, Muller W, Roers A, Eming SA (2010) Differential roles of macrophages in diverse phases of skin repair. J Immunol 184:3964–3977

Manjunath N, Shankar P, Stockton B, Dubey PD, Lieberman J, von Andrian UH (1999) A transgenic mouse model to analyze CD8(+) effector T cell differentiation in vivo. Proc Natl Acad Sci U S A 96:13932–13937

Mempel TR, Pittet MJ, Khazaie K, Weninger W, Weissleder R, von Boehmer H, von Andrian UH (2006) Regulatory T cells reversibly suppress cytotoxic T cell function independent of effector differentiation. Immunity 25:129–141

Mirza R, DiPietro LA, Koh TJ (2009) Selective and specific macrophage ablation is detrimental to wound healing in mice. Am J Pathol 175:2454–2462

Murata T, Honda T, Miyachi Y, Kabashima K (2013) Morphological character of pseudoxanthoma elasticum observed by multiphoton microscopy. J Dermatol Sci 72:199–201

Natsuaki Y, Egawa G, Nakamizo S, Ono S, Hanakawa S, Okada T, Kusuba N, Otsuka A, Kitoh A, Honda T et al (2014) Perivascular leukocyte clusters are essential for efficient activation of effector T cells in the skin. Nat Immunol 15:1064–1069

Nestle FO, Di Meglio P, Qin JZ, Nickoloff BJ (2009) Skin immune sentinels in health and disease. Nat Rev Immunol 9:679–691

Ng LG, Hsu A, Mandell MA, Roediger B, Hoeller C, Mrass P, Iparraguirre A, Cavanagh LL, Triccas JA, Beverley SM et al (2008) Migratory dermal dendritic cells act as rapid sensors of protozoan parasites. PLoS Pathog 4:e1000222

Ng LG, Qin JS, Roediger B, Wang Y, Jain R, Cavanagh LL, Smith AL, Jones CA, de Veer M, Grimbaldeston MA et al (2011) Visualizing the neutrophil response to sterile tissue injury in mouse dermis reveals a three-phase cascade of events. J Invest Dermatol 131:2058–2068

Nowotschin S, Hadjantonakis AK (2009) Use of KikGR a photoconvertible green-to-red fluorescent protein for cell labeling and lineage analysis in ES cells and mouse embryos. BMC Dev Biol 9:49

Onishi Y, Fehervari Z, Yamaguchi T, Sakaguchi S (2008) Foxp3+ natural regulatory T cells preferentially form aggregates on dendritic cells in vitro and actively inhibit their maturation. Proc Natl Acad Sci U S A 105:10113–10118

Ono S, Kabashima K (2015) Proposal of inducible skin-associated lymphoid tissue (iSALT). Exp Dermatol 24:630–631

Overstreet MG, Gaylo A, Angermann BR, Hughson A, Hyun YM, Lambert K, Acharya M, Billroth-Maclurg AC, Rosenberg AF, Topham DJ et al (2013) Inflammation-induced interstitial migration of effector CD4(+) T cells is dependent on integrin alphaV. Nat Immunol 14:949–958

Phillipson M, Kubes P (2011) The neutrophil in vascular inflammation. Nat Med 17:1381–1390

Romani N, Clausen BE, Stoitzner P (2010) Langerhans cells and more: langerin-expressing dendritic cell subsets in the skin. Immunol Rev 234:120–141

Runnels JM, Zamiri P, Spencer JA, Veilleux I, Wei X, Bogdanov A, Lin CP (2006) Imaging molecular expression on vascular endothelial cells by in vivo immunofluorescence microscopy. Mol Imaging 5:31–40

Sanchez Rodriguez R, Pauli ML, Neuhaus IM, Yu SS, Arron ST, Harris HW, Yang SH, Anthony BA, Sverdrup FM, Krow-Lucal E et al (2014) Memory regulatory T cells reside in human skin. J Clin Invest 124:1027–1036

Sawada Y, Honda T, Hanakawa S, Nakamizo S, Murata T, Ueharaguchi-Tanada Y, Ono S, Amano W, Nakajima S, Egawa G et al (2015) Resolvin E1 inhibits dendritic cell migration in the skin and attenuates contact hypersensitivity responses. J Exp Med 212:1921–1930

Sen D, Forrest L, Kepler TB, Parker I, Cahalan MD (2010) Selective and site-specific mobilization of dermal dendritic cells and Langerhans cells by Th1- and Th2-polarizing adjuvants. Proc Natl Acad Sci U S A 107:8334–8339

Sica A, Mantovani A (2012) Macrophage plasticity and polarization: in vivo veritas. J Clin Invest 122:787–795

Tanaka A, Sakaguchi S (2017) Regulatory T cells in cancer immunotherapy. Cell Res 27:109–118

Tomura M, Honda T, Tanizaki H, Otsuka A, Egawa G, Tokura Y, Waldmann H, Hori S, Cyster JG, Watanabe T et al (2010) Activated regulatory T cells are the major T cell type emigrating from the skin during a cutaneous immune response in mice. J Clin Invest 120:883–893

Tsai TH, Jee SH, Dong CY, Lin SJ (2009) Multiphoton microscopy in dermatological imaging. J Dermatol Sci 56:1–8

Vignali DA, Collison LW, Workman CJ (2008) How regulatory T cells work. Nat Rev Immunol 8:523–532

Witherden DA, Havran WL (2011) Molecular aspects of epithelial gammadelta T cell regulation. Trends Immunol 32:265–271

Wollenberg A, Wagner M, Gunther S, Towarowski A, Tuma E, Moderer M, Rothenfusser S, Wetzel S, Endres S, Hartmann G (2002) Plasmacytoid dendritic cells: a new cutaneous dendritic cell subset with distinct role in inflammatory skin diseases. J Invest Dermatol 119:1096–1102

Chapter 27
Development of Upright CT and Its Initial Evaluation: Effect of Gravity on Human Body and Potential Clinical Application

Masahiro Jinzaki

27.1 X-Ray Imaging of the Human Body

The first images of the human body's interior date back to 1895, when Roentgen discovered X-rays (Röntgen 1896). An X-ray of his wife's hand provided the first image of a human internal structure. Unfortunately, the contrast produced by X-rays was not sufficient to visualize internal organs, such as the liver, spleen, kidney, or urinary bladder (Fig. 27.1).

To compensate for the weakness of low-contrast X-rays, a contrast material was developed in 1896, 1 year after the discovery of X-rays (Haschek 1896). Thereafter, iodinated contrast material (CM) was developed and has been widely used ever since (Brooks 1924; Wallingford 1953). CM enables the visualization of the vascular system, urinary tract system, biliary tract system and alimentary tract system during projection imaging using X-rays (Fig. 27.2).

27.2 Cross-Sectional Imaging of Human Body

In 1972, Hounsfield developed a technology called computed tomography (CT) that enabled cross-sectional imaging in humans (Hounsfield 1973). Since then, the scanning time has improved with the development of single-helical scans in 1990 (Kalender et al. 1990) and a four-row detector CT in 1999 (Hu 1999), and the scanning time was drastically improved by the development of a 64-detector CT in 2004. This development also enabled thinner slice images with a slice thickness of less

M. Jinzaki (✉)
Department of Diagnostic Radiology, Keio University, School of Medicine, Shinjuku, Tokyo, Japan
e-mail: jinzaki@rad.med.keio.ac.jp

Y. Toyama et al. (eds.), *Make Life Visible*,
https://doi.org/10.1007/978-981-13-7908-6_27

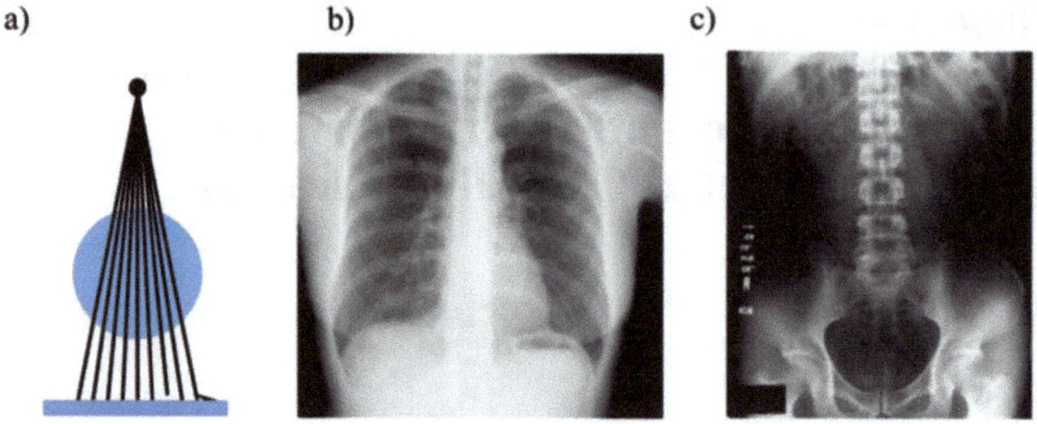

Fig. 27.1 Scheme of X-ray and X-ray images. (**a**) Scheme of X-ray (**b**) Chest X-ray images (**c**) Abdominal X-ray image
An X-ray image is a form of projection image. Unfortunately, the contrast of X-ray images is insufficient to visualize internal organs such as the mediastinum, liver, spleen, kidney, and bladder

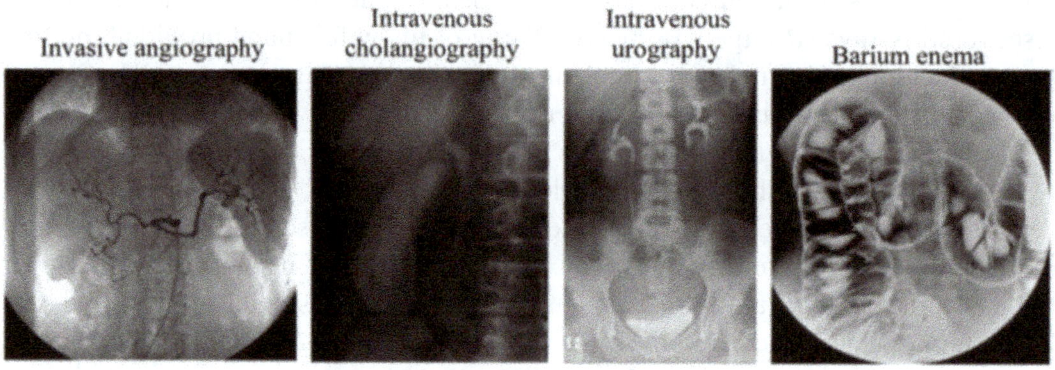

Fig. 27.2 X-ray images with contrast material

than 2 mm to be routinely obtained in clinical medicine. In turn, these thinner slice images enabled more detailed three-dimensional (3D) images to be created. 3D CT imaging has since replaced X-ray examinations using CM (Fig. 27.3). For example, CT angiography has replaced invasive angiography (Jinzaki et al. 2009), CT urography has replaced intravenous urography (McTavish 2002; Jinzaki et al. 2011), CT cholangiography has replaced intravenous cholangiography, and CT colonography has replaced Barium enemas (Halligan et al. 2013). These replacements have not only enabled less invasive imaging procedures, but have also improved the efficacies of diagnostic algorithms. CT examination alone, which provides both cross-sectional images and 3D images, can potentially replace multiple examinations that are often required for evaluation purposes. We have devoted considerable time studying the replacement of X-ray examinations requiring CM with the application of 3D CT examinations (Jinzaki et al. 2009; McTavish 2002; Jinzaki et al. 2011).

Although X-ray examinations using CM have been replaced by 3D CT, simple X-ray examinations remain widely used for two reasons. One reason is that most simple X-ray examinations are performed with the subject in a standing position. Prior to 2000, several minutes were required to obtain a whole body image using

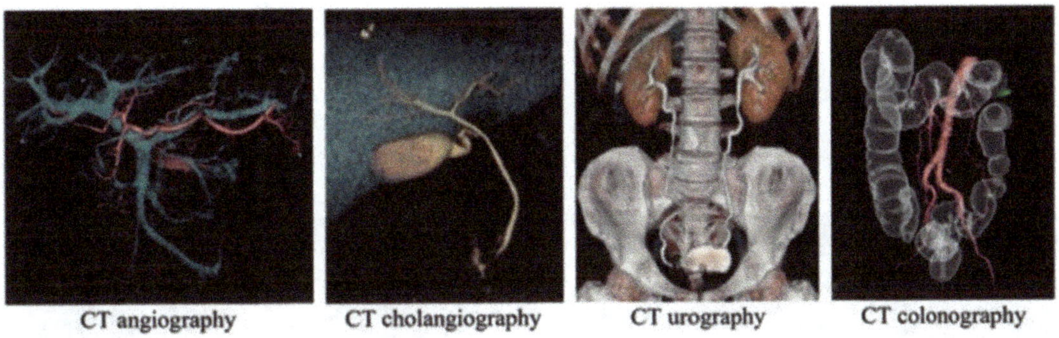

Fig. 27.3 Three-dimensional CT images
3D CT has replaced X-ray examinations with CM

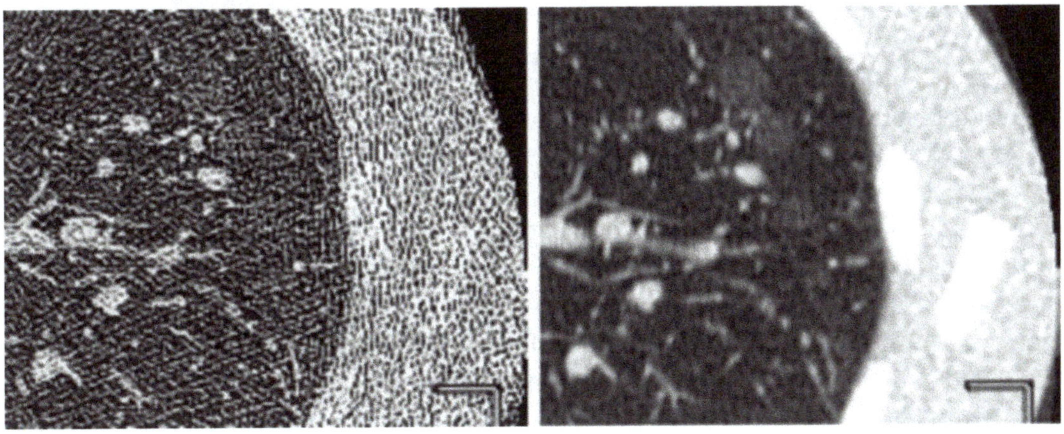

Fig. 27.4 Improvement of CT image quality using iterative reconstruction techniques
Left: An image obtained using 0.12 mSv, which is almost equal or less than the dose associated with a simple chest X-ray examination. The image quality is very low
Right: An image reconstructed from the 0.12 mSv image using an iterative reconstruction technique. The image quality has become acceptable

CT. Slight movements of the body are inevitable with longer CT scanning times, and these movements cause motion artifacts. The second reason is that the radiation dose required during CT examinations is significantly higher than that required during a simple X-ray examination. However, with the development of a 64-detector CT in 2004, the whole body trunk can now be scanned in less than 20 s. Also, with the re-emergence of new reconstruction techniques around 2010 (Hara et al. 2009), the radiation dose required by CT to maintain good image quality has gradually decreased. For example, CT images obtained at a dose of 0.12 mSv, which is almost equal to or less than the dose associated with a simple chest X-ray examination, have now become acceptable in terms of image quality thanks to the use of new reconstruction techniques (Yamada et al., 2012a, b) (Fig. 27.4).

Furthermore, a 320 detector CT device was developed in 2007, enabling a longitudinal coverage of 16 cm in one rotation (Rybicki et al. 2008). Repetitive acquisitions at the same position using a wider range of acquisition during one rotation has enabled four dimensional (4D) imaging (Fujiwara et al. 2013; Sakamoto et al. 2015)

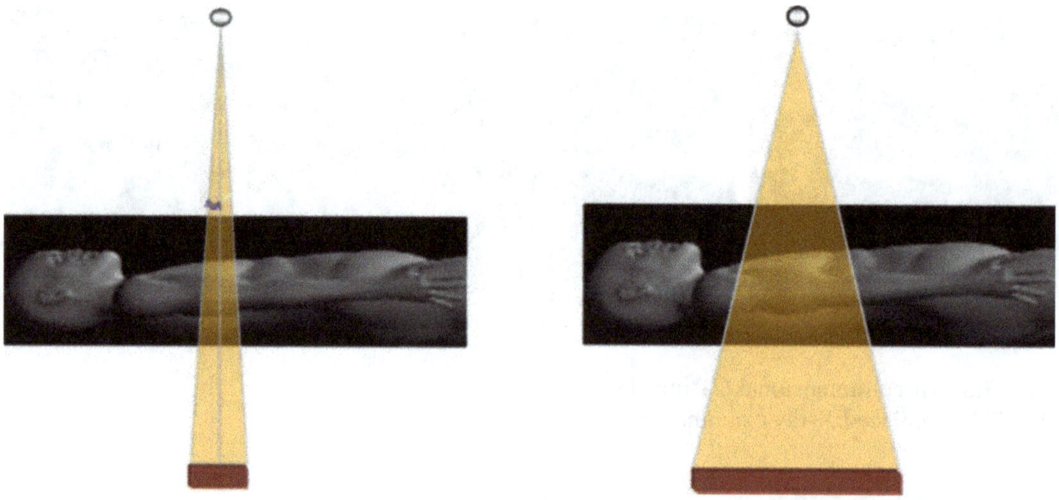

Fig. 27.5 Difference in coverage during one rotation between a 64-detector CT device and a 320-detector CT device
Left: 64-detector CT. The width of one rotation was 3.2 cm
Right: 320-detector CT. The width of one rotation was 16 cm

(Fig. 27.5). While 3D images, which have been used since 2004, provided mainly morphological information, the new 4D CT images can also provide functional information. However, many functions of the human body that occur with the subject in an upright position, such as swallowing, voiding, and walking, cannot be evaluated using CT machines that requiring the subject to be in a supine position.

27.3 Development of Upright CT

Upright CT devices offer substantial advantages: (1) they have the potential to replace poorer quality X-ray examinations, (2) they enable the visualization of cross sections of the entire human body (including soft tissue) while the body is subjected to a load or gravity, and (3) they enable functional imaging using 4-D scanning.

We presented a proposal for an upright CT device to Toshiba Medical Systems (presently Canon Medical Systems). To assuage company concerns regarding clinical indications and profitability, we listed several conceivable clinical applications and gathered information regarding the needs and benefits of such a device from various medical fields to convince the company of the wide applications of such a device. The "Upright CT Project" was finally approved in 2014.

The most difficult task was to achieve a high-speed, high-precision vertical rotation while minimizing the vibration, since even miniscule amounts of vibration cause motion artifacts, degrading image quality. Several advanced technologies were introduced to solve this problem. The second task was to create various aids to enable the subject to maintain a stable standing position. We also created a knee-high acrylic wall that encircles the subject's body to help prevent falls.

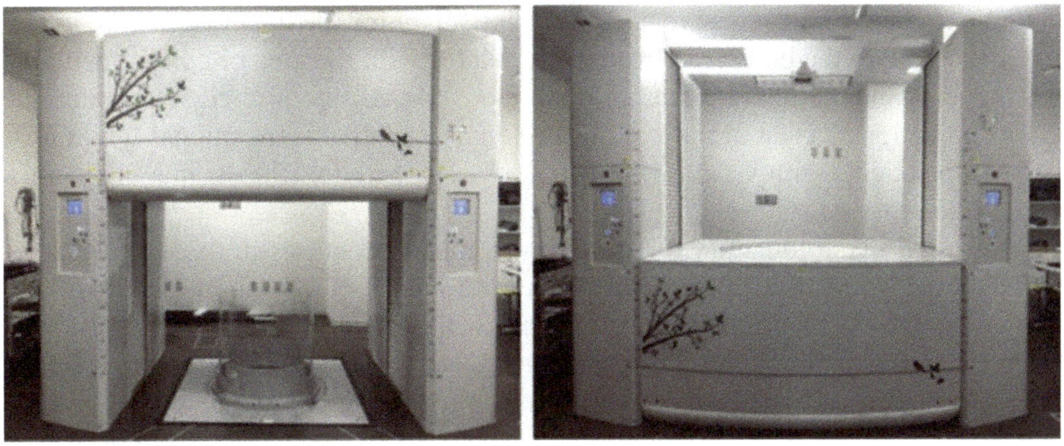

Fig. 27.6 The first upright CT machine, introduced at our institute
Left: The gantry is in the up position
Right: The gantry is in the down position

The resulting upright CT system enables vertical movements of a transverse 320 row-detector gantry (detector size, 0.5 mm) with a 0.275-s gantry rotation speed at its best performance (Fig. 27.6). This machine was approved by the Japanese Pharmaceuticals and Medical Devices Agency in March 2017.

27.4 Physical Properties and Clinical Data Analysis

After the introduction of an upright CT device for whole body imaging at our institute, we first evaluated several physical properties using a phantom to confirm whether the vertical movements of the gantry degraded the image quality. Spatial resolution, noise, and low contrast resolution were analyzed using a modulation transfer function, noise-power spectrum and visual inspection, respectively. As a result, each factor of the upright CT was comparable to conventional 320-detector row CT scanner.

During scans of volunteers, we noticed that the workflow for upright CT examinations proceeds very smoothly, compared with conventional scans. In an upright CT examination, the patient enters the CT room and proceeds directly into the gantry space; the scan begins immediately thereafter. In a conventional CT examination, however, the patient must first lie down on the scanner bed and the examiner must then raise the bed and position the bed within the gantry.

A quantitative analysis of clinical data revealed that the structure of the brain is slightly descended when the subject is in an upright position, compared with a supine position, although the brain was previously thought not to move. We also found that gravity differentially affects the volume and shape of the vena cavae depending on position, while those of the aorta remain constant regardless of the position. The lung volume was larger in an upright position than in a supine position, and the amount of change was larger for the lower lobe than for the upper or middle lobes. The centerline of the body was strongly correlated with the area of contact between the hip joint and the femoral head. Furthermore, we also confirmed that an upright CT examination can reveal more remarkable findings than conventional CT examinations in patients with various diseases, such as spondylolisthesis, inguinal hernia and pelvic prolapse.

We would like to quantify all human anatomical structures in three-dimensions while the subject is in an upright position and to quantify the effect of gravity on the human body by comparing CT images taken while the subject is in either a supine or upright position. Upright CT has the potential to become a powerful tool for both functional evaluations and evaluations of pathogenesis in the human body.

References

Brooks B (1924) Intra-arterial injection of sodium iodide. JAMA 82:1016

Fujiwara H, Momoshima S, Akiyama T et al (2013) Whole-brain CT digital subtraction angiography of cerebral dural arteriovenous fistula using 320-detector row CT. Neuroradiology 55:837–843

Halligan S, Wooldrage K, Dadswell E et al (2013) Computed tomographic colonography versus barium enema for diagnosis of colorectal cancer or large polyps in symptomatic patients (SIGGAR): a multicentre randomised trial. Lancet 381(9873):1185–1193

Hara AK, Paden RG, Silva AC, Kujak JL, Lawder HJ, Pavlicek W (2009) Iterative reconstruction technique for reducing body radiation dose at CT: feasibility study. AJR Am J Roentgenol 193:764–771

Haschek H, Lindenthal OT (1896) A contribution to the practical use of the photography according to Röntgen. Wien Klin Wschr 9:63

Hounsfield GN (1973) Computerized transverse axial scanning (tomography). Part 1. Description of system. Br J Radiol 46:1016–1022

Hu H (1999) Multi-slice helical CT: scan and reconstruction. Med Phys 26:5–18

Jinzaki M, Sato K, Tanami Y et al (2009) Diagnostic accuracy of angiographic view image for the detection of coronary artery stenoses by 64-detector row CT: a pilot study comparison with conventional post-processing methods and axial images alone. Circ J 73:691–698

Jinzaki M, Matsumoto K, Kikuchi E et al (2011) Comparison of CT urography and excretory urography in the detection and localization of urothelial carcinoma of the upper urinary tract. AJR Am J Roentgenol 196:1102–1109

Kalender WA, Seissler W, Klotz E, Vock P (1990) Spiral volumetric CT with single-breath-hold technique, continuous transport, and continuous scanner rotation. Radiology 176:181–183

McTavish JD, Jinzaki M, Zou KH et al (2002) Multi-detector row CT urography: comparison of strategies for depicting the normal urinary collecting system. Radiology 225:783–790

Röntgen WC (1896) On a new kind of rays. Science 3:227–231

Rybicki FJ, Otero HJ, Steigner ML et al (2008) Initial evaluation of coronary images from 320-detector row computed tomography. Int J Cardiovasc Imaging 24:535–546

Sakamoto Y, Soga S, Jinzaki M et al (2015) Evaluation of velopharyngeal closure by 4D imaging using 320-detector-row computed tomography. J Plast Reconstr Aesthet Surg 68:479–484

Wallingford VH (1953) The development of organic iodide compounds as X-ray contrast media. J Am Pharm Assoc (Scientific Edition) 42:721–728

Yamada Y, Jinzaki M, Tanami Y et al (2012a) Model-based iterative reconstruction technique for ultralow-dose computed tomography of the lung: a pilot study. Investig Radiol 47:482–489

Yamada Y, Jinzaki M, Hosokawa T et al (2012b) Dose reduction in chest CT: comparison of the adaptive iterative dose reduction 3D, adaptive iterative dose reduction, and filtered back projection reconstruction techniques. Eur J Radiol 81:4185–4195

Chapter 28
The Future of Precision Health & Integrated Diagnostics

Sanjiv Sam Gambhir

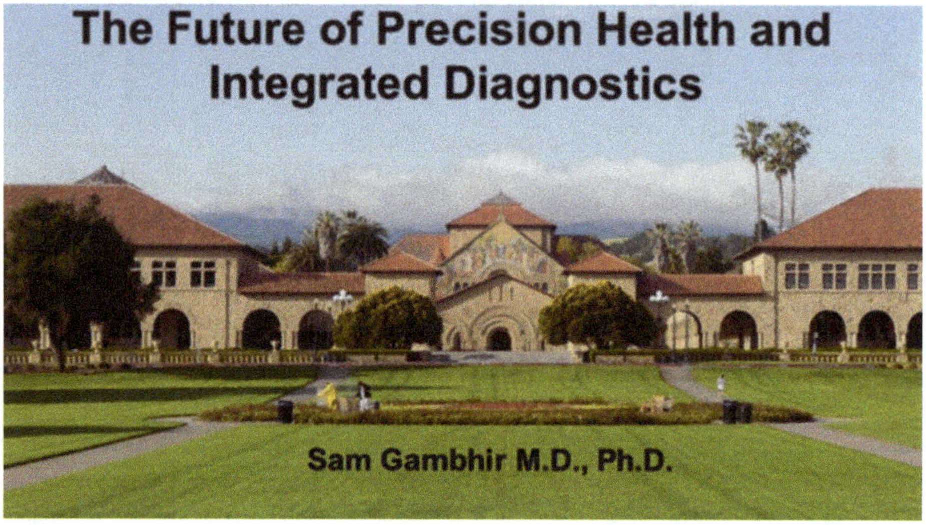

Disclosures

Relevant to this Talk

Endra Inc. – Founder, Visualsonics – SAB
Bracco – Consultant, MagArray – SAB

Others

ImaginAB, Click Diagnostics, Nine-Point Medical, GE Medical, Bayer, Site-One Therapeutics, Rio Inc., Sanofi Aventis, Piramal MI, Novartis, CellSight, Cytomx

Electronic Supplementary Material The online version of this chapter (https://doi.org/10.1007/978-981-13-7908-6_28) contains supplementary material, which is available to authorized users.

S. S. Gambhir (✉)
Stanford University, Stanford, CA, USA
e-mail: sgambhir@stanford.edu

Y. Toyama et al. (eds.), *Make Life Visible*,
https://doi.org/10.1007/978-981-13-7908-6_28

Most of the world's health care systems are focused on patients after they present with disease, and not before. While precision medicine uses personalized information to more effectively treat disease, the emerging field of precision health is situated to help assess disease risks, perform customized disease monitoring, and facilitate disease prevention and earlier disease detection. Currently an individual's health is evaluated only a few times a year if at all, making it difficult to gather the amount of information needed to implement precision health. The emergence of continuous health monitoring devices with combined in vitro and in vivo(integrated) diagnostics, worn on the body and used in the home, will enable a clearer picture of human health and disease. However, challenges lie ahead in developing and validating novel monitoring technologies, and in optimizing data analytics to extract meaningful and actionable conclusions from continuous health data. This presentation will show some of the emerging technologies for diagnostics with a focus on cancer and the challenges to making precision health a reality in the decades to come (Gambhir et al. 2018) (Slides 28.1, 28.2, and 28.3).

Summary

- The focus needs to shift to earlier detection of disease away from late stage disease
- Scientists working on *in vitro* technologies need to work closely with those who work on molecular imaging
- Strategies for signal amplification to detect fewer numbers of cells or their by-products are needed
- Strategies for continuous sensing and wearable/implantable diagnostics need further development
- Technology remains ahead of the biology

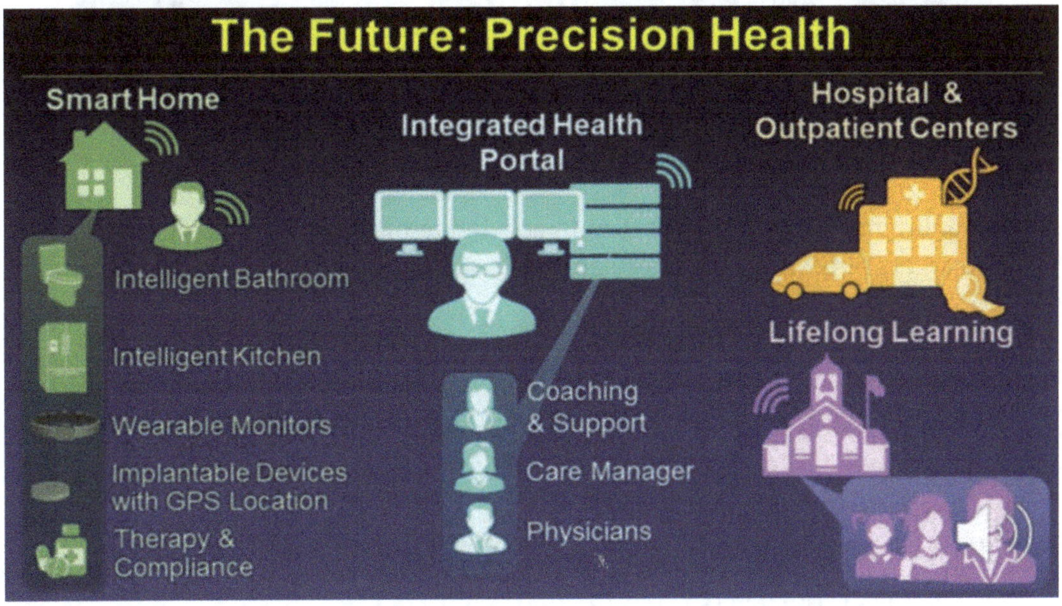

Slide 28.1 The future: precision health

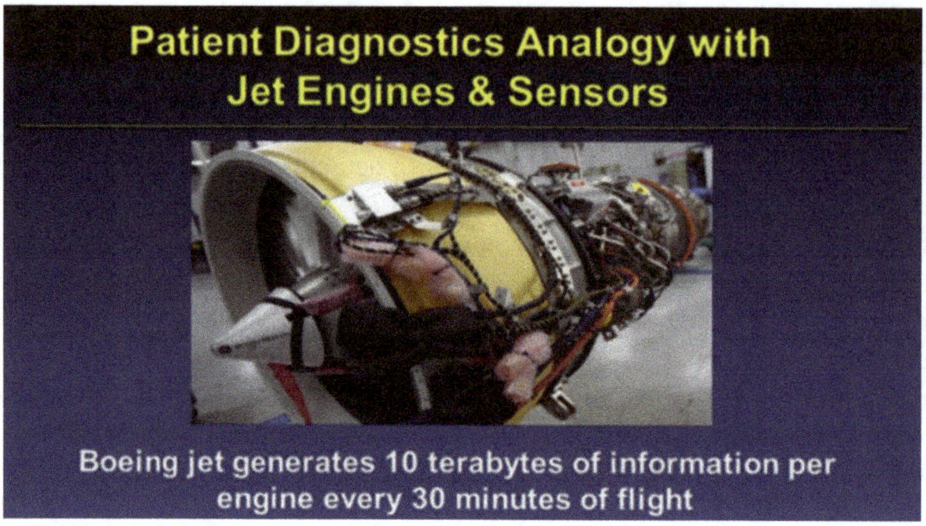

Slide 28.2 Patient diagnostics analogy with jet engines & sensors

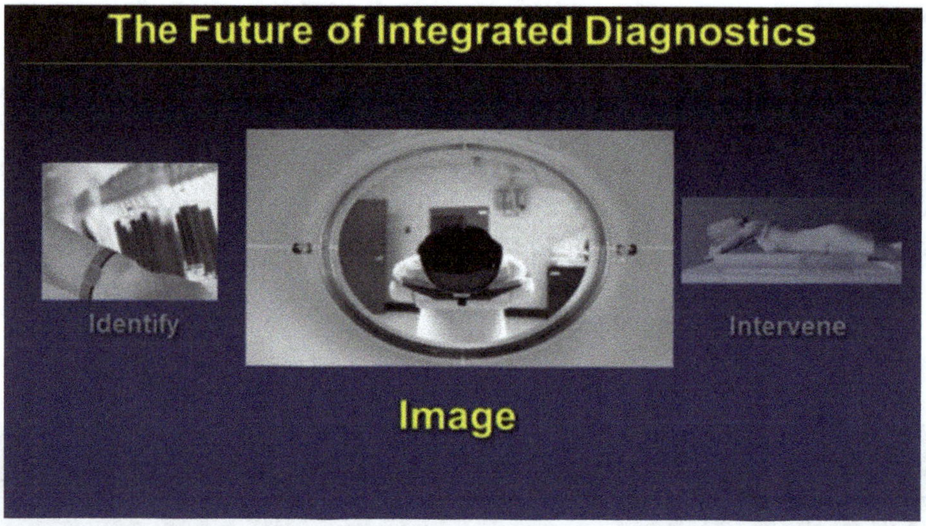

Slide 28.3 The future of integrated diagnostics

- Technology needs to be developed to accelerate biological discovery
- Biomarkers of EARLY disease need accelerated discovery and validation through novel nanotechnologies
- Lower cost solutions are key from a global economic perspective
- Collaboration between academics, government funding agencies, industry, foundations, and the FDA will help to test these approaches in pilot clinical trials

Special Thanks

- Patients & Healthy Volunteers
- National Cancer Institute
  - CCNE U54, PSOC U54, ICMIC P50, NTR U54
  - EDRN U01, ICBP U54, RO1's, R21's, R25T, T32's

- Canary Foundation
- Ben & Catherine Ivy Foundation
- Sir Peter Michael Foundation
- GE/Bayer/Bracco/Google Life Sciences
- Visualsonics/Endra/Optosonics
- Fred Hutchinson Cancer Center
- Molecular Imaging Program at Stanford (MIPS)

Reference

Gambhir SS, Ge TJ, Vermesh O, Spitler R (2018) Toward achieving precision health. Sci Transl Med 10(430):eaao3612. https://doi.org/10.1126/scitranslmed.aao3612. Review. PMID: 29491186

Chapter 29
Imaging and Therapy Against Hypoxic Tumors with ^{64}Cu-ATSM

Yasuhisa Fujibayashi, Yukie Yoshii, Takako Furukawa, Mitsuyoshi Yoshimoto, Hiroki Matsumoto, and Tsuneo Saga

29.1 Radiolabeled Cu-ATSM as a Hypoxia Imaging Agent for PET

In tumors, hypoxia frequently occurs due to poor vascularization and tight packing of cancer cells. Tumor hypoxia is associated with adverse prognosis due to failures in radiotherapy and chemotherapy and to tumor metastasis (Brown 1999). It is thus important to develop methods for diagnosis and therapy of hypoxic tumors. Noninvasive methods to detect hypoxic tumor have been intensively developed (Padhani et al. 2007).

Electronic Supplementary Material The online version of this chapter (https://doi.org/10.1007/978-981-13-7908-6_29) contains supplementary material, which is available to authorized users.

Y. Fujibayashi (✉) · Y. Yoshii
National Institute of Radiological Sciences, National Institutes for Quantum and Radiological Science and Technology, Chiba, Japan
e-mail: fujibayashi.yasuhisa@qst.go.jp; y-fujibayashi@cmi-jpn.co.jp; yoshii.yukie@qst.go.jp

T. Furukawa
Department of Radiological and Medical Laboratory Sciences, Nagoya University Graduate School of Medicine, Nagoya, Japan
e-mail: furukawa@met.nagoya-u.ac.jp

M. Yoshimoto
Division of Functional Imaging, National Cancer Center Hospital East, Kashiwa, Japan
e-mail: miyoshim@ncc.go.jp

H. Matsumoto
Research Centre, Nihon Medi-Physics Co., Ltd., Sodegaura, Japan
e-mail: hiroki_matsumoto@nmp.co.jp

T. Saga
Department of Diagnostic Radiology, Kyoto University Hospital, Kyoto, Japan

Y. Toyama et al. (eds.), *Make Life Visible*,
https://doi.org/10.1007/978-981-13-7908-6_29

We have developed a novel positron emission tomography (PET) imaging agent, Cu-diacetyl-bis (N^4-methylthiosemicarbazone) (Cu-ATSM), which can target tumor hypoxia with over-reduced conditions. Cu-ATSM can be labeled with several Cu radioisotopes, such as ^{60}Cu, ^{62}Cu and ^{64}Cu (Dehdashti et al. 2008; Fujibayashi et al. 1997, 1999; Lewis et al. 2001; Obata et al. 2001, 2005; Yoshii et al. 2012). Cu-ATSM is reported to accumulate in hypoxic environments in many kinds of tumor cells *in vitro* (Obata et al. 2005; Lewis et al. 1999; Burgman et al. 2005). Distribution of Cu-ATSM in tumor tissues differs from that of ^{18}F-fluorodeoxyglucose (^{18}FDG), a commonly used PET imaging tracer of glucose uptake (Obata et al. 2003; Tanaka et al. 2006). Cu-ATSM shows its high uptake in regions that are hypovascular, undergoing cell cycle arrest but little necrosis, while ^{18}FDG accumulates regions of hypervascularity and cell proliferation going to necrosis (Obata et al. 2003; Tanaka et al. 2006). The mechanism of Cu-ATSM accumulation in hypoxic regions has been reported (Fujibayashi et al. 1997; Obata et al. 2001; Burgman et al. 2005; Dearling et al. 2002; Holland et al. 2009). Cu-ATSM, a rigid complex of Cu(II) and ATSM, is easily divided by reduction of Cu(II) to Cu(I) and trapped into the cells under highly reduced intracellular conditions such as hypoxia (Fujibayashi et al. 1997; Obata et al. 2001; Burgman et al. 2005; Dearling et al. 2002). Cu-ATSM rapidly diffuses into cells and tissues even in low perfusion areas and is trapped within cells under highly reduced conditions such as hypoxia (Fujibayashi et al. 1997, 1999; Obata et al. 2001; Yoshii et al. 2012; Holland et al. 2009; Bowen et al. 2011). Preclinical studies have revealed that Cu-ATSM uptake increases with higher intracellular levels of the biological reductant NAD(P)H, which is associated with hypoxia and mitochondrial dysfunction, and activity of NAD(P)H-dependent reductive enzymes, rather than oxygenic conditions (Obata et al. 2001; Yoshii et al. 2012; Holland et al. 2009; Bowen et al. 2011).

In recent years, clinical PET studies using radiolabeled Cu-ATSM have been conducted for many types of cancers throughout the world. In Japan, our institute produced a generator system of ^{62}Cu and multicenter clinical studies of ^{62}Cu-ATSM PET have been conducted using our system. These clinical studies have shown that Cu-ATSM uptake is associated with therapeutic resistance, metastatic potential, and poor prognosis in several types of cancer (Dehdashti et al. 2008; Dietz et al. 2008; Lewis et al. 2008; Sato et al. 2014; Tateishi et al. 2013). Cu-ATSM uptake is correlated with high HIF-1α expression in patients' glioma (Tateishi et al. 2013). These clinical studies have demonstrated that tumor hypoxia assessed by Cu-ATSM uptake is associated with the tumors' malignant behaviors (Dehdashti et al. 2003, 2008; Dietz et al. 2008; Grigsby et al. 2007).

29.2 ^{64}Cu-ATSM as a Theranostic Agent

^{64}Cu-ATSM can be used as a "theranostic" agent. Namely, this agent can be applied not only as a PET imaging agent but also as an internal radiotherapy agent against tumors, since ^{64}Cu shows β^+ decay (0.653 MeV, 17.4%) as well as β^- decay

(0.574 MeV, 40%) and electron capture (42.6%). The photons from electron-positron annihilation can be detected by PET, while the β^- particles and Auger electrons emitted from this nuclide can damage tumor cells (Lewis et al. 2001; Obata et al. 2005; Yoshii et al. 2011; Yoshii et al. 2016). In addition, the half-life of ^{64}Cu ($t_{1/2}$ = 12.7 h) is appropriate for both diagnostic and therapeutic use. ^{64}Cu is a practical nuclide for the use of both diagnosis and therapy, because it can be readily produced with an in-hospital small cyclotron. The therapeutic effect of ^{64}Cu-ATSM has been demonstrated in both *in vitro* (Obata et al. 2005) and *in vivo* studies (Lewis et al. 2001; Aft et al. 2003). ^{64}Cu-ATSM reduces the clonogenic survival of tumor cells under hypoxia by inducing post-mitotic apoptosis (Obata et al. 2005). This is caused by heavy damage to DNA via high-linear energy transfer (LET) Auger electrons emitted from ^{64}Cu (McMillan et al. 2015). An *in vivo* study using tumor-bearing hamsters demonstrated that ^{64}Cu-ATSM treatment increased survival time without severe toxicity (Lewis et al. 2001). These previous studies supported the feasibility of ^{64}Cu-ATSM treatment against hypoxic tumors with high-LET radiation.

29.3 ^{64}Cu-ATSM Theranostics for Cancer Stem Cells

We have demonstrated that ^{64}Cu-ATSM preferentially localizes in intratumoral regions with a high density of CD133$^+$ cells, which show characteristics of cancer stem cells or cancer stem cell-like cells (CSCs) and showed therapeutic effect against CSCs in a mouse colon carcinoma (Colon-26) and human colon carcinoma (HT-29) models (Yoshii et al. 2011; Yoshii et al. 2016; Yoshii et al. 2010). In these studies, ^{64}Cu-ATSM treatment inhibited tumor growth, and the percentage of CD133$^+$ cells and metastatic ability in ^{64}Cu-ATSM treated tumors were decreased compared to that in non-treated control tumors. ^{64}Cu-ATSM accumulated in the cells under hypoxic conditions and incorporation of ^{64}Cu-ATSM under hypoxia caused cell death in both CD133$^+$ and CD133$^-$ cells. We have demonstrated that the intratumoral ^{64}Cu-ATSM high-uptake regions exhibited upregulation of DNA repair, which results in therapeutic resistance. ^{64}Cu-ATSM high-uptake regions showed upregulation of pathways related to DNA repair along with nucleic acid incorporation (bromodeoxyuridine uptake). In addition, combination use of nucleic acid antimetabolites, such as a pyrimidine analog 5-fluorouracil, a purine analog 6-thioguanine, and a folate analog pemetrexed, enhanced the efficacy of ^{64}Cu-ATSM internal radiotherapy by inhibiting DNA repair and effectively reduced %CD133$^+$ CSCs. Therefore, our study suggested that co-administration of ^{64}Cu-ATSM and nucleic acid antimetabolites could have a potential to cure tumor malignant environment and CSCs.

29.4 Biodistribution and Dosimetry of ^{64}Cu-ATSM

We have examined biodistribution of ^{64}Cu-ATSM using mice and performed dosimetry analysis. Relatively high accumulation of ^{64}Cu was observed in the liver, small intestine, and large intestine among normal organs. ^{64}Cu were mainly excreted in the feces, but little urinary excretion was observed. Our dosimetry analysis demonstrated that the liver, ovaries, and red marrow should be considered as dose-limiting organs in ^{64}Cu-ATSM internal radiotherapy. For clinical applications, we have developed a strategy to reduce radiation doses to these critical organs while preserving tumor radiation doses by the appropriately scheduled administration of copper chelator penicillamine during ^{64}Cu-ATSM internal radiotherapy (Yoshii et al. 2014). In this method, penicillamine was orally administered at 1 h after ^{64}Cu-ATSM injection, when radioactivity was almost cleared from the blood and tumor uptake had plateaued. Using this method, penicillamine decreased ^{64}Cu accumulation in the critical organs, while maintaining tumor uptake.

29.5 This Project

Anti-VEGF antibody bevacizumab is an antiangiogenic agent in widespread clinical use for cancer. Despite the initial positive effect of this treatment, continued use of bevacizumab induces hypoxia and makes tumors malignant. Thus, additional strategies to treat the hypoxia during bevacizumab therapy are needed. In this project, we are developing a method to detect and treat tumors that became malignant by acquiring decreased vascularity and hypoxia, during antiangiogenic bevacizumab treatment, with ^{64}Cu-ATSM.

29.6 Development of a Method to Detect Vascularity and Hypoxia In Vivo

Recently, an imaging technology with single-photon emission computed tomography/positron emission tomography/computed tomography (SPECT/PET/CT) to obtain simultaneous images using two different tracers labeled with SPECT and PET nuclides with CT has been developed. By applying the SPECT/PET/CT technology, we developed a method to simultaneously visualize vascularity and hypoxia with ^{99m}Tc-labeled human serum albumin (^{99m}Tc-HSA) to detect blood pool, and ^{64}Cu-ATSM to detect hypoxia (Adachi et al. 2016). In this study, we performed in vivo imaging experiments using the VECTor SPECT/PET/CT small-animal

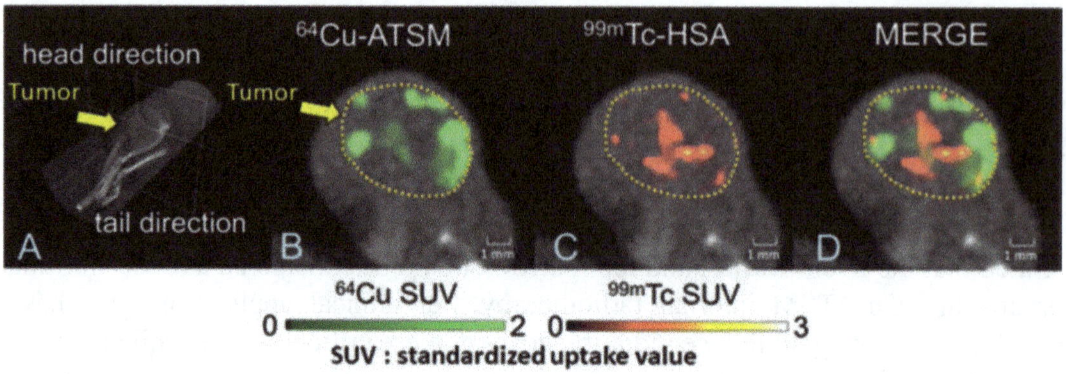

Fig. 29.1 In vivo SPECT/PET/CT imaging with ^{64}Cu-ATSM and ^{99m}Tc-HSA

scanner (MILabs) with HT-29 tumor-bearing mice. ^{64}Cu-ATSM (37 MBq) and ^{99m}Tc-HSA (18.5 MBq) were intravenously injected into a mouse at 1 h and 10 min, respectively, before scanning for 20 min. The ^{99m}Tc/^{64}Cu dual-isotope SPECT/PET/CT images were then obtained. In vivo SPECT/PET/CT imaging with ^{64}Cu-ATSM and ^{99m}Tc-HSA visualized distribution of each probe and showed that ^{64}Cu-ATSM high-uptake regions barely overlapped with ^{99m}Tc-HSA high-uptake regions within non-treated HT-29 tumors (Fig. 29.1).

To obtain a bevacizumab-treated tumor model, HT-29 tumor-bearing mice were treated with bevacizumab (5 mg/kg twice a week) for 3 weeks. Using this model, dual-isotope SPECT/PET/CT imaging with ^{99m}Tc-HSA and ^{64}Cu-ATSM was performed to check tumor vascularity and hypoxia. For comparison, un-treated tumors that showed similar size to bevacizumab-treated tumor model, were used. From imaging study, bevacizumab-treated tumors showed reduced vascularity and increased proportion of hypoxic areas within tumors.

29.7 ^{64}Cu-ATSM Therapy

For treatment study, ^{64}Cu-ATSM (37 MBq) or saline was intravenously injected into mice with bevacizumab-treated mice (bevacizumab+^{64}Cu-ATSM or bevacizumab group). For comparison, a group without bevacizumab-treatment (^{64}Cu-ATSM alone) and un-treated control were also examined. Bevacizumab+^{64}Cu-ATSM group showed the greater inhibition of tumor growth, compared with bevacizumab group, ^{64}Cu-ATSM alone group, and un-treated control, without side effect. Therefore, our data demonstrated that ^{64}Cu-ATSM therapy effectively inhibited tumor growth in bevacizumab-treated HT-29 tumors. ^{64}Cu-ATSM therapy could be a novel approach as an add-on to antiangiogenic therapy with bevacizumab (Fig. 29.2).

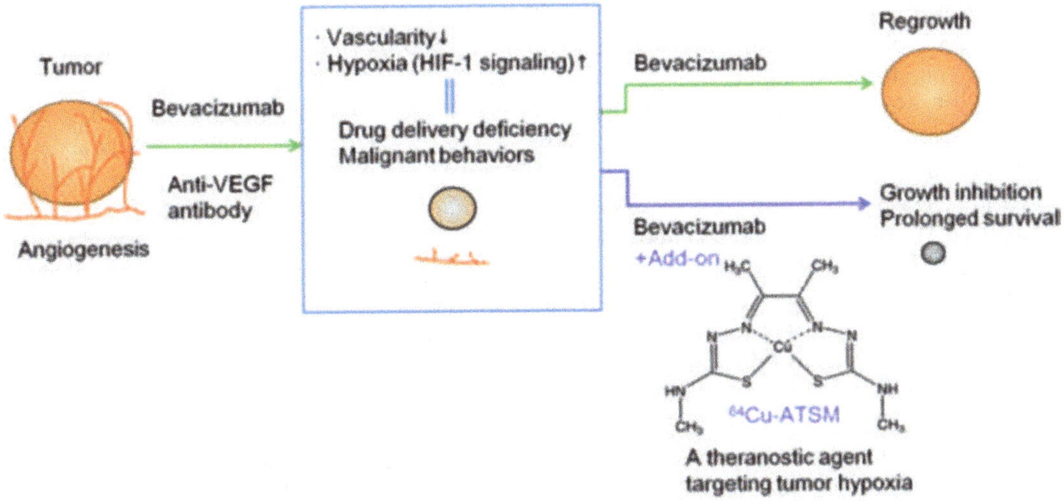

Fig. 29.2 ^{64}Cu-ATSM therapy as an add-on to antiangiogenic therapy with bevacizumab

29.8 Conclusion

We have seen that ^{64}Cu-ATSM is a promising theranostic agent targeting tumor hypoxia, which is related to tumor malignant behaviors, such as therapy resistance, metastatic potential, existence of cancer stem cells. ^{64}Cu-ATSM has unique characteristics to target tumor malignant behaviors. Therefore, ^{64}Cu-ATSM would be useful to cure malignant tumors due to hypoxia.

References

Adachi N, Yoshii Y, Furukawa T, Yoshimoto M, Takeuchi Y, Inubushi M, Wakizaka H, Zhang MR, Tsuji AB, Takahashi M, Fujibayashi Y, Saga T (2016) In vivo simultaneous imaging of vascular pool and hypoxia with a HT-29 tumor model: the application of dual-isotope SPECT/PET/CT. Int J Sci 25:26–39

Aft RL, Lewis JS, Zhang F, Kim J, Welch MJ (2003) Enhancing targeted radiotherapy by copper(II)diacetyl- bis(N^4-methylthiosemicarbazone) using 2-deoxy-D-glucose. Cancer Res 63:5496–5504

Bowen SR, van der Kogel AJ, Nordsmark M, Bentzen SM, Jeraj R (2011) Characterization of positron emission tomography hypoxia tracer uptake and tissue oxygenation via electrochemical modeling. Nucl Med Biol 38:771–780

Brown JM (1999) The hypoxic cell: a target for selective cancer therapy – eighteenth Bruce F. Cain Memorial Award lecture. Cancer Res 59:5863–5870

Burgman P, O'Donoghue JA, Lewis JS, Welch MJ, Humm JL, Ling CC (2005) Cell line-dependent differences in uptake and retention of the hypoxia-selective nuclear imaging agent Cu-ATSM. Nucl Med Biol 32:623–630

Dearling JL, Lewis JS, Mullen GE, Welch MJ, Blower PJ (2002) Copper bis(thiosemicarbazone) complexes as hypoxia imaging agents: structure-activity relationships. J Biol Inorg Chem 7:249–259

Dehdashti F, Grigsby PW, Mintun MA, Lewis JS, Siegel BA, Welch MJ (2003) Assessing tumor hypoxia in cervical cancer by positron emission tomography with ^{60}Cu-ATSM: relationship to therapeutic response-a preliminary report. Int J Radiat Oncol Biol Phys 55:1233–1238

Dehdashti F, Grigsby PW, Lewis JS, Laforest R, Siegel BA, Welch MJ (2008) Assessing tumor hypoxia in cervical cancer by PET with ^{60}Cu-labeled diacetyl-bis(N^4-methylthiosemicarbazone). J Nucl Med 49:201–205

Dietz DW, Dehdashti F, Grigsby PW, Malyapa RS, Myerson RJ, Picus J, Ritter J, Lewis JS, Welch MJ, Siegel BA (2008) Tumor hypoxia detected by positron emission tomography with ^{60}Cu-ATSM as a predictor of response and survival in patients undergoing neoadjuvant chemoradiotherapy for rectal carcinoma: a pilot study. Dis Colon Rectum 51:1641–1648

Fujibayashi Y, Taniuchi H, Yonekura Y, Ohtani H, Konishi J, Yokoyama A (1997) Copper-62-ATSM: a new hypoxia imaging agent with high membrane permeability and low redox potential. J Nucl Med 38:1155–1160

Fujibayashi Y, Cutler CS, Anderson CJ, McCarthy DW, Jones LA, Sharp T, Yonekura Y, Welch MJ (1999) Comparative studies of Cu-64-ATSM and C-11-acetate in an acute myocardial infarction model: ex vivo imaging of hypoxia in rats. Nucl Med Biol 26:117–121

Grigsby PW, Malyapa RS, Higashikubo R, Schwarz JK, Welch MJ, Huettner PC, Dehdashti F (2007) Comparison of molecular markers of hypoxia and imaging with ^{60}Cu-ATSM in cancer of the uterine cervix. Mol Imaging Biol 9:278–283

Holland JP, Giansiracusa JH, Bell SG, Wong LL, Dilworth JR (2009) In vitro kinetic studies on the mechanism of oxygen-dependent cellular uptake of copper radiopharmaceuticals. Phys Med Biol 54:2103–2119

Lewis JS, McCarthy DW, McCarthy TJ, Fujibayashi Y, Welch MJ (1999) Evaluation of ^{64}Cu-ATSM in vitro and in vivo in a hypoxic tumor model. J Nucl Med 40:177–183

Lewis JS, Laforest R, Buettner T, Song S, Fujibayashi Y, Connett J, Welch M (2001) Copper-64-diacetyl-bis(N^4-methylthiosemicarbazone): an agent for radiotherapy. Proc Natl Acad Sci U S A 98:1206–1211

Lewis JS, Laforest R, Dehdashti F, Grigsby PW, Welch MJ, Siegel BA (2008) An imaging comparison of ^{64}Cu-ATSM and ^{60}Cu-ATSM in cancer of the uterine cervix. J Nucl Med 49:1177–1182

McMillan DD, Maeda J, Bell JJ, Genet MD, Phoonswadi G, Mann KA, Kraft SL, Kitamura H, Fujimori A, Yoshii Y, Furukawa T, Fujibayashi Y, Kato TA (2015) Validation of ^{64}Cu-ATSM damaging DNA via high-LET Auger electron emission. J Radiat Res 56:784–791

Obata A, Yoshimi E, Waki A, Lewis JS, Oyama N, Welch MJ, Saji H, Yonekura Y, Fujibayashi Y (2001) Retention mechanism of hypoxia selective nuclear imaging/radiotherapeutic agent cu-diacetyl-bis(N^4-methylthiosemicarbazone) (Cu-ATSM) in tumor cells. Ann Nucl Med 15:499–504

Obata A, Yoshimoto M, Kasamatsu S, Naiki H, Takamatsu S, Kashikura K, Furukawa T, Lewis JS, Welch MJ, Saji H, Yonekura Y, Fujibayashi Y (2003) Intra-tumoral distribution of ^{64}Cu-ATSM: a comparison study with FDG. Nucl Med Biol 30:529–534

Obata A, Kasamatsu S, Lewis JS, Furukawa T, Takamatsu S, Toyohara J, Asai T, Welch MJ, Adams SG, Saji H, Yonekura Y, Fujibayashi Y (2005) Basic characterization of ^{64}Cu-ATSM as a radiotherapy agent. Nucl Med Biol 32:21–28

Padhani AR, Krohn KA, Lewis JS, Alber M (2007) Imaging oxygenation of human tumours. Eur Radiol 17:861–872

Sato Y, Tsujikawa T, Oh M, Mori T, Kiyono Y, Fujieda S, Kimura H, Okazawa H (2014) Assessing tumor hypoxia in head and neck cancer by PET with ^{62}Cu-diacetyl-bis(N^4-methylthiosemicarbazone). Clin Nucl Med 39:1027–1032

Tanaka T, Furukawa T, Fujieda S, Kasamatsu S, Yonekura Y, Fujibayashi Y (2006) Double-tracer autoradiography with Cu-ATSM/FDG and immunohistochemical interpretation in four different mouse implanted tumor models. Nucl Med Biol 33:743–750

Tateishi K, Tateishi U, Sato M, Yamanaka S, Kanno H, Murata H, Inoue T, Kawahara N (2013) Application of ^{62}Cu-diacetyl-bis (N^4-methylthiosemicarbazone) PET imaging to predict highly malignant tumor grades and hypoxia-inducible factor-1alpha expression in patients with glioma. AJNR Am J Neuroradiol 34:92–99

Yoshii Y, Furukawa T, Kiyono Y, Watanabe R, Waki A, Mori T, Yoshii H, Oh M, Asai T, Okazawa H, Welch MJ, Fujibayashi Y (2010) Copper-64-diacetyl-bis (N^4-methylthiosemicarbazone) accumulates in rich regions of CD133+ highly tumorigenic cells in mouse colon carcinoma. Nucl Med Biol 37:395–404

Yoshii Y, Furukawa T, Kiyono Y, Watanabe R, Mori T, Yoshii H, Asai T, Okazawa H, Welch MJ, Fujibayashi Y (2011) Internal radiotherapy with copper-64-diacetyl-bis (N^4-methylthiosemicarbazone) reduces $CD133^+$ highly tumorigenic cells and metastatic ability of mouse colon carcinoma. Nucl Med Biol 38:151–157

Yoshii Y, Yoneda M, Ikawa M, Furukawa T, Kiyono Y, Mori T, Yoshii H, Oyama N, Okazawa H, Saga T, Fujibayashi Y (2012) Radiolabeled Cu-ATSM as a novel indicator of overreduced intracellular state due to mitochondrial dysfunction: studies with mitochondrial DNA-less rho0 cells and cybrids carrying MELAS mitochondrial DNA mutation. Nucl Med Biol 39:177–185

Yoshii Y, Matsumoto H, Yoshimoto M, Furukawa T, Morokoshi Y, Sogawa C, Zhang MR, Wakizaka H, Yoshii H, Fujibayashi Y, Saga T (2014) Controlled administration of penicillamine reduces radiation exposure in critical organs during ^{64}Cu-ATSM internal radiotherapy: a novel strategy for liver protection. PLoS One 9:e86996

Yoshii Y, Furukawa T, Matsumoto H, Yoshimoto M, Kiyono Y, Zhang MR, Fujibayashi Y, Saga T (2016) Cu-ATSM therapy targets regions with activated DNA repair and enrichment of CD133 cells in an HT-29 tumor model: sensitization with a nucleic acid antimetabolite. Cancer Lett 376:74–82

www.ingramcontent.com/pod-product-compliance
Lightning Source LLC
LaVergne TN
LVHW082119200926
848484LV00008B/1984